T0331799

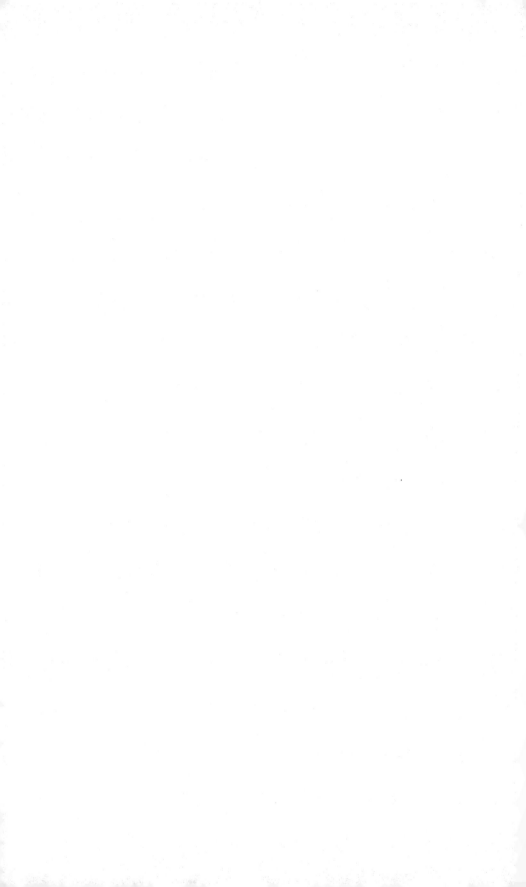

Moral Leadership in Medicine

Building Ethical Healthcare Organizations

Moral Leadership in Medicine

Building Ethical Healthcare Organizations

Suzanne Shale
Senior researcher, Health Experiences Research Group, University of Oxford;
Senior ethics tutor, Guy's, King's and St Thomas' School of Medicine, King's College London, UK

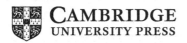

CAMBRIDGE
UNIVERSITY PRESS

CAMBRIDGE
UNIVERSITY PRESS

University Printing House, Cambridge CB2 8BS, United Kingdom

One Liberty Plaza, 20th Floor, New York, NY 10006, USA

477 Williamstown Road, Port Melbourne, VIC 3207, Australia

314-321, 3rd Floor, Plot 3, Splendor Forum, Jasola District Centre, New Delhi - 110025, India

79 Anson Road, #06-04/06, Singapore 079906

Cambridge University Press is part of the University of Cambridge.

It furthers the University's mission by disseminating knowledge in the pursuit of education, learning and research at the highest international levels of excellence.

www.cambridge.org
Information on this title: www.cambridge.org/9781107006157

© Suzanne Shale 2012

First published 2012

A catalogue record for this publication is available from the British Library

Library of Congress Cataloging in Publication data
Shale, Suzanne.
Moral leadership in medicine : building ethical healthcare organizations /
Suzanne Shale.
    p. ; cm.
Includes bibliographical references and index.
    ISBN 978-1-107-00615-7 (Hardback)
    1. Medical ethics–Great Britain.   2. Health services administration–Moral
and ethical aspects–Great Britain.   3. Leadership–Great Britain.   I. Title.
    [DNLM: 1. Ethics, Medical–Great Britain.   2. Delivery of Health
Care–ethics–Great Britain.   3. Health Facility Administrators–ethics–
Great Britain.   4. Leadership–Great Britain.   5. Moral Obligations–Great
Britain.   6. Physician-Patient Relations–ethics–Great Britain. W 50]
    R724.S454 2012
    174.20941–dc23
                                                        2011024205

ISBN 978-1-107-00615-7 Hardback

....

Every effort has been made in preparing this book to provide accurate and up-to-date information which is in accord with accepted standards and practice at the time of publication. Although case histories are drawn from actual cases, every effort has been made to disguise the identities of the individuals involved. Nevertheless, the authors, editors and publishers can make no warranties that the information contained herein is totally free from error, not least because clinical standards are constantly changing through research and regulation. The authors, editors and publishers therefore disclaim all liability for direct or consequential damages resulting from the use of material contained in this book. Readers are strongly advised to pay careful attention to information provided by the manufacturer of any drugs or equipment that they plan to use.

Contents

Preface

This book has been gestating a long time; almost exactly thirty years in fact. I can trace its beginnings to 1981, the year that racial tension erupted into riots in the Brixton area of London. I was a political activist at the time, heavily involved in campaigning against racism and for greater social equality. I was also working my way through law school, and I used to cycle off at 5 a.m. every weekday morning to an ill-paid job cleaning government offices. On the day in question I was half-way through emptying wastebaskets, scouring coffee cups and wiping ashtrays (they still smoked in offices back then) in a messy typing pool (they still had typing pools too) when my supervisor sidled over and announced that he had a new assignment for me. He was white, and I am white, and those facts have relevance to my story. He escorted me to a different office, evidently kept spankingly clean by its occupants, and explained that from now on my entire morning round would consist of this pristine domain alone. I appraised it with an office cleaner's eye and calculated that the new assignment would give me at least an extra hour in bed. Then he said – and this is the point – 'we have to look after our own you know'. And what did I do? I did not upbraid him for his discriminatory attitude. I did not question his management decision. I did not reject his offer. But I did spend the rest of the week feeling guilty and uncomfortable, so much so that I went out and found myself another job. And I've spent a lot of time since then thinking about why I didn't live up to my deeply held convictions, and what gets in the way of other people living up to theirs.

Of course one of the reasons we don't always do what we think is right is that self-interest gets in the way. It would be ridiculously naive not to acknowledge that. But it's not the whole answer. In my case, I was already going out of my way – incurring personal disadvantage – to act in opposition to racial inequality. And I ended up walking away from the benefit that had been handed to me on a plate. I genuinely didn't want it. So why couldn't I do what I thought was right there and then, on the spot? It was partly because I was taken by surprise, and could not immediately make sense of what he said. I was pretty sure I'd got it right, but I was also worried that maybe I'd got it wrong and was making a horrible misjudgement. And my reaction was partly because when I was sure I knew what he was hinting at, I simply couldn't think of what to say that would actually alter his outlook. And finally, it was because although I loathed his attitude he hadn't hitherto done anything to make me loathe him; and I didn't want to offend him by spurning his gift.

After the events of that summer I went on to become a legal scholar and got rather distracted by other questions. But eventually I worked my way back towards questions about moral action, and added to them some questions about medical leadership that had arisen along the way. The immediate stimulus to this book came when I took a highly regarded year-long course in medical ethics and realized that by the end of it I still had very little idea of what doctors, patients, ethicists or others were actually doing when they did something they thought of as 'ethical'. I was also puzzled by the peculiar absence of organizations, and the activity of managing them, from the core medical ethics literature. Medical ethics seemed to deal almost exclusively with doctors and patients, and they apparently encountered one another in a moral space independent of the institutions of healthcare. But I was now providing ethics and educational support in healthcare organizations, and every time I walked into one I confronted problematic structures, differing professional moralities, convoluted regulatory mechanisms, conflicting collegial loyalties, morally controversial organizational incidents, and groups of health and management professionals working together to make sense of it all. I knew that much of medical organizational life was missing from medical ethics, and that in these missing places there were people finding it difficult, sometimes, to do the right thing.

Three aspects of moral action have intrigued me over the years, and I have tried to account for how they play out in the 'backrooms' of medicine in forthcoming pages. How do we make sense of situations 'on the fly', so that we respond in ways that are consistent with our moral beliefs? What do we do to generate ideas about what can be done, and, alongside that, what sorts of behaviours signal fidelity to important moral values? And how do we learn and teach the sort of moral resourcefulness that really makes a difference to how people conduct themselves in their work? Perhaps because I already had enough familiarity with moral failure on my own part, I decided when I was planning this research to try and capture the components of moral success. Because I was interested in the moral life of organizations, talking to those responsible for leading them seemed a good place to start. I have looked at the question of what 'doing ethics' of healthcare organization actually is at present, and what 'doing ethics' of healthcare organization ought to be.

I argue in Chapter 1 that medicine is a global business, and that health systems and medical leaders everywhere face some common challenges. There are clearly dramatic national differences too, but I firmly believe in the value of comparative study. So I have aimed to make the book useful to readers around the world who will – like most of us in the UK – know little about the internal workings of the British National Health Service. National Health Service organizations are constantly mutating, and they were doing so during the writing of the book. What changes far less frequently is the underlying issues confronting medical leaders. If they do not emerge in one familiar guise, they almost invariably pop up in another.

I have written the book for clinicians thinking about leadership; for ethicists; for readers interested in healthcare organizations and how they work; for medical educators, trainees, or graduate students; and for anyone intrigued by the question of what the day-to-day practice of ethics in professional organizations looks like. I hope I have made it possible to read it without having to know anything much about ethical theory. The moral leaders who contributed to this study rarely, if ever, used the argot of religious or secular ethics to describe or justify their actions. That they nevertheless had compelling grounds for behaving in the manner that they did will be clear as the text unfolds.

During the period of writing the book I have been working as an ethicist with senior doctors, nurse leaders, and management professionals who are facing together just the sorts of issues I discuss in forthcoming chapters. They have been relieved to know that other leaders experience the same sense of being pulled between apparently incompatible moral commitments, and they have found it useful to think about how certain sorts of behaviour can help them to maintain a satisfactory moral equilibrium. Healthcare organizations are complex, demanding, morally febrile institutions that concern themselves with the best and the worst that human beings can do for one another. I hope this book will contribute to our understanding of the sort of leadership these institutions need, and throw new light on how to support the people entrusted with providing it.

Acknowledgements

This book is about the confidence and trust that we place in medical practice. As I have been writing it, I have had cause to reflect on how deeply we are affected by our experiences of medical care. When they go well we can be left with a profound and enduring sense of gratitude, the knowledge that we owe a debt that can never be repaid. In my case, I am indebted to Dr. Geoffrey Marsh, who made a visit to my childhood home in Norton-on-Tees way back in the early 1960s, and saved my life by promptly diagnosing acute appendicitis. Dr. Marsh went on became a leader in the field of general practice, but it is for that 'ordinary' act of care I should like to thank him here.

A different debt is owed to the medical leaders who were participants in this study. They all took time to reflect upon their moral lives and in interviews spoke with candour and insight about difficult issues and continuing doubts. Some gave additional support and advice at the conclusion of the study. All were promised anonymity, so sadly I cannot thank them by name however much I would like to.

There are many other colleagues I am glad to be able to acknowledge personally however. I am particularly grateful to Professor Alan Cribb, who has contributed more to my research than seems fair. He has nurtured my ideas, shared his own, questioned my analyses, bolstered my confidence and made me laugh. Professor Jonathan Glover supported the initial research proposal, and Professor Soren Holm and Professor Richard Ashcroft were encouraging in their appraisal of my findings and arguments. Dr. Kenji Watanabe and Dr. Greg Plotnikoff gave me an early opportunity to present my research at Keio University, and Professor Akira Akabayashi and his colleagues at Tokyo University graciously allowed me to continue the interesting conversations in Japan. I have benefited from the insights offered by participants at seminars hosted by the Centre for Ethics in Medicine at the University of Bristol, and by the Department of Primary Care and Public Health at Brighton and Sussex Medical School. Dr. Lindsay Hadley, Dr. Clare Penlington and Dr. Adrian Bull invited me to discuss moral medical leadership with several audiences of medical managers and senior management professionals, and the book was enriched through these conversations. Miss Kate Evans and Dr. Rosemary Field read and commented on parts of the manuscript. Dr. Deborah Bowman has been a warm and thoughtful inquirer into the book's central themes, and shared her knowledge of Mary Gentile's work with me. My father heroically read an entire early version; I only wish I could write as clearly as he would like, and tell a story as entertaining as the ones my mother has told. Rachel Warren supplied vital research assistance, bringing energy, insight, and commitment to the task of preparing the book for publication.

This research was supported in the early years by a grant from the Wellcome Trust, and the Daiwa Foundation has kindly supported my visits to Japan. I am very grateful to those organizations. Further financial subsidy has come from my own ethics consultancy. Rev. Peter Haughton kindly invited me to teach on the intercalated BSc in Medical Ethics and Law at King's College London. I have enjoyed his intellectual companionship alongside that of Roger Higgs, Carolyn Johnston, Paquita de Zulueta and Susan Bewley and I have benefited from the challenge and insight of our clever and committed students. The Kent, Surrey and Sussex Deanery has for several years given me interesting work and stimulating colleagues. Kath Sullivan has been a particularly supportive co-mentor and collaborator. The University of Oxford and www.healthtalkonline.org made the final stages of preparing the book far less stressful by offering me a fascinating assignment and agreeing to allow me to finish the manuscript before I started it. Thomas the Tank Engine – for reasons that will become apparent in a moment – was also a vital source of support.

I have seen far too little of my friends Jackie Fosbury and Hazel Hagger, but have relied on their affection and their understanding of the importance of meaningful work. Kerry Shale is a brilliant storyteller and has been a brilliant editor when I have been wise enough to ask him for help. Kerry's ability to create characters convincing to the eye and to the ear (from Swifty Lazar in Frost/Nixon to the Fat Controller in Thomas the Tank Engine) has helped to fund my extended foray into medical ethics. Most important of all his infinite capacity for love reminded me that while it was worth persevering, understanding moral leadership wasn't all that mattered.

Why medicine needs moral leaders

A certain day became a presence to me;
there it was, confronting me – a sky, air, light:
a being. And before it started to descend
from the height of noon, it leaned over
and struck my shoulder as if with
the flat of a sword, granting me
honor and a task. The day's blow
rang out, metallic or it was I, a bell awakened,
and what I heard was my whole self
saying and singing what it knew: *I can.*

*By Denise Levertov, from Breathing the
Water, copyright © 1987 by Denise Levertov.
Reprinted by permission of New Direction
Publishing Corp and Bloodaxe Books.*

This book is about the moral challenges that confront medical leaders running the complex healthcare institutions on which we all rely. In the chapters to come I shall be discussing the issues that medical leaders have found to be morally troubling, what they have done to orchestrate an organizational response to their moral concerns, and the impact that leading healthcare organizations has upon them personally. In the course of my analysis of their experience I shall be suggesting a framework to conceptualize ethical action, discussing ways of understanding the ethics of healthcare organization, and proposing a new approach to developing ethical leadership.

Preventing or responding to medical harm, and associated worries about the capability or trustworthiness of colleagues, rank among medical leaders' foremost moral concerns. In the case of medical harm they know that they have important moral work to do, but also that however well they do it they cannot change what has happened. It falls to medical leaders to patch things together in the aftermath, to repair something irrevocably broken, and to endeavour to prevent the same harm happening again. In the case of colleagues, medical leaders are troubled by how to prove suspected poor clinical performance, how to weigh evidence that is contradictory, and what to do about unverifiable allegations that doctors deny. They are concerned about doctors who act contrary to clinical protocols but apparently get good results, and about doctors who deliver a good service to individual patients but take so long or spend so much that other patients suffer. They worry that their judgement of colleagues might be based on grounds of prejudice, or in questionable cultural assumptions about how doctors should behave; they wonder whether they are siding with colleagues or failing to give them support, whether their standards are too low or too high and if they have 'drawn the line' in the right place. They sometimes take action knowing that colleagues are at risk of suicide, or aware of how colleagues' families will pay the price for professional disrepute.

But medical harm and the performance of colleagues are not medical leaders' only moral concerns. When I set out on this research, academic colleagues almost invariably predicted that medical leaders' main moral burden would be problems around resource allocation. (The healthcare professionals I work with who aspire to leadership roles more often anticipate that medical harm and colleagues' performance will be major sources of moral trouble.) Much moral challenge does arise from the perennial problem of stretching finite capacity over infinite demand, but this is a conundrum that is not just about money. There are far broader questions about matching assets to demand, because a health economy's assets comprise people, knowledge, buildings, infrastructure, cultures, systems, reputation, goodwill, and trust. Medical leaders have to consider all of these.

Sometimes an issue is (more or less) straightforwardly to do with money. Medical leaders see funds moving around the health system in ways that are not always responsive to patient needs, and it falls to them to use money wisely where they can. They face difficult questions about how to allocate drug budgets, resource new therapies, and pay for improvement projects, how to service organizational debts, reduce expenditure while not withdrawing services, and how to marry funded national or regional initiatives to unfunded local health demands.

The wider set of issues concerns systems, infrastructure, buildings and cultures. Medical leaders spend years negotiating priorities with different agencies so that, for example, elderly patients' health is accorded no less importance than that of people of working age, care for chronic disease is treated as no less important than acute care, and access to healthcare is improved for traditionally excluded groups. They look for ways of using information technologies to support patient care, but worry about privacy and confidentiality. They lead change in the face of public disquiet when plans for reorganizing hospitals and clinics involve modifying popular services. They are the object of anger and mistrust when they propose reorganizing services that are not as good as they ought to be. They simultaneously dislike and defend the moral necessity of fair bureaucracy, and they view corporate loyalty as both an asset and a potential liability.

An important dimension of moral leadership is making sense of all of this: creating a moral narrative that explains to the people whom leaders lead, and the people whom leaders serve, why it is better and not worse to do things in the ways that are eventually settled upon. Such moral narratives are not just explanations. They are also the form in which the knowledge of colleagues is pooled, the way in which situations come to be understood for what they are, the approach by which moral resolve is mobilized, the shape in which action is orchestrated, and the avenue through which organizations and individuals are rendered accountable.

Who this book is for

I hope I have made it possible to read this book without having to know anything at all about ethical theory, or anything about the internal machinery of the British National

Health Service. There are very few people who are familiar with both. The book is for clinicians thinking about leadership; for ethicists; for readers interested in healthcare organizations and how they work; for medical educators, trainees, or graduate students; and for those interested in what the day-to-day practice of professional ethics might look like.

The risk in trying to satisfy so many different audiences is, of course, failing to satisfy any. I have tried to set out my argument in such a way that it will make sense to anyone who comes to the question of moral leadership in medicine without a background in healthcare ethics, medical sociology, or medical management. Readers may therefore find that less is taken for granted than is usual in texts firmly located in a single discipline. Ethicist readers will no doubt find it odd that I identify 'Bernard Williams' as a 'philosopher'. UK clinical leaders may find it equally odd to encounter an explanation of the familiar nuts and bolts of medical managerial life in the British National Health Service (henceforth, NHS). I hope that these peculiarities will be forgiven.

Most of the chapters in the book are concerned with explaining what I think moral leadership in medicine consists of, where we observe it, and how we might think about it. My hope is that morally thoughtful people working in healthcare will recognize their world in these chapters, and will also find the arguments helpful for thinking about how to refine their own ethical expertise. For those who observe healthcare from some external vantage point, I hope that the portrait of moral leadership I present here will afford insight into the moral challenges that clinicians face, and the intellectual and emotional resources they invest in resolving them.

This book is, I think, a sympathetic portrayal of clinicians' worlds. It is one that may not satisfy critics distrustful of the power of the professions. But I have tried to understand what moral challenge looks like to clinicians who genuinely believe they hold their patients' best interests in mind, are committed to running fair and effective public organizations, and who are endeavouring to do what good they can in frequently difficult circumstances.

Some parts of the book offer more detailed theoretical arguments than clinicians or students will find edifying, and I expect that readers will choose to focus on sections relevant to their interests and needs. Philosophers, ethicists, educators and the sociologically inclined may find the fuller argument helps to resolve doubts about the force of my claims, helps to point up my arguments' implications, or helps to iron out conceptual difficulties.

How this book came to be written

My portrait of moral leadership draws on research into the moral experience of medical directors leading hospitals and primary care organizations in the NHS.

I carried out detailed, in-depth interviews with NHS medical directors, purposively selected from a range of healthcare organizations. These organizations were of different sizes, some large and some small. They had different sorts of patients, from affluent, settled, predominantly white, middle-class town and countryside populations to poor, transient, predominantly minority ethnic, working-class, city dwellers. The organizations had different public profiles, some with long-standing support from their local communities and others with reputations that had had to be rebuilt after well-publicized failures of care. They were located in different geographical regions across the UK.

My sample of twenty-four organizational leaders was tiny – microscopic – by comparison with the number of subjects recruited to a clinical trial and the number of respondents required for quantitative social research. However, the sample size is not unusual in qualitative research. More to the point, it is about twenty-four times the size of the average sample used in philosophical theorizing, which depends heavily upon the philosopher's own experience and intuitions. Taking as its focus the moral experience of medical leaders across a wide range of different organizations, this is in fact one of the most extensive in-depth studies of moral leadership in medicine to date.

Interviewees were promised anonymity and almost all spoke very frankly about sensitive and contentious issues. This has entailed some care in discussing data containing confidential information [1–3].[1] A degree of artifice has been used to conceal the identity of participants and those to whom they referred. In some of the cases that I discuss in forthcoming chapters I have withheld telling detail, and in other cases I have changed it.

The most problematic detail to change is the sex of interviewees. The majority of UK medical directors are men, and interviewees recruited from among the minority of women were potentially far more easily identifiable. My sample of twenty-four medical directors included five women. In order to conceal my female participants' identities, I retained roughly the same proportion of men and women when reporting the data but have arbitrarily changed the gender identity of interviewees. Doctors may be male or female as their names suggest, but equally they may not. Interview transcript should never, therefore, be read as an example of specifically male or female thought, speech or action.

The interesting question that is raised through making such a change is whether male and female medical directors had a different outlook or were inclined to do things differently. I came to the conclusion that the medical leaders I interviewed did not differ significantly in their approach. This is partly because the men in my study reasoned and acted in ways that are consistent with theories of morality that – ironically – were initially based in understandings about how women's moral experience differed from men's. I touch on this point again in Chapter 6, when I consider how the data in this study inform our understanding of moral practice.

A list of the participants' pseudonyms and a description of the type of organization they worked for is included as an addendum at the end of this chapter.

What morality and leadership mean in this book

The words moral, ethical, leader and leadership will appear throughout this book with almost tiresome frequency, so it would be as well to make clear from the start how I intend to use them. Getting at the meaning of these common words is no simple matter, however.

The philosopher Bernard Williams described an ethical consideration as one that 'relates to us and our actions the demands, needs, claims, desires, and, generally, the lives of other people' [4(p12)]. To an ethicist, this vague and expansive definition makes some sense. But for newcomers to the field it simply begs the question 'so what exactly are we talking about when we talk about morals and ethics?' In the following section I hope to give a reasonably lucid account of what people mean when they use these words, and how I will use them, before I go on to explain how morals and ethics apply to leaders and leadership in medicine.

---

[1] On privacy, see reference 1. On cases in bioethics, see references 2 and 3 .

What 'moral' and 'ethical' mean

The moral philosopher turned bioethicist Judith André once observed that confusion and disagreement in bioethics is fuelled by the illusion that all who come to the debate share a common academic language [5(p42)]. Clinicians, social scientists, lawyers and philosophers all enter the fields variously known as clinical ethics, medical ethics or bioethics schooled in their own disciplines. One problem that then arises is that the use of the words of 'morality' and 'ethics' are different in medicine, sociology, law and moral philosophy.

I start with common usage among doctors who were, after all, the main subject of this inquiry. Use of the term morality or ethics in medical circles generally follows informal conversational conventions. 'Morality' refers to issues such as abortion that wider society conventionally treats as 'moral' issues. But when these same issues involve professionals, as they do in managing patients' requests for termination of pregnancy, 'ethics' is the preferred term. Practitioners speak of 'professional ethics' rather than 'professional morals'; and generally label poor professional behaviour 'unethical' rather than 'immoral'. However, particularly depraved behaviours attract the epithet 'immorality' all the better to register deep disapproval or disgust. Overall, then, 'ethics' seems to be thought more suitable for what doctors ought to do because they occupy special roles, while 'morality' is preferred for talking about fundamental and enduring human concerns or for uttering strong condemnation.

'Ethics' may thus mean any of the following to medical professionals: medical-ethical principles and concepts; professional codes; the practices that implement medical-ethical conventions; and the personal values carried into the professional domain. To work through one example, the ethical principle of 'respect for autonomy' is said to account for the ethical concept of 'informed consent'; requirements of informed consent are embedded in professional and organizational codes; there are ethical practices around 'consenting patients', which can be performed for better or for worse, and about which judgements of performance can be made; and professionals may experience moral satisfaction when they 'consent' their patient well.

In the social sciences, the terms 'morality' and 'ethics' are used to refer to the conventions or conventional behaviours that a particular group treats as 'good' or 'correct'. Social theorists themselves rarely advocate any particular code of conduct. They are by and large more concerned with understanding how groups settle what is 'good' or 'right' among themselves.

The social phenomenon of 'morality' and 'ethics' interests social theorists because it is a distinctive means of governing individual and group behaviour. Members of social groups – and hence also social theorists – typically distinguish between behaviour procured by force, behaviour that is compliant with formal codes such as law, behaviour that is produced by informal codes such as morality or etiquette, and behaviour that comes from merely wanting to be nice to one another. How groups distinguish between force, law, morality, friendship and altruism is a complex matter, not least because the boundaries between the various categories overlap and are apt to move around. What is morality one day may become law the next, what some treat as a rule of etiquette may look to others like ethics, and so on.

What is special about morals and ethics, however, is that when groups label certain issues as 'moral' or 'ethical' these issues assume a particular gravity. 'Moral' and 'ethical' discussions are believed to be about matters of great import. Moreover, when issues are thought to be 'moral' or 'ethical' in nature, they elicit and give licence to strong sentiments of approval and disapproval.

From a social scientific perspective, however, so-called 'moral' conflicts may be no more than factional disagreements between social groups and sub-groups. The business comes to be badged as 'morality' because one side in a conflict sees some advantage in persuading themselves and others that there is something particularly precious at stake. 'Claiming the moral high ground' turns ordinary disagreements into righteous crusades. Writing about ethics in nursing, for example, sociologist Daniel Chambliss argued that ethics talk is frequently an expression of conflict between powerful interest groups such as doctors and nurses, or nurses and managers: 'what could be described as political arguments or turf battles are translated into moral terms and become "ethical problems"' [6].

Finally, moral philosophy starts its inquiry into morality with questions about the form that morality takes. Moral philosophers treat morality as a special case. What makes 'morality' different from other aspects of human experience and relationships? For moral philosophers, what is special about 'morality' is that it concerns what we *ought* to do in relation to others, and thus also how we reason about what is right or good. Moral philosophy has tended to treat morality as rule-like, with moral considerations applying in similar fashion to all rational persons who find themselves in similar situations.

Kant gave 'morality' a very restrictive definition, at least in terms of the form that it took. He argued that true morality was a conscious decision to do the right thing, solely out of a concern to do one's duty. Moral philosophers after Kant have, however, been rather more liberal in their definitions of the form morality takes. The issue continues to be debated, but most moral philosophers converge on seeing morality as guidance on important domains of human behaviour, guidance that is rational, primarily concerned with lessening harm or evil, and binding on everyone [7].

If we are all of us bound by the same moral considerations, working out exactly what our moral obligations are becomes a critically important, and highly contentious, task. In this context, the word 'ethics' takes on a quite specific meaning: it is reasoning about the content of our moral obligations, where it has already been agreed that morality is a rational code binding on everyone. Ethics is the study of the question of what exactly our moral code of conduct ought to be, and why. For example, ought we to do only what produces the most pleasure and the least pain for the largest number of people, or should we unwaveringly follow absolute rules, such as always telling the truth, regardless of the consequences?

However, a significant group of philosophers, Bernard Williams among them, have also argued that ethics should be treated as a much more wide-ranging inquiry into the question 'how should one live?' Ethics, they argue, should not be treated as parasitic upon definitions of morality.[2] They question the assumption that the question 'how should one live?' is always best answered by referring to universal moral obligations or general moral duties. Instead, they invite us to consider a multitude of possible reasons for acting. Because so many different reasons may be brought to bear, these philosophers are inclined to accept the possibility that different people may justifiably decide to do different things for different reasons in roughly similar circumstances.

Which brings us – at last – to what I mean by 'moral' and 'ethical' in this book.

---

[2] I am referring here to a broad group including virtue ethics, narrative ethics, care ethics, feminist ethics and responsibility ethics.

First, I follow the conventions familiar to clinicians and social scientists and will be using 'moral' and 'ethical' as almost – but not quite – interchangeable.

Second, I am sidestepping difficult questions posed by moral philosophers about whether there are some 'universal' moral propositions and what deserves to be labelled 'moral', simply because for current purposes it is not necessary to answer them. This book is about the issues that medical leaders identified as the morally troubling stuff of medical management. That some managerial troubles are *experienced* as moral or ethical troubles is in my view a good enough reason to include them in a study of moral leadership.

In very large part, what was troubling about the issues medical leaders discussed was that they entailed attempting to realize conflicting and equally important values. Some medical leaders' moral troubles concerned life and death decisions about patients, and would probably be viewed as 'moral' issues by most observers. Other troubles could undoubtedly be mapped onto their organizational turf battles. But while I think it is helpful to be aware of how 'claiming the moral high ground' can be a useful tactic in turf wars, I am disinclined to redefine particular moral arguments as 'really' turf warfare, or 'really' anything else. Whether issues are 'truly' moral issues is a matter of interpretation: a matter about which philosophers, social theorists, clinicians, and managers may quite legitimately differ.

All of the moral issues that I write about in forthcoming chapters fall easily within Bernard Williams's sense of the 'ethical'. They also fit well with philosopher Margaret Walker's explanation of what makes certain responsibilities 'moral responsibilities' below:

> [W]e are most likely to invoke the notion of moral responsibility in cases where the stakes are high, or cases where dependability or dereliction is apt to reflect on character, or cases where we know we are relying entirely on the informal system . . . where there are no official judiciaries or enforcers. [8]

Third, and perhaps most importantly, what I am really interested in is what medical leaders *do* when moral trouble is in the offing. A great deal of the discussion in medical ethics is about what people should *decide* when they are confronted with a moral fork in the road. But that is not what it is like in medical management, as we shall see. Medical leaders have to realize that there is a problem, work out what it is, and come up with potential solutions, before they can make momentous decisions about what might be the optimally ethical option to pursue. And then, the truly difficult moral work often starts after decisions have been made about which way to go, in seeing the whole business through to its end. How decisions come to be necessitated, and how they are subsequently implemented, may be what matters most to building ethical healthcare organizations.

What 'moral leadership' means

Whatever their formal position, all healthcare professionals have an interest in understanding moral leadership, and sometimes an obligation to undertake it.

It is an unoriginal (but nonetheless accurate) observation that officially designated leaders frequently fail to lead well, or indeed lead at all. Equally, people who are not officially designated leaders may play a significant leadership role, visible in the way that they steer groups towards accomplishing desirable goals. It is helpful to keep in mind this distinction between the position of leader and the activity of leadership. When I use the term moral leader and moral leadership in this book I mean to refer to people doing the activity of moral leadership. Some will be formal leaders, doing moral leadership. Others will become informal moral leaders, because in the absence of anyone else stepping up to the mark their own moral leadership is all there is.

Moral leadership in medicine does not mean being a doctor. Potentially any member of a healthcare professional group is liable to be called upon to play a moral leadership role. Neither does it mean having a senior role in the professional hierarchy. Junior staff may sometimes have to confront moral problems unseen or ignored by their seniors. And finally, moral leadership in medicine does not mean being the doctor who is best able to do 'applied ethics'. It will become clear why this is so from Chapter 2 onwards, when we begin to look at the processes through which ethical commitments come to be enacted.

Moral, or indeed ethical, medical leadership means being astute to the moral connotations of all that is involved in providing care, determining where action is needed, identifying situations where action is needed to improve or maintain the moral quality of care, and orchestrating the activity of other people to provide a morally appropriate response when one is required. Moral leaders will frequently orchestrate by example: creating the ethical tone of an organization through the quality of their moral awareness, and the quality of their response to morally challenging situations.

This book is based on research into the moral experience of doctors who were, in fact, the officially designated leaders of the medical workforce within their organization. I studied them because it was the most practical way of researching the phenomenon of moral leadership. But this approach does invite a tricky question: were the leaders I talked to *able* moral leaders, those to whom one should look for examples of medical leadership?

The difficulty in answering one way or another is that we have no agreed criteria against which to measure them, or indeed anyone else. To judge competence, or even better, expertise, is to judge the skill exhibited within a particular practice. To judge the skill, we have to understand the practice. But I undertook this research precisely because we do not fully understand the practice of moral leadership.

So what claims can I make about the quality of the moral leadership I discuss here? One alone: the features of moral leadership that I consider in forthcoming chapters have been distilled from leaders' reflections on their moral experience. These leaders were respected by other leaders for their moral wisdom. Their reflections have supplied us with a useful framework for thinking about how to do moral leadership. They do not, however, supply a ready reckoner on how to be good.

Why medicine is a (fairly) special case of morality and leadership

It is said to have been St. Basil of Caesarea who founded the first 'proper' hospital around AD 360 [9]. Hospices, hospitals, clinics, 'polyclinics', community health centres, local surgeries, managed care organizations, medical aid networks – healthcare organizations of remarkable diversity – have since grown up to serve medicine's ends. For centuries, care organizations have been potent symbols of our frailty, of our determination to overcome our afflictions, and of the attitudes that societies hold towards assisting some of their most vulnerable members.

The medical care that organizations exist to provide is nothing if not (to recall Bernard Williams) a response to 'the demands, needs, claims, desires, and, generally, the lives of other people' [4(p12)]. Medicine is, on this reading, an intrinsically moral activity. As bioethicist John Harris noted, the ways in which we provide care 'demonstrate the value that we place on one another's lives and display the respect that we believe we owe to each other'

[10(p1)]. There is almost nothing that happens in medicine that is not a moral issue. Even interventions freely chosen by competent healthy adults – cosmetic surgery, contraception, genetic testing for example – are fit topics for moral analysis. There is a sense, then, in which medicine and morality are so inseparable that leadership in medicine is, for better or worse, inevitably a form of moral leadership.

If to lead in medicine is to lead a moral enterprise, it is also, often, to lead a moral enterprise in which the everyday moral world is turned upside down. As sociologist Daniel Chambliss observed,

> In the hospital it is the good people, not the bad, who take knives and cut people open; here the good stick others with needles and push fingers into rectums and vaginas, tubes in to urethras, needles into the scalp of a baby; here the good, doing good, peel dead skin from a screaming burn victim's body and tell strangers to take off their clothes .... The layperson's horrible fantasies here become the professional's stock in trade. [6(p12)]

Many ordinary moral understandings – about what is permissible, what is shameful, what is perverse, what is pleasurable, what is cruel and what is kind – must simply be set aside for the purposes of conceptualizing medical care. The special moral understandings that apply to medicine suggest that moral leadership here is a special case. It is perhaps akin to moral leadership in a war zone, another arena where ordinary moral understandings are temporarily suspended.

The need to sidestep conventional moral thinking in order to provide medical treatment affects healthcare professionals in two, paradoxically opposite, ways.

One reaction is to become impervious. Professionals who deal with death, disorderly bodies and unruly minds on a daily basis might be forgiven for forgetting how odd the moral world of medicine is. The assumptions that dominate life outside it – about what is dignified, who is in control, what is valuable, who is vulnerable – can all too easily disappear from view. The opposite reaction is to become hyper-vigilant in relation to moral concerns. Consciously or otherwise, healthcare professionals counter the risk of going morally adrift by looking for moral anchorage. This can come in the form of dogmatic reliance on some basic moral principles, in anxious scanning of the environment to identify moral trouble, and sometimes both. Counterintuitively, perhaps, some people seem to adopt both of those strategies at once: becoming both impervious to day-to-day indignities, and also intensely aware of the scope of their moral responsibilities.

In the peculiar moral world of medical care what the moral issues are may not always be obvious; potential moral troubles are obscure; and potential moral troubles are everywhere abundant.

Moral leadership is about doing, not just deciding

This book is not just about making moral decisions. It is about doing moral behaviour to build ethical organizations.

This focus on enactment sets it apart from the mainstream of medical ethical discussion. Normative medical ethics is concerned with what decisions ought to be made; and empirical medical ethics mostly looks at how professionals approach decisions. This is of course to simplify a much more intricate picture. My point, though, is that most medical ethics treats moral decisions as the chief object of interest. Discussion concentrates on what people should, or could, or did, decide about something morally important. In the case of empirical ethics, discussion may start with how people come to a decision, and it may end with how they communicate it. But 'big' moral decisions remain the core concern.

I am not uninterested in big decisions and how they are justified. But if we think of morality as being mostly about making decisions we risk overlooking all of the surrounding, equally important, aspects of moral life in which moments of decision are embedded. If we overlook these elements, we will fail to ask and answer some important questions. What does it take to notice that 'something moral' is going on? How do people make sense of the 'something moral' that is going on? What is the range of possible responses to the 'something moral'? How do we narrow them down? How does one decision lead to another? How does the way we *act out* our decisions affect their 'moral goodness'? How do we influence the moral actions of others? How do we manage our moral identity? These questions are all part of my account of moral leadership.

Although it is not a particularly endearing word, in forthcoming chapters I use the term 'enactment' and its variants (enacting, enacted) to refer to the totality of the moral or ethical process. I think of 'enacting' as a form of 'moral artistry', a creative process that relies upon perception, knowledge, social skill, and creative imagination. The process starts with sensing that something 'moral' may have to be dealt with, right through to assessing whether one is a morally good person for having done things as one did [11–13].[3]

On charismatic, transformational, distributed, and connective leadership

What is a good leader? There is already a vast literature on leadership in general, and a burgeoning literature dealing with ethical leadership in particular. The search for an answer to the question of leadership has produced a regal parade of new 'leadership paradigms'. In recent decades the medical leadership industry has rejected 'charismatic' leadership, embraced 'transformational' leadership, moved to favour 'distributed' or 'shared' leadership and flirted with 'connective' leadership. So what can this book offer that is different?

This book is an account of only one dimension (moral) of one kind of leadership (medical). I am not convinced that it is helpful to treat every aspect of leaderly activity, across the gamut of human endeavour, as a single behavioural phenomenon captured in description of a single paradigm – leadership. Moral leadership may not be the same phenomenon as strategic leadership, and leadership in medicine may not be the same phenomenon as leadership in banking. Whether or not I am right to be sceptical about the existence of the phenomenon of leadership-in-general, I do think it is worth trying to understand the phenomenon of moral-leadership-in-medicine. So that is where I start.

Each of the paradigms that I listed has elements in common with the model of moral leadership that I describe. None of them tells us in concrete terms, however, what moral leadership is about or how it actually gets done. That is exactly what this book sets out to explain. It addresses the issues that medical leaders identified as being the stuff of moral leadership. And it looks in detail at exactly how moral leadership appears to work, paying attention to the actual behaviours that supported the pursuit of moral goals. I have argued that morality in medicine is a special case of morality, and I suspect that so too is medical leadership a special case of moral leadership. I have argued that what is of critical importance is what we do about moral challenge, not just what we decide.

---

[3] The term enactment is also used by Cribb; see reference 11. Since MacIntyre the notion of enactment has been used in narrative ethics, but the meaning often left unspecified: see reference 13 for Macintyre and 13, p. 5, for one example.

My focus on the medical context, together with my focus on doing, sets this book apart from other discussions of ethical leadership.

Why this book focuses on organizational ethics

Mountains of paper and terabytes of data have been consumed by debate over the ethical principles governing doctors' relationships with patients. Almost as much resource has been invested in defining national, global and humanitarian medical-ethical obligations. There has been far less ethical analysis of the responsibilities that arise at the middle levels of healthcare, that is, where discrete care organizations exist.

This is in some respects surprising because care for patients is almost always provided through care organizations, ranging from small provider partnerships to vast care networks. But social and ethical theorists have generally been slow to recognize the moral dimensions of institutions – or the institutional dimensions of morality – and it is only in recent years that a literature on institutional responsibility in general has emerged [14,15]. This has been matched by growing discussion of the organizational dimension of medical ethics, as clinicians, managers, ethics committees and academics have recognized how organizations shape the problems that they confront. In the past decade there has been wider recognition of the several dimensions of responsibility that care organizations owe: towards the users they serve, towards the community at large, towards the environment, and towards the staff who work in them. Healthcare organizational ethics as a field deals with what these moral responsibilities are, and how they should be discharged (I discuss this literature in Chapter 7).

Healthcare organizations have to decide whom they ought to treat, what conditions should be treated, how they should be treated, and when to turn away people to whom they perceive they have no obligation. They have to decide how to reward those who provide care, how to pay for buildings and equipment, what a dignified environment for care requires, and what part of their budget should be spent on emotional or moral goods such as uplifting art or dignified burial of the dead. Organizations have to ensure that caregivers and care systems are worthy of the trust that patients place in them, and if things go wrong they have to protect patients without doing injustice to the caregivers. And when harm occurs – inevitably, eventually, it will – moral relations must somehow be repaired, and confidence restored. National or local health economies, and leaders in the organizations that plan for them, have to weigh in the balance different demands: to cure people who are sick and care for those who are incurable; to provide care that compensates for the limitations imposed by disability, accidental injury, or genetic bad luck; to prevent illness in people who are currently healthy. Making and implementing such choices, and many more besides, is what healthcare organizational ethics and medical management are about.

We frequently look to the law and to regulators to define a host of organizational responsibilities. But legal responsibilities and regulatory rules are not exhaustive of moral responsibilities. We take it for granted that doctors' responsibilities towards patients go beyond the minimal standards set by law and regulation. The same principle applies at organizational level. Mere compliance with the law or regulatory requirements does not satisfy the moral expectations we have of organizations.

We can see this by working through a familiar example. When a doctor's care causes harm to patients for reasons that are not legally blameworthy – as when a known side effect, which the doctor had explained to the patient, materializes – the law does not demand any further action from the doctor. Medical ethics does. At the very least, an ethical doctor will acknowledge the harm that has occurred, deal with the patient's distress, and generally do what is required to repair the situation. It works the same way at organizational level. When a patient complains to an organization about care that was poor, but not legally blame-worthy, the law does not impose any obligation to respond. Organizational ethics does. At the very least, in an ethical organization an appropriate person who has been appointed to act as the organization's representative will acknowledge the harm, and take steps to ensure that it does not happen again.

It may by now be obvious why organizational ethics has been chosen as the focus for a discussion of medical moral leadership. While medical-ethical issues often require leader-ship, organizational-ethical issues always involve leaders and will always entail leadership. Putting it the other way around, clinicians with formal medical leadership responsibilities will always be doing organizational ethics, whether they know it or not.

How this book isn't just about the British National Health Service

This book is based on a study of medical leaders in the British National Health Service. So is it of relevance to anyone else? The answer is, emphatically, yes. There are two reasons why.

First, healthcare systems around the world are all managing changes characteristic of an era of 'network medicine'. Medicine is a globally organized, protocol-driven, politically contentious welfare industry. These features of medicine have implications for how it is locally organized in every country. Second, healthcare systems around the world are all confronting moral challenges that are integral to medicine itself, however care is organized. One such challenge includes managing medical harm, a key theme in the forthcoming discussion.

Although the NHS supplied the settings in which data were collected, the moral themes that have emerged from this study are highly relevant to medical leaders in other countries.

The new era of 'network medicine': industrialization, institutionalization and diffusion of the health agenda

American bioethicist George Khushf noted over a decade ago that advances in technology and society were transforming the delivery of healthcare in Europe and America; and that comparative scholarship made an important contribution to understanding these global changes [16–20]. The trends he discussed affect healthcare systems across all developed and developing countries. There are three developments to note: global industrialization of medical production; institutionalization of medical procedures; and 'diffusion of the health agenda' across social support systems. These are trends we might conveniently gather together under the rubric of 'network medicine'.

Medicine was once a cottage industry that could be practised by solo physicians and local apothecaries. No longer. Medicine is now a global industry that relies upon complex local, regional, national, and supra-national networks to plan, manage and provide care, and to safeguard public health. Practitioners who work alongside one another in the same locality depend on a global commerce in research, knowledge transfer, pharmaceuticals, medical equipment, and international outsourcing of services such as medical imaging.

Public images of medicine tend to conceal quite how far care has become an industrial process. Ideals of personalized, artisanal medical care have proved remarkably tenacious. Care is often depicted as an interaction between a single doctor and a single patient, albeit against a very high-tech backdrop. This focus on the tip of the iceberg – doctor-patient interactions – tends to obscure the mass of local, national and international systems that are equally important to patients' experiences of care.

One effect of the global trade in medicine, and the escalating expectations that accompany it, is that all developed healthcare systems face similar rising demands, and similar difficulties in rationing services. The central problem of rationing – weighing individual needs and a collective good – permeates all levels of healthcare everywhere in the world to a greater or lesser degree. At the system level, public conviction that a price cannot be put on health or life comes up against the view that healthcare competes with other goods so that its costs ought to be contained [21–23].[4] At an organizational or network level, resources have to be stewarded in such a way that community obligations, service priorities, appropriate standards of care, service improvement, and professional education can all be served. At an individual level healthcare practitioners have to balance that part of their role requiring they act as a patient advocate, with that part requiring they act as gatekeepers to resources [21(Ch8),24–32].[5] Moral leadership is, then, called for at every level.

Worldwide, the joint forces of industrialization, evidence-based medicine and increased awareness of human error have promoted 'institutionalization' – the widespread adoption of care protocols and standardized procedures. These aim to regulate professional practice, reduce the scope for undesirable variability, and avoid accidental harm. The overall effect of institutionalization is to undercut idiosyncratic 'medical artistry', which, whatever its benefits, is worryingly resistant to measurement and evaluation. In place of artistry is an expectation of compliance with protocol, a process which is altogether more amenable to inspection and control [33–36].

With medical processes and health outcomes subject to far greater external scrutiny, there is an increasingly prominent quality management role for both medical leaders and healthcare organizations. A further consequence is the impact of institutionalization on notions of medical professional responsibility. Arguably it will result in 'deprofessionalization' of the medical workforce, with all that this implies for the task of moral leadership.

A growing focus on preventive health measures has resulted in a process bioethicist Alan Cribb dubbed 'the diffusion of the health agenda' [11]. As health outcomes are shown to depend on a range of social factors, so public welfare, self-care, health promotion and social care all assume greater prominence. Doctors and healthcare organizations thereby come to be (no more than) equal partners in a network of providers supporting health and wellbeing. 'Network' style healthcare relies upon many non-medical occupations – in education, social care, welfare and local government organizations – to produce health benefits.

Creating 'seamless' pathways of support across a network of agencies, each with different aims, requires providers both to be clear about what they can contribute and to be adaptable to new demands. In this context, clarity of mission, organizational integrity, effective communication, and meaningful negotiation – all of which call for moral medical leadership – are increasingly important.

In the USA the accelerated move away from fee-for-service payment and health insurance plans, towards 'managed care' health packages, has been in part a response to

---

[4] See, for example, references 21–23.
[5] See, for example, references 21 and 24–32.

industrialization, institutionalization and diffusion of the health agenda. Managed care health plans approach health provision as an industrial process that is in principle amenable to efficiencies of scale, rationalization, managerial control and incentivization.

The criticism, resentment and ethical debate that managed care has provoked reflects the discomfort that arises when artisanal work processes are industrialized [20,37–39].[6] Doctors are in conflict with insurance companies and hospital administrators, acute healthcare organizations in conflict with long-stay facilities, and patients in conflict with them all. Much of this conflict has assumed a moral tone, in arguments about entitlement to care, support, choice, and life itself. Although the immediate reason for of all of this is managed care, the underlying cause is the changing nature of medicine.

In the UK the growth of professional management in the NHS owes much to the era of 'network medicine'. The expansion in the number of NHS managers since the mid-1980s, and the perceived need for well-qualified general managers in senior strategic roles, is frequently ascribed to meddlesome governments. It is better understood as a consequence of industrialization, institutionalization and diffusion of the health agenda. In rather the same way as managed care became the villain in the USA, so too has general management – with its rationing, controlling, bureaucratizing remit – become a target of derision in the UK. Whether network medicine can do without general management, or which general management roles can in fact be better carried out by medical leaders, are questions that still remain to be answered.

Managing medical harm

Medical care carries within itself the ever-present threat of medical harm. The Roman physician Galen, a follower of Hippocrates, recognized this in his command *primum non nocere*: first do no harm. But however hard individual doctors and their organizations work to avoid it, the tragic inevitability of medical harm remains. When it happens, what, morally, must be done?

Ethics is concerned with the question 'what ought I to do?' But as Margaret Walker observed, this

> seems to imply a set of choices on a fresh page. One of our recurrent ethical tasks, however, is better suggested by the question 'What ought I – or better *we* – to do *now*?' after someone has blotted or torn the page by doing something wrong. [40]

When a patient is harmed during medical care, it will not necessarily be because someone has done something wrong. Even when someone has, there are often several people involved, and faulty systems may be equally to blame. But whatever the reason for the harm, the moral order of medicine – an endeavour that aims to make health better, not worse – has been overturned. Moral order must therefore be restored.

Managing medical harm was central to the moral experience of medical leaders interviewed for this book. It is surely central to the moral experience of medical leaders everywhere. One way or another, moral leadership in medicine will always involve moral repair: in the aftermath of medical accidents, treatment errors, equipment failure, catastrophic omissions, unwanted side effects, unanticipated outcomes, organizational dysfunction

---

[6] There is an extensive literature. Agich, Emmanuel and Morreim have been influential in shaping the debate.

and management disasters. For this reason, detailed discussion of morally managing medical harm occupies Chapter 2 and Chapter 5.

How medical leaders described medical management

I have already made plain that moral leadership is not the exclusive preserve of doctors with additional managerial responsibility. But my account of moral leadership is based on a study of medical leaders who were also almost full-time medical managers. If we are to understand something of the complexity of moral leadership in medicine as they experience it, we need to understand something of the complexity of medical management. The picture I sketch below is obviously a portrait of one particular healthcare system but its central features are characteristic of medical management anywhere [41].

Doctors have always been involved in managing healthcare. Whatever the nature of the venture, care has had to be planned, promoted and delivered within available means. But as medical enterprises have become larger and more complex, and the pace of scientific and social change has accelerated, the need for expert medical managers has grown. Moreover, the managerial component present in all medical roles has become more apparent.

The defining feature of medical management is the presence of competing, and sometimes conflicting, values and goals. Medical leadership entails resolving the tension between competing values and goals when such tension is capable of being resolved; and containing the tension when conflict between competing values and goals is not capable of resolution.

The hard choices that NHS medical leaders grapple with will be familiar to colleagues around the world, because human wants will always challenge available healthcare expertise and resources. The need to provide core services at reasonable cost to a large population of patients conflicts with the desire to offer flexible, personalized services that maximize individual choice. The goal of locating complex clinical interventions in well-equipped facilities, where practitioners carry out sufficient procedures to become and remain expert, runs counter to offering accessible services in small facilities close to the homes of potential users. The goal of being responsive to the health needs of local communities, which differ hugely in terms of age, wealth, employment, education, and housing quality, is in conflict with the aim of uniform and equitable standards of provision across regions or nations. A rule of rescue that demands expenditure on expensive treatments for life-threatening conditions in the here and now vies for priority with a rule of prevention demanding expenditure on public health strategies to reduce the burden of ill-health in the communities of the future [42]. And so it goes on.

The organizational background in the UK

In the next paragraphs, I outline medical management roles in the NHS for those who may not be familiar with them. In the section that follows I go on to identify four value conflicts that pervade these roles, and which account for some of the unease with which many doctors view medical management.

Hospital medicine

For those managing hospital medicine in the UK, a turning point took place in the middle of the 1980s when 'general management' was urged upon the NHS. Created in 1948 the NHS had, by that time, existed for a little less than four decades. But it had yet to find an answer to the seemingly insoluble problem of how best to divide managerial powers and responsibilities between doctor leaders, nurse leaders, administrators and financial managers. The upshot, according to the business leader commissioned by the UK government in 1983 to review the situation, was inertia and indecision. His report notoriously observed 'if Florence Nightingale were carrying her lamp through the corridors of the NHS today she would almost certainly be searching for the people in charge'. His proposals, one of which was for robust 'general management' at organizational level, inaugurated a new approach [43–45].

'General management' was meant to result in clear, purposeful leadership. Identifiable managers were to have authority, responsibility and accountability for management decisions at every level of the organization. But the new generation of general managers were confronted with – to put it mildly – a role of considerable complexity and challenge.

There was, of course, the wholly predictable resistance to significant organizational change and reallocation of power. Added to this, general management assumed its place in the NHS just as healthcare systems around the world started to experience the changing medical and political environment I discussed above [46–49].[7] The intransigent problems of resource allocation, cost management, service design and delivery of national policy objectives, ever present in healthcare systems, were as much exacerbated as alleviated by globalization, institutionalization and diffusion of the health agenda.

The difficulties facing general management were compounded by the place of 'lay' managers in professional hierarchies [50–53].[8] It is all too easy for professionals to question the expertise and commitment of lay managers, and for lay managers to question the expertise and commitment of doctors, when disagreements arise about how things should be done [54–59].[9] Medical leaders, many of them observed, are important mediators between the worlds of management and medicine, as the following example suggests.

> [Imagine] you have a doctor who has taken over the role from their predecessor, and doesn't want to take on the predecessor's workload because a chunk of that workload, they don't believe they're trained or competent to deliver. That immediately gives the manager a problem ... I'm in there saying [to the doctor], 'Well actually you're wrong, I think you should be doing that. In fact you're telling the manager that you're not qualified to do that or it's not appropriate for you to do that, and it's really because it's boring and you don't want to do it'. Or I'm coming in there and saying [to the manager] 'Well they're right, and we're going to have to find a different solution because this person's not [appropriately] trained' ... I suppose you can see the medical director role there being used in those two directions. You're there to stop medical staff being pressurized by the management into doing things which are inappropriate or wrong; and you're there to not allow the management to be hoodwinked by the medical staff into doing things.
>
> (Dr. Alex Adrien, Greenborough Hospital Trust)[10]

As general management structures matured, new clinical directorates started to emerge with the aim of improving financial controls and better developing service provision. By the

---

[7] For comparative accounts of doctor manager relationships in the UK and other countries, see references 46–48. An excellent comparative account of the current state of medical management in Europe is to be found in reference 49.

[8] See references 50–53 for articles on bureaucratization and professional management.

[9] For articles discussing doctor-manager relationships, see references 54–59.

[10] The study participants' pseudonyms, together with a description of the type of organization they worked for, are listed at the end of this chapter.

middle of the 1990s, consistent with the requirements of the 1990 NHS Act, NHS hospitals had created clinical directorates. These were formally led by clinicians with the support of general managers, and based around clinical specialties. The clinical director role typically includes recruiting and appraising medical staff, reviewing and improving the quality of services and overseeing the directorate budget. The hospital medical director, an executive member of the board of the organization, sits at the apex of this directorate structure.

Medical directors in secondary care have an extensive portfolio of responsibilities, but they vary from organization to organization. Common to all, though, is one of the most significant moral challenges: managing the performance of individual doctors. Medical directors rarely do this directly, delegating the oversight that is necessary to their clinical directors. But the medical director's desk is where the buck stops, and it is medical directors who must ultimately ensure that the performance of individual doctors is kept under review. This may be done through day-to-day organizational routines, such as ensuring that appraisal is implemented, reviewing clinical governance data, and also through dealing with difficult situations such as patient complaints or disciplinary proceedings. As we shall see, medical directors also rely upon their informal networks, corridor rumours and sometimes their own clinical practice to get 'early warning signs' that colleagues' performance may be cause for concern.

Medical directors will have a major new role to play from 2012, when UK doctors will be required to 'revalidate' their licence to practice every five years. Prior to the introduction of revalidation, UK doctors, once certified, were certified for life. Their licence to practice could be suspended or revoked if they were found guilty of a range of misdemeanours, but there was no requirement to renew their licence on a routine basis. Under the new arrangements all doctors will be obliged to compile a portfolio of evidence demonstrating that they are fit to continue in their role, submitting this to appraisal by a senior clinician on an annual basis. Once every five years, a 'Responsible Officer' will advise the General Medical Council, the profession's regulatory body, whether the doctor's licence should be renewed. As the lead clinician, most hospital medical directors will be the designated 'Responsible Officer' for the doctors who work in their employing organization. This process is unlikely to diminish the scale or scope of the performance issues that medical leaders must manage. It will, however, alter the form in which they arise.

Along with their responsibility for keeping the performance of doctors under review, all hospital medical directors participate in agreeing budgets at Board level. Many become involved in contentious hospital development plans. Some medical directors fulfil the role of the 'Caldicott Guardian', ensuring that personal information about patients and employees is properly safeguarded. Many participate in appointing consultant colleagues, head patient safety or clinical change projects, guide the development of practice protocols, direct investigations into clinical incidents and intervene in disputes over treatment of specific patients.

General practice

In primary care, things are naturally rather different. Although General Practitioners in the UK receive most of their income from public funds, and are branded as NHS providers, general practices are still small businesses run by the practice partners. They generally employ no more than a handful of other clinicians, and are supported by a proportionate office staff. Patterns of authority, responsibility and accountability are clearer within these general practice partnerships. Roughly speaking the partners are co-leaders who all have an equal interest in holding each other accountable for the clinical and financial performance of the practice [60–62].[11]

This simpler picture of medical management in primary care becomes more complex as primary care doctors move into leadership roles at local, regional and national levels. In past decades, most GPs performing leadership roles for the NHS have been doing so within committees, where they advise on the provision of both primary and secondary care within their locality. Some GPs – those interviewed for this book – had taken on full-time leadership positions as medical directors in local Primary Care Trusts. These bodies were responsible for planning and procuring (that is, commissioning) all the NHS care supplied by general practices and hospitals across the local health economy; they also had responsibility for local regulation of GP services. Commissioning responsibilities are due to transfer from Primary Care Trusts to GP-led commissioning consortia in 2012. The moral challenges that lay before a small group of medical leaders involved with Primary Care Trusts at the time of this research will, in future, tax a much wider group of General Practitioners.

The work undertaken by medical directors in primary care reflected the role of the Primary Care Trusts. As those bodies were responsible for commissioning healthcare, and for local regulation of primary care physicians, medical directors were heavily involved in advising on the pattern of local services, and assuring the quality of primary care in their locality. Many participated in decisions on funding 'exceptional' treatment, such as non-routine pre-implantation genetic diagnosis, or drugs not yet approved for use in the NHS. Many were involved in serious incident inquiries. And some had specific responsibilities as directors of public health.

As the government looks to English GPs to take charge of the business of commissioning healthcare in England, their responsibilities are set to become considerably more complicated and morally complex. The GP community has anticipated many of these moral difficulties in its response to the government's proposed changes. There are passionate advocates of GP commissioning, who share the government's view that doctors are those best placed to commission care on behalf of their patients. But many fear that actual conflicts of interest, or perceived conflicts of interest, will compromise the role and status of doctors. This division in the profession reflects the enduring tension in medical management, a tension between focussing on care for individuals and making management decisions for populations.

Commissioning brings with it some vexatious moral responsibilities. A host of moral questions surrounding resource allocation have to be answered in the process of commissioning. They include entitlement to morally controversial therapies (such as those using human gametes and other tissue); the proper limits of NHS provision (IVF for example); difficult decisions around limiting the kinds of treatment that the NHS in a particular locality will provide (a trade-off between what is desirable and what is affordable); justifying the pattern of clinical services, for example trading-off large centres offering clinical excellence against smaller, less sophisticated local services; and holding colleagues to account for their clinical and organizational performance. The changes to commissioning mean that these and similar questions will in future fall to be answered not by 'faceless bureaucrats'

---

[11] For discussion of clinicians as managers, see references 60–62.

but by family doctors. We may begin to wonder which is best, and whether faceless bureaucrats don't after all provide a rather useful service to medicine.

'It's not just about the stethoscope': the pleasures and pitfalls of medical management

One view of modern medicine is that management tasks are integral to it because managing people, and engineering systems, is what secures good care for patients. On this view of medicine as manufacture, the doctor who is not managing is not doing his job. A different view – perhaps more traditional but still widely held – is that management is a dark art that jeopardizes the integrity of clinicians who dabble in it. On this view of medicine as craft, the doctor who is doing more management than is the minimum necessary stands to lose both his honour and his clinical identity. Most medical directors are firmly of the first view, medicine as manufacture. Medicine is not, in the words of one, 'just about the stethoscope'. It simply cannot be done without participating in institutions, organizations, networks, policies, strategies, protocols, guidelines and all the other paraphernalia of planning and control.

Mastery of managerial processes is, for doctors who fall into the first category, a source of considerable satisfaction. If offers the opportunity to have an impact on the experience of a much wider group of patients than they could ever do as a clinician. It is a chance to promote or manage change in organizations so that they work better in the interests of patients, as these doctors understand patients' needs to be; and perhaps to make organizations more responsive to the demands of clinical colleagues too. Formal medical leadership roles bring with them the general pleasures of power, influence, trust and responsibility. But for doctors persuaded that medicine is a craft or art, medical management carries some quite negative connotations. The world of medical management is redolent of much that these doctors resent: bureaucracy, constraint on medical artistry in the form of protocols and policies, inflexible targets, meddlesome lay managers, indifference to individual patients' needs, refusal of clinicians' demands, and so on.

To understand the distaste, and indeed distrust, that medical management sometimes seems to elicit, it helps to see the way in which corporate objectives and expectations can rub up against a cherished ethic of individual professional responsibility. This friction discourages some doctors from taking on managerial roles altogether, and is source of continuing role tension for those who do.

'Playing the percentage game'

It is an everyday fact of life that doctors are obliged to juggle attending to the needs of the patient in front of them with attending to the needs of other patients waiting to be seen, either now or in the more distant future. Medical professional ethics attaches overriding importance to the duty of care that practitioners owe to individual patients in need in the here and now [17,63,64]. In medical management, however, the focus of attention is reversed. Pursuing organizational strategies and implementing health policies is all about tending to the needs of the wider group of future patients.

To play the percentage game – in the memorable phrase used by one of the medical leaders in the study – is to pursue a broadly utilitarian ethic that cuts across ideals of person-focussed care. It invites the medical manager to calculate how a group might benefit from a proposed course of action, and then to proceed with that course of action if the benefits to the group as whole outweigh individual losses. Playing the percentage game is one of the most commonly remarked upon 'pinch points' in medical management. Health-care professionals of all kinds – not just doctors – are trained to make the interests of patients their first concern. Professionals who are drawn to medical management roles because they want to do the best by a group of patients inevitably find themselves making decisions that disadvantage some individuals.

The percentage game is at its most evident in policies aimed at making best use of resources. An obvious example is the local formulary, the list of drugs approved for use within a particular organization (in the UK) or a particular drug benefit plan (in the USA). The most uncomfortable decisions concern marginal benefits to very sick patients gained at considerable cost: say, achieving a few extra days, weeks or months of life for terminally ill patients through costly medication. Few doctors would deny that individual patients could benefit from extra days at the end of life, but most medical managers would be driven to conclude that it served the interests of the population as a whole to exclude it from the formulary and spend the money on something else.

A somewhat different version of the percentage game often emerges around decisions to modernize clinical facilities. Re-arranging small, old-fashioned, less cost-effective clinical units into large, modern, more efficient services means trading-off losses to a group that values the services it currently enjoys, for overall gains to a larger community. This version of the game is often rather more palatable to clinicians. Although few relish the task of justifying to patients a decision to withdraw certain services, most favour the centres of clinical excellence that are created by doing so.

'Giving the best coverage overall'

A second aspect of medical management that discomfits practitioners is the way in which it places communal, corporate needs ahead of specialty allegiances.

All doctors, including those who specialize in general practice, train in specialties, work in specialties and to a significant degree think in specialties. Doctors enter a specialty because they believe it is worthwhile, as well as interesting. Medical leaders rely on doctors' commitment to pursue excellence within their specialty, and to promote, develop and defend their specialty on behalf of their own group of patients. But the job of those leading organizations is to organize services for different groups of patients so as to achieve, as Dr. Chalcraft put it, 'the best coverage overall'.

Specialty interests – in costly equipment, expensive treatments, increased numbers of trainees, more trained doctors – may have to be sacrificed in order to achieve 'the best coverage overall' for the patients the organization serves. Which specialty interests ought to be forfeited, though, for the good of all? Most specialties can establish a good moral claim to the importance of their work. To be communal or corporate in one's thinking requires specialists to moderate their allegiance to their own specialty without, in the view of some, any very compelling reason to do so [65,66].[12] Moreover, medical leaders must be careful not just to moderate, but also to be seen to moderate, their own specialty and directorate allegiances. But in doing so they stand to lose some of the fellowship upon which they may have come to rely. Medical leaders who succumb to favouring their own specialty lose the moral support of the wider group of colleagues. Conversely, doctors harbouring

---

[12] A vivid example of this phenomenon of specialty loyalties is apparent in reference 65.

expectations of favourable treatment from a medical director who is 'one of their own' may well find themselves ruefully disappointed.

Some commentators have argued that specialty allegiances may in the long run give way to a differently ordered professional hierarchy. Observing medical management in the USA, where a cadre of executive medical leaders is further consolidating its position, Montgomery and Freidson have both suggested that traditional divisions along specialty lines may in future be less significant than those produced by extra-clinical roles [67,68]. They prognosticate that professional status distinctions will be drawn according to whether clinicians provide care (the producers), conduct research and education (a knowledge elite) or are involved in managerial activities (an administrative elite). In the here and now, however, specialty allegiances remain. This difficult issue of negotiating collegial expectations leads us to consideration of the third reason many doctors are wary of medical management: 'the standoff thermometer'.

'The stand-off thermometer'

Medical leadership rests on a precarious balance of clinical and managerial credibility. Medical leaders are appointed from the ranks of clinicians who are respected by their colleagues; and bonds of collegiality are almost inseparable from professional respect. Indeed, such bonds are a compelling reason to appoint clinicians as leaders, capable as they are of commanding the loyalty as well as the esteem of peers. But it may then be a hazardous business for medical leaders to go against the interests of the clinician community, as that community sees it.

'The stand-off thermometer' was another term coined by Dr. Chalcraft, which described his estimate of colleagues' reactions to his decisions and actions. Medical leaders may meet with a ferociously heated response, or indeed an icy chill, when they participate in management decisions with which clinician colleagues disagree. Medical leaders are permanently at risk of jeopardizing the bond they enjoyed with clinical colleagues by being seen to side with management; they are equally at risk of losing the respect of management by being seen to be too overtly concerned with the sectional interests of doctors.

'The standoff thermometer' may read particularly hot or cold when medical leaders encounter the definitive point in their leadership career that many remember with particular clarity. This is the shining moment when they propose or defend a course of action that defines them as a corporate leader, not a 'mere' clinician. Such a course of action may well be one in which the needs of the organization, and a wider group of patients, are placed ahead of the needs of a particular specialty, or a smaller group of patients. In other words, it will often be 'the percentage game' or 'getting the best coverage overall' that sets medical leaders at odds with their peers.

Medical directors spoke of how they felt there was no turning back from this point: they felt that their ties with their fellows had changed once and for all. It is, I suggest, a moment at which medical leaders open a new chapter in the narrative of their moral identity. Some doctors, and in indeed medical leaders, may not relish the prospect or realization of this new sense of self.

Accountability 'to God and the patient in front of me'

Holding colleagues to account for the quality of care an organization provides is, morally speaking, one of the most important obligations of medical leadership. It is certainly one of the most demanding, and often troubling. It is relevant to our discussion of 'pinch points' in medical management because some doctors who hold the 'craft' view of medicine chafe at the notion that they are accountable to organizations and to organizational officers.

Accountability to the organization is problematic for those who cleave to a Hippocratic ethic of individual responsibility that predates, by some two and a half thousand years, the organizational structures within which they now work. On one hand are medical managers who are accountable for the clinical performance of the doctors they lead, and who expect doctors in turn to be accountable to them. On the other are doctors whose view is that they are accountable first and foremost to their own patients, then to their profession, and ultimately, in the minds of some, to God. Adherents to these two very different views of accountability may find each other's outlook equally exasperating as well as morally insupportable. As Dr. Breedon told it:

> Some of the most impossible people I've dealt with, they look you in the eyes and say: 'But . . .' and you say, 'Who do you think you're accountable to?' And one of them said, 'I'm accountable to God and the patient in front of me'. 'The taxpayer?' 'Nope'. 'Me?' 'Nope'. 'The Chief Executive, the Board of Directors?' 'Nope'. 'Government?' 'Nope'. It's *really* difficult . . . .
>
> (Dr. Breedon, Barton Dene Hospital)

The adherent to individual responsibility may see himself as the defender of patients' interests, defiant in the face of an overweening bureaucracy bent upon playing the percentage game. The adherent to corporate responsibility may see himself as the promoter of public good, resolutely overriding sectional or individual self-interest. It is unlikely that both will have their way, however compelling each believes their moral position to be.

A synopsis of the book's argument

We are nearly at the end of this introductory chapter, and the time has come to set out the argument that I shall be pursuing in the rest of the book.

I propose that the best way to conceptualize moral leadership in medicine is as the process of orchestrating organizational moral narratives. Organizational moral narratives are created through the interactions of members of an organization with one another, with members of other organizations, and with the people they serve. Organizational moral narratives are the form in which groups express their moral values, and realize their moral decisions. Moral leaders in organizations play a significant role in the emergence of such narratives: instigating, investigating, sense-making, influencing, supporting, promoting and enforcing groups' story-making activities.

For the most part I shall be using the term narrative in preference to story in forthcoming discussion, because narrative has a rather wider meaning (see Chapter 6). Although defining the essence of moral leadership runs the risk of reducing the interesting-sounding process of 'story-making' into a dull and colourless formula, readers may find it helpful to have the following definition in mind: moral leadership is the active promotion of collaborative efforts to formulate, test, modify, and express a fitting moral narrative.

There are three phases in the group enterprise of making an organizational moral narrative. In the first phase, moral leaders become aware of the need for moral action, through starting to make moral sense out of the data of everyday experience. During a second phase, moral leaders involve others in their group in understanding what is going on, and making a deeper moral sense of the situation. In the third and final phase, moral leaders encourage their group to continue to develop and act out their agreed moral narrative. These three phases do not always progress in an orderly manner. Phases may overlap, earlier phases may be revisited, and phases may be skipped. Most often, activity will spiral through the phases, with each phase being revisited and the moral narrative being modified at each turn of the circle.

As individual moral leaders and their groups go about creating and enacting their moral narrative, they conduct themselves in ways that are quite distinctive. Such behaviours are not exclusive to 'morality' but taken together, as a set of values, beliefs, and practices, they are identifiable as moral practices. These moral practices include general 'practices of responsibility' as well as specific practices of 'propriety'.

In adopting the term 'practices of responsibility', I am drawing on the work of philosopher Margaret Walker. She views practices of responsibility as behaviours and cultural arrangements that play 'a fundamental and critical role in trying to secure certain states of affairs ... especially those consisting in or bearing on harms and benefits to other people . . . . It is an important end of these arrangements that certain things get done, and that people and valued things be kept out of unnecessary harm's way' [8(p100–1)]. Walker invites those interested in understanding morality to give greater consideration to the concrete practices that sustain moral relations in society. Practices of responsibility are common and widely recognizable social behaviours, geared towards promoting collective interests and protecting one another from harm.

Walker comments that practices of responsibility are 'as marvellously intricate as philosophical accounts of responsibility have tended to be austere' [8(p100)]. They run the gamut from A to W, if not quite to Z: they include such behaviour as apologizing, blaming, conciliating and excusing; through praising, quizzing or reprimanding; to voicing one's values and whistleblowing [69].[13] We would expect to find in medicine a special subset of practices of responsibility, practices geared towards protecting particularly vulnerable people from harm. Our interest in this book is even more specialized, however; what we shall be considering are that particular subset of practices of responsibility apparent in medical leadership.

I have used the term propriety to identify the central practices of responsibility that medical leaders in this study described. Distinctive patterns of moral thought and action became quite apparent in their accounts of leadership. My argument is that such patterns (in my terms 'proprieties') express insoluble moral tensions present at the heart of medical management. I discuss five such proprieties: fiduciary propriety, bureaucratic propriety, collegial propriety, inquisitorial propriety and restorative propriety. What generates the moral tension is that each of these proprieties gives priority to different needs and values, and in the course of medical management they inevitably come into conflict with each other.

'Fiduciary propriety' will perhaps need least introduction. Doctors stand in a fiduciary relationship to their patient beneficiaries, and the essence of the fiduciary role is to promote the beneficiary's interests. Fiduciary propriety thus exhibits in action the principle that attending to their patients' needs must be doctors' first priority. Learning the skills of fiduciary propriety begins in medical school, and developing them is a life's work.

Fiduciary propriety fuels noble dreams and selfless endeavour. It has motivated courageous action on behalf of patients around the world: patients stigmatized by HIV/AIDS, mutilated during war, incarcerated by state authorities, abandoned by their families. In the normal run of things however, fiduciary propriety is most evident in how it grants

---

[13] The practice of voicing values refers to Gentile; see reference 69.

a licence to speak very assertively on behalf of patients; indeed, to speak in ways that would be thought unacceptable if interests other than those of patients were at stake. It is fiduciary propriety that frequently underpins rhetorical sorties into 'shroud-waving' or other regions of the moral high ground.

'Bureaucratic propriety' has as its first concern the needs of the organization, in so far as the organization is the repository of collective interests. Bureaucracy might seem an unlikely place to go looking for moral goodness. But bureaucracy has a legitimate purpose and a positive ethical intent, in the form of supporting equitable, efficient and effective distribution of community goods such as healthcare. A virtuous bureaucracy serves us very much better than nepotism, for example. Equally, vicious bureaucracy can do great evil. The difference between the two is, to some degree, dependent upon whether bureaucrats act with bureaucratic propriety or bureaucratic impropriety.

The hallmarks of bureaucratic propriety are the behaviours of the good bureaucrat: impartiality in deed and in demeanour, transparency and a willingness to be held to account, abnegation of personal interests and moral predilections, support for rules and protocols as a way of distributing public goods, conscientiousness in office. These practices do not come naturally. They have to be learned, and it takes self-discipline to exercise them, especially in the face of provocation.

'Collegial propriety' is a way of behaving suited to an enterprise in which participants rely not upon hierarchy, but upon goodwill and cooperation, to meet their professional and moral responsibilities. No healthcare professional can meet the needs of their patients single-handedly, nor can they do so without the moral support of others. Collegial propriety is a bond that sustains the medical professional community, and in doing so it also serves patients.

The bonds of collegiality have been the subject of sustained criticism from commentators critical of self-serving professional alliances and their tendency to operate, in George Bernard Shaw's memorable phrase, as a 'conspiracy against the laity' [70]. In the positive form of collegial propriety, we see behaviours that help doctors to understand what they can reasonably ask of others, to express what they owe to each other, and see where they stand in relation to their professional community of practice. Collegial propriety is visible in values and practices such as fellowship, reciprocity, support for and mentoring of juniors, service to a professional body such as a Royal College, arbitration of clinical standards and empathy with fellow professionals.

'Inquisitorial propriety' is a set of moral practices called upon when allegations of harmful treatment, poor performance or misconduct arise. Misconduct, misbehaviour and medical mistakes presented many of the medical leaders in the study with their most intractable moral troubles. The informal and formal inquiries that follow in the wake of actual or alleged misconduct, and actual or alleged mistakes, call for active moral leadership. Inquisitorial propriety facilitates the expression of 'proper behaviour' by everyone involved in an investigation. Medical leaders will typically have experience of several inquiries, while individual doctors or witnesses will be unlikely to experience more than one. Leaders therefore become the repository of understandings of how things ought morally to be done, and their own practice of inquisitorial propriety encourages others to comply.

For the person leading an investigation, 'inquisitorial propriety' suggests demeanours such as objectivity, neutrality and openness to 'hearing the other side'. For the person under investigation, 'inquisitorial propriety' calls for candour, regret and, where appropriate, frank confession. In a complainant, 'inquisitorial propriety' demands truthfulness and, if not forgiveness, then mercy towards the transgressor. Inquiries are capable of either rebuilding or destroying patient trust, collegial relationships, clinician self-confidence, team dynamics and respect for medical management. The answers to apparently pragmatic questions such as who should be told about an allegation, and when, carry a significant moral load: telling the wrong people at the wrong time in the wrong way can cause real injustice.

'Restorative propriety' is the fifth and final propriety. It is conduct that seeks to restore moral relations after harm and it turns on acknowledgement: acknowledging that a harm has occurred, acknowledging that certain persons or bodies are responsible, acknowledging that a complaint is legitimate, acknowledging that the person who was harmed has a 'moral right' to define the situation in their terms, acknowledging that steps must be taken to respond.

'Restorative propriety' is a familiar element in our everyday lives, apparent in such behaviours as contrition, the performance of apologies, or making financial restitution. Restorative propriety becomes much more problematic in institutional settings. In organizations, it raises questions such as who has standing to 'perform' gestures such as apology, whether there is sincere regret, whether and what changes to practice may be made, and how such changes can be monitored.

One of the most potent sources of moral anxiety in medical leadership roles is that these five proprieties not infrequently conflict with one another. Each propriety promotes a particular moral good, permitting – to recall Walker – 'people and valued things to be kept out of unnecessary harm's way' [8(p100–1)]. But precisely because each propriety gives priority to a singular good, medical leaders find the proprieties pulling in different directions. They may find they have to choose between enacting the good of partiality towards their own patients in fiduciary propriety or enacting the good of impartiality towards patients in general in bureaucratic propriety; between enacting the good of fellowship in collegial propriety and enacting the good of neutrality in inquisitorial propriety; or between enacting the good of 'hearing the other side' in inquisitorial propriety and enacting the good of acknowledging a patient's perception of harm in 'restorative propriety'.

Medical leaders have many overlapping moral responsibilities: to individual patients, to the general population, to their political masters, to their colleagues, and to those who may be or become the victims of medical harm. Switching between 'proprieties' may be even more demanding than choosing between moral principles. This is because the proprieties are not necessarily consciously recognized forms of behaviour. Whatever knowledge medical leaders have of the proprieties tends to be tacitly held. This means that the basis for a strongly felt decisional bias may not always be apparent; and that a customary behaviour may take hold of the situation before there is any conscious deliberation about how best to proceed.

The medical leaders I interviewed for this study described moral leadership in ways that pose important questions about what we mean when we talk about 'morality'. I noted earlier that Kant placed the capacity to reason, and compliance with moral duty, at the centre of his account of morality. For Kant, being 'moral' meant to align one's actions with universal and absolute moral laws. If this meant unwillingly surrendering to the demands of moral duty, against one's inclinations, so much the better [71,72].[14] This rather austere view encouraged Kant to argue that

---

[14] For a helpful exposition see reference 72.

'accessibility, affability, politeness, refinement, propriety, courtesy, and ingratiating and captivating behaviour ... call for no large measure of moral determination and cannot, therefore, be reckoned as virtues.' [73]

I think that Kant's emphasis on reason and duty tends to narrow the scope of morality and virtue too far. I propose a broader view. It is one that includes social behaviours that could appear, superficially, to be no more than accessibility, politeness, refinement and so on. In the form of propriety, such behaviours constitute highly disciplined moral accomplishments that help to build ethical healthcare organizations. Propriety is the medium through which important values and principles find expression and have consequences. My argument in this book is not that norms, obligations, reasons, duties or, on occasion, universal moral laws are unimportant. My point, rather, is that these are not the only moral artefacts that are important. I shall be arguing throughout that understanding the behaviours through which we express our commitment to duties, responsibilities, obligations and so on is at least as important as debating the norms themselves.

How the book is organized

We shall shortly start to consider the stories of moral leadership that are at the heart of the book. My analysis of them proceeds as follows.

The narratives begin in Chapter 2, where readers get an overview of the cycle of moral leadership in healthcare organizations by following two medical directors managing the aftermath of serious failures of care. Chapter 2 looks at how moral issues come to the attention of medical leaders, how they make sense of the circumstances they find themselves in, and how they go about orchestrating a response to moral troubles. In this chapter I aim to make intelligible the definition of moral leadership as the active promotion of collaborative efforts to formulate, test, modify and express a fitting moral narrative.

Chapter 3 then follows up the concerns of Chapter 2, focussing on the 'normative expectations' that medical directors hold. The concept of normative expectations is an important one that is introduced for the first time in Chapter 2 and then re-emerges throughout subsequent chapters. In Chapter 3 I explore normative expectations by looking at several more of the stories that medical leaders told about the moral challenges of their role. As we examine further examples we gain greater understanding of how medical leaders think about appropriate standards of behaviour in organizations, and how they become alert to potential moral troubles.

A Prologue to Chapters 4 and 5 introduces the concept of propriety that is the focus of those chapters. In Chapters 4 and 5 I examine the fine grain of moral leadership, looking at how propriety works to structure moral behaviours and give expression to distinctive clusters of belief and value. In Chapter 4 I analyse fiduciary, bureaucratic and collegial proprieties through the lens of organizational moral narratives concerning service redesign and resource management. In Chapter 5 I explore inquisitorial and restorative propriety in the context of organizational moral narratives seeking to repair confidence, trust and hope following medical harm. In these two chapters I show how moral leadership entails seeking an appropriate balance between what are seemingly contradictory needs and ideals. In the Epilogue to Chapters 4 and 5 I then look at some important general questions about the proprieties. I discuss here how the concept of propriety emerged from the research, how medical leaders learn it, and how it differs from notions of virtue.

Chapter 6 returns to theoretical concerns, examining the theoretical basis for the concept of organizational moral narrative. I look here at how my model of moral narrative relates to other domains of scholarship in narrative ethics and narrative social research. This chapter therefore clarifies what is meant in the book by narrative, and it supplies a theoretical underpinning to claims made about the nature of narrative in earlier chapters. This chapter is not entirely abstract, however. It contains further examples of the organizational moral narratives that medical leaders recounted.

In Chapter 7 I draw together the strands of earlier discussion to consider how my account of moral leadership relates to the emerging field of healthcare organizational ethics, and how it might contribute to it. I consider here some continuing controversies about approaches to bioethics in general, and the new directions suggested by the 'expressive-collaborative' model of morality that has been proposed by Margaret Walker. In the final part of Chapter 7 I consider how educators can help to develop the ethical expertise that healthcare organizations need. I argue that we need to balance our efforts to promote sound individual normative reasoning with efforts to enhance the performance of collaborative moral practice. There are no easy answers, especially given how much we already ask medical students and trainees to learn, but I hope here to stimulate a dialogue with other educators so that we can find a way forward together.

Readers who wish to review the conduct of the research will find it described in Appendix 1. A summary of the performance management framework for individuals and organizations in the NHS is included for reference in Appendix 2. Readers who have no familiarity with the ethical frameworks commonly used for doing applied ethics in medicine may find the short guide in Appendix 3 to be useful. I would emphasize again, however, that it is quite possible to understand what medical leaders were doing without knowing anything about applied ethics or moral philosophy.

Addendum: the study participants

Who were the participants in this study and in what contexts did they work? The medical directors were drawn from three types of NHS organization: general and specialist hospital trusts, mental health trusts and primary care trusts. They are introduced by their pseudonyms below, with a brief description of their employing organization. I named participants alphabetically by random selection of surname and first name in the order in which they were interviewed. For convenience each was allocated the same initials for the first and last name (Dr. A.A, Dr. B.B, and so on). This alliterative conceit aimed to make it easier to recognize each participant but might become tiresome for the reader. For this, apologies are offered in advance.

The pseudonyms suggest that all of the participants were of white British origin. This is consistent with the interview sample, and it reflects the ethnic origin of the overwhelming majority of current NHS medical directors. The names also indicate that about one-fifth of the sample were women. Although twenty-four participants were interviewed, twenty-five names are listed. This is because one interview has been split into two parts, so as to protect the participant's anonymity when reporting sensitive data.

Doctor	Name and type of organization
1. Alex Adrien	Greenborough Hospital Trust, a district general hospital on the outer fringes of a large city.
2. Ben Breedon	Barton Dene Hospital, a general hospital serving an economically disadvantaged metropolitan district.
3. Christopher Chalcraft	The Royal Metropolitan Infirmary, a major inner-city teaching hospital.
4. Daniel Dillon	Five Bridges Mental Health Trust, a large organization serving part of a major city.
5. Edward Evans	Brickvale Hospital NHS Trust, a general hospital serving an old industrial area of a major city.
6. Francis Fox	The Three Spires Hospital, a large general hospital based in a prosperous county town.
7. George Gulvin	Stoneyhill and District NHS Trust, a group of hospitals and health centres serving a major city.
8. Henry Hutchinson	Evenlode Park NHS Trust, a large mental health organization in a major city.
9. Ingrid Iliffe	Graveldene NHS Trust, a thriving district general hospital.
10. Jonathan Jay	The Charter NHS Trust, a specialist hospital.
11. Katie Kingsley	Cityside NHS Trust, a hospital and several community facilities serving part of a large city.
12. Luke Lister	Long River Hospital NHS Trust, a large city teaching hospital.
13. Matthew McGregor	Remembrance Hospitals Trust, a major teaching hospital.
14. Nathan Nugen	Former medical director in more than one large city hospital.
15. Oliver Oxley	Goldenshire Primary Care Trust, based in a prosperous county.
16. Patrick Phelps	Valleyshire University Hospitals Trust, a group of city teaching hospitals.
17. Quentin Quinn	Bankside Hospitals NHS Trust, a group of hospitals serving a large city and its surrounding area.
18. Richard Rosenberg	St. Frideswide Hospitals NHS Trust, a group of hospitals serving an urban conurbation.
19. Samuel Seddon	Saxonvale University Hospitals Trust, a group of teaching hospitals serving a major city and its surrounding area.
20. Thomas Thirtle	Parkside Primary Care Trust, based in a vibrant, economically and racially diverse inner-city area.
21. Ursula Usborne	Churchland Primary Care Trust, based in a deprived inner city area with a predominantly minority ethnic population.
22. Vivian Vaisey	Riverdale Primary Care Trust, based in a mixed agricultural and industrial county.
23. William Woodhouse	Meadborough Primary Care Trust, located in an economically and ethnically mixed inner city area.

Doctor	Name and type of organization
24. Yvonne Young	Urban Marshes Primary Care Trust, serving a large industrial conurbation.
25. Anne Archer	The Royal City Hospital NHS Trust, a large teaching hospital.

Further reading

Hartley J, Benington J. *Leadership for Healthcare*. Bristol: The Policy Press; 2010.

Cribb A. *Health and the Good Society: Setting Healthcare Ethics in Social Context*. Oxford: Clarendon Press; 2005.

Boyle PJ, DuBose ER, Ellingson SJ, Guinn DE, McCurdy DB. *Organizational Ethics in Health Care: Principles, Cases, and Practical Solutions*. San Francisco, CA: Jossey-Bass and AHA Press; 2000.

The NHS Handbook. London: NHS Confederation; published annually.

Tallis R. *Hippocratic Oaths: Medicine and its Discontents*. London: Atlantic Books; 2004.

References

1. Peshkin GC. *Becoming Qualitative Researchers: An Introduction*. New York: Longmans; 1992.

2. Chambers T. *The Fiction of Bioethics: Cases as Literary Texts*. New York: Routledge; 1999.

3. Davis D. Rich cases: the ethics of thick description. *Hastings Center Report*. 1991;**21**:12–7.

4. Williams B. *Ethics and the Limits of Philosophy*. Kermode F, ed. London: Fontana Paperbacks and William Collins; 1985.

5. André J. *Bioethics as Practice*. Chapel Hill: University of North Carolina Press; 2002.

6. Chambliss DF. *Beyond Caring: Hospitals, Nurses, and the Social Organization of Ethics*. Chicago: Chicago University Press; 1996.

7. Gert B. The definition of morality. In: Zalta EN, ed. *The Stanford Encyclopedia of Philosophy*. Stanford: Metaphysics Research Lab; 2008.

8. Walker MU. *Moral Understandings: A Feminist Study in Ethics*. 2nd edn. New York: Oxford University Press; 2007.

9. Crislip AT. *From Monastery to Hospital: Christian Monasticism and the Transformation of Health Care in Late Antiquity*. Ann Arbor: University of Michigan Press; 2005.

10. Harris J. *The Value of Life*. London: Routledge; 1985.

11. Cribb A. *Health and the Good Society: Setting Healthcare Ethics in Social Context*. Oxford: Clarendon Press; 2005.

12. MacIntyre A. *After Virtue*. 3rd edn. London: Duckworth; 2007.

13. Greenhalgh T, Hurwitz B, eds. *Narrative Based Medicine*. London: BMJ Books; 1998.

14. Thompson DF. *Restoring Responsibility: Ethics in Government, Business, and Healthcare*. Cambridge: Cambridge University Press; 2005.

15. Williams G. 'Infrastructures of responsibility': the moral tasks of institutions. *Journal of Applied Philosophy*. 2006;**23**(2):14.

16. Khushf G. The case for managed care: reappraising medical and socio-political ideals. *Journal of Medicine and Philosophy*. 1999;**24**:415–33.

17. Khushf G. The value of comparative analysis in framing the problems of organizational ethics. *HEC Forum*. 2001; **13**(2):125–31.

18. Cribb A. Reconfiguring professional ethics: the rise of managerialism and public health in the U.K. National Health Service. *HEC Forum*. 2001;**13**(2): 111–24.

19. Rodwin MA. *Medicine, Money and Morals.* New York: Oxford University Press; 1993.

20. Morreim H. *Balancing Act; The New Medical Ethics of Medicine's New Economics.* Washington DC: Georgetown University Press; 1995.

21. Daniels N. *Just Health: Meeting Health Needs Fairly.* New York: Cambridge University Press; 2008.

22. Daniels N, Sabin J. *Setting Limits Fairly: Can We Learn to Share Medical Resources?* New York: Oxford University Press; 2002.

23. Menzel PT. Justice and the basic structure of health-care Systems. In: Battin MP, Rhodes R, Silvers A, eds. *Medicine and Social Justice: Essays on the Distribution of Health Care.* New York: Oxford University Press; 2002.

24. Angell M. The doctor as double agent. *Kennedy Institute of Ethics Journal.* 1993;3 (3):279–86.

25. Menzel PT. Double agency and the ethics of rationing health care: a response to Marcia Angell. *Kennedy Institute of Ethics Journal.* 1993;3(3):287–92.

26. Beach MC, Meredith LS, Halpern J, Wells KB, Ford DE. Physician conceptions of responsibility to individual patients and distributive justice in health care. *Annals of Family Medicine.* 2005;3(1):53–9.

27. Tauber AI. Medicine, public health and the ethics of rationing. *Perspectives in Biology and Medicine.* 2002;45(1):16–30.

28. Alexander GC, Hall MA, Lantos JD. Rethinking professional ethics in the cost-sharing era. *The American Journal of Bioethics.* 2006;6(4):17–22.

29. Weingarten MA, Guttman N, Abramovitch H, Margalit RS, Roter D, Ziv A, et al. An anatomy of conflicts in primary care encounters: a multi-method study. *Family Practice.* 2010;27(1):93–100.

30. Spece R, Shimm D, Buchanan A. *Conflicts of Interest in Clinical Practice and Research:* Oxford University Press; 1996.

31. Murray TH. Divided loyalties for physicians: social context and moral problems. *Social Science & Medicine.* 1986;23(8):827–32.

32. Morar S. Ethical aspects of the physician-society relationship (Aspecte etice ale relaţiei medic-Societate). *Revista Romana de Bioetica.* 2007;5(2):37–42.

33. Timmermans S, Berg M. *The Gold Standard: The Challenge of Evidence-Based Medicine and Standardization in Health Care.* Philadelphia: Temple University Press; 2003.

34. Timmermans S, Mauck A. The promises and pitfalls of evidence-based medicine. *Health Affairs.* 2005;24(1):18–28.

35. Timmermans S, Epstein S. A world of standards but not a standard world: toward a sociology of standards and standardization. *Annual Review of Sociology.* 2010;36(1):69–89.

36. Mykhalovskiy E, Weir L. The problem of evidence-based medicine: directions for social science. *Social Science & Medicine.* 2004;59(5):1059–69.

37. Agich GJ. The Importance of management for understanding managed care. *Journal of Medicine and Philosophy.* 1999;24:518–34.

38. Emanuel EJ. Medical ethics in the era of managed care: the need for institional structures instead of principles for individual cases. *Journal of Clinical Ethics.* 1995;6:335–8.

39. Bondeson WB, Jones JW, eds. *The Ethics of Managed Care: Professional Integrity and Patient Rights.* Dordrecht: Kluwer; 2002.

40. Walker MU. *Moral Repair: Reconstructing Moral Relations after Wrongdoing.* Cambridge: Cambridge University Press; 2006.

41. Žydžiūnaite V, Suominen T, Åstedt-Kurki P, Lepaite D. Ethical dilemmas concerning decision-making within health care leadership: a systematic literature review. *Medicina (Kaunas)* 2010;46(9):595–603.

42. Klein R. What does the future hold for the NHS at 60? *BMJ.* 2008;337:a549.

43. Griffiths R. *NHS Management Inquiry Report.* London: Department of Health and Social Security; 1983.

44. Harrison S, *et al*. *Just Managing: Power and Culture in the National Health Service*. London: Macmillan; 1992.

45. Watkins S. Medicine and government: partnership spurned. In: Harrison AGS, ed. *Governing Medicine: Theory and Practice*. Maidenhead: Open University Press; 2004.

46. Fitzgerald L, Dufour Y. Clinical management as boundary management: a comparative analysis of Canadian and U.K health-care institutions. *Journal of Management in Medicine* 1998;**12**(4–5):199–214

47. Rundall TG, Davies HT, Hodges CL. Doctor-manager relationships in the United States and the United Kingdom. *J Healthcare Management* 2004;**49**(4): 251–68; discussion 68–70.

48. Kirkpatrick I, Jespersen PK, Dent M, Neogy I. Medicine and management in a comparative perspective: the case of Denmark and England. *Sociology of Health & Illness*. 2009;**31**(5):642–58.

49. Neogy Indareth KI. *Medicine in Management: Lessons Across Europe*. Leeds: Centre for Innovation in Health Management, University of Leeds; 2009.

50. Kitchener M. The bureaucratization of professional roles: the case of clinical directors in U.K hospitals. *Organization*. 2004;**7**(1):129–54.

51. Fitzgerald L, Lilley C, Ferlie E, Addicott R, McGivern G, Buchanan D. *Managing Change and Role Enactment in the Professionalised Organisation*: National Co-ordinating Centre for NHS Service Delivery and Organisation R & D (NCCSDO); 2006.

52. Waring J, Currie G. Managing expert knowledge: organizational challenges and managerial futures for the UK medical profession. *Organization Studies*. 2009;**30**(7):755–78.

53. Ewa Wikström LD. Contemporary leadership in healthcare organizations: fragmented or concurrent leadership. *Journal of Health Organization and Management*. 2009;**23**(4):411–28.

54. Davies H, Harrison S. Trends in doctor-manager relationships. *BMJ*. 2003;**326**:646–9.

55. Davies H, Hodges C, Rundall T. Views of doctors and managers on the doctor-manager relationship in the N.H.S. *BMJ*. 2003;**326**:626–8.

56. Huw Davies C-LH, Thomas Rundall. Consensus and contention: doctors' and managers' perceptions of the doctor-manager relationship. *British Journal of Healthcare Management*. 2003;**9**(6):202–8.

57. Marshall MN. Doctors, managers and the battle for quality. *Journal of the Royal Society of Medicine* 2008;**101**(7):330–1.

58. Kirkpatrick IS, Shelly M, Dent M, Neogy I. Towards a productive relationship between medicine and management: reporting from a national inquiry. *The International Journal of Clinical Leadership*. 2008;**16**(1):27–35.

59. Harrison S, Hunter D, Marnoch G, Politt C. *Just Managing: Power and Culture in the National Health Service*. Basingstoke: Palgrave Macmillan; 1992.

60. Llewellyn S. 'Two-way windows': clinicians as medical managers. *Organization Studies*. 2001;**22**(4):593–623.

61. Iedema R, Degeling P, Braithwaite J, White L. 'It's an interesting conversation I'm hearing': the doctor as manager. *Organization Studies*. 2003;**25**(1):15–33.

62. Witman Y, Smid GAC, Meurs PL, Willems DL. Doctor in the lead: balancing between two worlds. *Organization*. 2011;**18**(4):477–95.

63. GMC. *Good Medical Practice: General Medical Council*; 2006. Available from: http://www.gmc-uk.org/guidance/good_medical_practice.asp; http://www.gmc-uk.org/static/documents/content/GMP_0910.pdf

64. GMC. *Management for Doctors: General Medical Council*; 2006. Available from: http://www.gmc-uk.org/guidance/ethical_guidance/management_for_doctors.asp; http://www.gmc-uk.org/Management_for_doctors_2006.pdf_27493833.pdf.

65. Gibson JL, Martin DK, Singer PA. Priority setting in hospitals: Fairness, inclusiveness, and the problem of institutional power differences *Social science & medicine*. 2005;**61**:2355–62

66. Gibson JL, Martin DK, Singer PA. Evidence, economics and ethics: resource allocation in health services organizations. *Healthcare Quarterly*. 2005;**8**(2):50–9, 4.

67. Freidson E. *Professionalism Reborn: Theory, Prophesy and Policy*. Chicago: University of Chicago Press; 1994.

68. Montgomery K. Physician executives: the evolution and impact of a hybrid profession. *Advances in Healthcare Management*. 2001;**2**:215–41.

69. Gentile MC. *Giving Voice to Values: How to Speak Your Mind When You Know What's Right* New Haven and London: Yale University Press; 2010.

70. Shaw GB. *The Doctor's Dilemma*. London: Constable; 1911. xxii, Act 1: p. 28.

71. Kant I. *Fundamental Principles of the Metaphysic of Morals*. New York: Prentice Hall, Library of Liberal Arts Press; 1949.

72. Norman R. *The Moral Philosophers*. 2nd edn. Oxford: Oxford University Press; 1998, Ch. 6.

73. Kant I. *Lectures on Ethics 1875–1880*. Translated by L Infield. New York: Harper; 1963.

Creating an organizational narrative

Leadership ultimately involves an ability to
define the reality of others .... In managing
the meanings and interpretations assigned to
a situation, the leader in effect wields a form
of symbolic power that exerts a decisive
influence on how people perceive their
realities and hence the way they act ... [1]

In the skeleton argument I set out in Chapter 1, I proposed that moral leadership is a process of orchestrating a moral narrative that finds expression in group and organizational activity. This chapter is the first of four that will describe this sort of moral leadership in action. It supplies an overview of the process of creating moral narrative, from initial awareness that something troubling may be happening, through to full realization of a comprehensive and compelling narrative shaping organizational behaviour.

We will follow the moral narrative assembled by two clinicians who took action in response to their suspicions of potentially serious medical malpractice. Each of their narratives is unique to the circumstances that they confronted and, to some degree, themselves created. But these narratives have been selected as typical of the account medical leaders gave me of dealing with 'moral trouble' in general, and with this sort of 'moral trouble' in particular.

In Chapter 1 I introduced a definition of moral leadership that it would be as well to revisit here. When a group creates a good moral narrative in response to events, significant moral values come to be realized in group members' interaction with one another and moral decisions are acted out in group members' behaviour. Moral leaders are those who instigate, influence, orchestrate and support groups' narrative activities. I therefore defined moral leadership in medicine as the active promotion of collaborative efforts to formulate, test, modify and express a fitting moral narrative.

What is a 'moral narrative'? When I use the term I mean to connote two aspects of narrative.

The first aspect is the most familiar and obvious. Moral narrative is what we communicate about events we see as morally significant. Moral narrative is what we say or write has happened, the moral significance we ascribe to what has happened when we say or write about it, and what we argue ought to happen next. I use the term narrative here because

I share the view with other ethicists that our moral thought and communications tend to be organized in story-like fashion [2,3].[1]

The second aspect of moral narrative, the rather less familiar and less obvious use of the notion of narrative, is what we *do* about a morally significant event. Moral narrative is what we do in order to find out what has happened, how we behave to convey the moral meaning of events to one another, how we act by way of a response to moral challenge. I use the term narrative here because I share the view with other social theorists that we tend to organize many dimensions of social activity in a story-like way [4,5].[2] We do so not least because a great deal of what we are actually doing in social life is expressing ourselves through our behaviour.

We will see as we follow the narratives in this chapter how two leaders converted their moral anxiety into ethical action; in other words, how they enacted moral leadership. Caught up in the rush, the clamour and the competing demands of medical management what arrests clinicians' moral attention? How do they make sense of events? What do they set out to do in response to events? How do they influence those around them? The two narratives will illustrate how moral leadership starts in the reasoning of individuals situated within a 'knowledge network', then how it proceeds through individuals influencing the behaviour of associates, and finally how it ends up in the cultural memory of organizations. In later chapters we will look more closely at the shape of activity within these basic processes, seeing how distinctive sets of moral ideas come to be expressed in matching patterns of moral behaviour.

Returning to my definition of moral leadership, exactly what 'the active promotion of collaborative efforts to formulate, test, modify and express a fitting moral narrative' involves, will no doubt seem somewhat opaque at present. It is the aim of this chapter to make it comprehensible. A more theoretical account of narrative and moral narrative, illustrated with examples from the study, appears in Chapter 7.

Three phases in moral leadership

In this chapter we meet two medical directors, to whom I have given the names Dr. Luke Lister and Dr. Ursula Usborne.

Dr. Lister stepped up to the role of medical director at the Long River Hospital NHS Trust just as evidence was emerging of serious failings in the care provided by one of his departments. So far as he could tell at the time, several patients appeared to have died entirely avoidable deaths as a direct result of poor care. An internal inquiry was instituted, external organizations became involved, the local press pursued the issue on behalf of aggrieved families, and the affair became the dominating concern of Dr. Lister's working life for the next two years.

Around the same period, Dr. Ursula Usborne took up her post as medical director in Churchland Primary Care Trust. At the time of this study, Primary Care Trusts (PCTs) had oversight of primary medical services across a geographical region. Reviewing the standards of performance by General Practitioners in primary care in her region, Dr. Usborne came to have doubts about almost thirty doctors. In her view, the care they provided was

---

[1] Notably references 2 and 3. Chapter 7 cites a number of authors writing from the perspective of narrative medicine and narrative medical ethics.

[2] See references in Chapter 7, and in particular 4 and 5 listed at the end of this chapter.

sufficiently poor that it warranted intervention by the PCT. Five years on, the result of her work was that almost half of those doctors were no longer in practice, either there or anywhere else; and, as importantly, General Practitioners across the region were aware that improving clinical standards was an overriding priority for the PCT.

The moral trouble we study in this chapter – managing actual and potential medical harm – is, in some respects, a highly specialized form of moral leadership. Studying the moral management of medical harm helps us to see, however, patterns of interaction that are common to many instances of moral leadership and enacted ethics. Just as importantly, it gives us some insight, right at the beginning of our inquiry into moral leadership, into a morally complex responsibility which troubled almost all medical leaders and affected many of them deeply. In this chapter our attention is focussed on the challenge of dealing with practitioners who have done harm because they may not be competent. When we return to the topic of medical harm in later chapters, we will look at how medical leaders respond to a wider range of harms to patients. These include innocent accidents, unavoidable complications and institutionalized indignities, as well as incompetent care.

Dr. Lister and Dr. Usborne found themselves managing situations that were in many respects very different. But their stories evidence three critical phases of activity that all moral leadership work has in common.

In a first phase, moral leaders recognize the need for moral action as they begin to make sense of an experience.

In a second phase, moral leaders involve others in making deeper moral sense of the situation.

In a third phase, moral leaders elicit the commitment of others who enact a shared vision.

The purpose of moral leadership is to bring about a state of affairs that manifests ethical aspirations. It is not enough to know one's own values, or to be able to make defensible moral decisions. What truly matters is that the course of action a group pursues exhibits values that are believed to be important. Enactment is what counts, and the role of the moral leader is to catalyse it. So these three phases of activity are phases through which a group 'enacts ethics' as well as being phases of moral leadership.

Whilst the three phases I describe are distinguishable, we should be careful not to treat them as a rigid sequence. Sometimes they will run concurrently, so that, for example, people begin to make a commitment to a solution while they are still trying to make sense of a situation. Sometimes there will be abrupt halts in the process or reversions to an earlier phase, as new events occur or when new information comes to light. Predictably, but importantly, any one of these three phases is capable of going awry; with the result that moral leadership fails to achieve its goal.

The background to the stories that follow

Dr. Luke Lister was appointed to the position of medical director at Long River Hospital NHS Trust having spent much of his career there. By the time we met he had worked for over thirty years within his demanding specialty, treating people who face mortifying, painful and potentially life-threatening conditions. As a clinician, he had built up a widely respected specialist treatment centre during some very lean years of Government under-investment in the NHS as well as earning a reputation for being a supportive and wise colleague. He was, in many respects, an obvious choice for the medical director role.

As the Trust's medical director, Dr. Lister led a consultant body based in several hospital sites and responsible for providing secondary care to a population of about half a million people. Many of his consultants also took tertiary care referrals (from specialists to other specialists) for patients from all over Britain and abroad. Long River Hospital Trust is, in addition, a significant provider of education and training for medical students and junior doctors, many from leading medical schools and among whom will undoubtedly be found future leaders of their profession.

Visitors to the most prominent of the Long River Trust's hospitals will find themselves in hard-edged, modernist buildings designed to declare, as well as to deliver, the promises of scientific healthcare. There are departments of national repute to be found behind an impressive frontage of concrete and steel and glass, and arrayed along colour-coded hallways. The Trust's other hospitals are older and still await redevelopment, and for the most part they are providing local services to local people. But although more modest in scale, they have in the past earned a well-deserved reputation for good care. Overall the Trust had much to be proud of at the time it ran into adversity.

Dr. Ursula Usborne worked in very different circumstances. At the time that I interviewed her, she had been the medical director of the Churchland PCT for about five years. From the outset of her career as a General Practitioner she had been a modernizer. She was an early adopter of 'new' information technologies, seeing their potential for monitoring and managing patients in primary care. She was involved in pilots to develop an NHS 'internal market', in which primary care practitioners would 'procure' NHS secondary care on behalf of their patients. And she was a keen observer of regulatory reform for the medical profession, supportive of efforts to increase the accountability of general practitioners in particular.

Churchland Primary Care Trust is headquartered in what was, in the days before the National Health Service, a hospital heavily dependent upon charity. The modest red-brick architecture and the plaques recording the generosity of long dead municipal grandees are a visible reminder of the philanthropic history of healthcare in the UK. Churchland itself is a neighbourhood much in need of philanthropy, having long been a deprived quarter of the city. Although there are remnants of past glory and scraps of gentrification among the general decay, Churchland today is a visibly post-imperial, post-industrial landscape. Its multi-racial population endures some of the worst poverty and poor health in the UK, and for many residents their expectancy of life will be well below the European average.

The scale of the task that Ursula Usborne faced when she arrived at Churchland becomes apparent if we set the outcome of her work there in context. Medical directors commonly quote a rough and ready assumption that about one in every twenty doctors working in the NHS may, for one reason or another, be failing to meet required standards of professional behaviour [6–14].[3] However, at the time of my meeting with her Dr. Usborne had halted the practice of more than a dozen doctors, and had a similar number working under some form of supervised, remedial practice. Had the doctors working in and around Churchland been a standard population of general practitioners, Dr. Usborne might have expected to encounter about six or seven experiencing

---

[3] The source of this statistic appears to be Donaldson's study entitled *Doctors with Problems in an NHS workforce*. See reference 7 for this study and references 6 and 8–13 for discussion of this research. See also reference 14.

performance problems.[4] Her numbers were some four times that. In order to preserve confidentiality, I have not given the exact figures for the numbers of doctors who were locally regulated by the Churchland Primary Care Trust, and it should be noted that Dr. Usborne's area was similar in size to at least fifty others. It is with some justification then, as well as rhetorical emphasis, that Dr. Usborne described what had been thought 'good enough' primary care for Churchland's residents in the past:

> Get some doctors in. Anyone will do .... And don't say boo in case they leave.

The cycle begins: moral leaders recognize the need for moral action

Moral leadership begins with a person being provoked into making moral sense out of the data of experience [15,16].[5] This is a contentious statement in philosophical terms. It invites questions about how persons have experiences, how persons make sense, and indeed whether we do freely decide how we will act. For current purposes we are obliged to bypass those difficulties, and the argument will proceed on the basis of the following assumptions.

First, moral leadership comes from persons. Every moral leader has a unique identity: beliefs about how the world works, values to which they commit with greater or lesser tenacity, cognitive capacity, a sense of self shaped by past experiences, a set of current role obligations, copious social and professional skills and knowledge, underlying character traits, and transient emotional states. These characteristics all function as perceptual filters. They affect what medical moral leaders will look for, notice and attend to in the dazzlingly complex world in which they work.[6]

Second, moral leadership has to attend to the particular situations in which persons find themselves. This presents would-be moral leaders with the not inconsiderable problem of ascertaining what the situation actually is. Life consists of many stubborn facts, but these give rise to multiple interpretive possibilities. Moral leaders have to perceive facts that have moral implications, perceive their moral salience and pay attention to potential moral trouble, often in situations where they are the only one who thinks at the outset that anything is amiss.

Third, because moral leaders take action on the basis of the sense that they make, the sense they make also 'makes' the world into what it becomes. We act on what believe to be true.

---

[4] The comparison has been made using the NHS Information Centre for Health and Social Care General and Personal Medical Services Census 30 September 2005. The census calculation included GP Registrars but excluded GP locums. The comparison locates Churchland within a range of 50 other PCTs.

[5] This account of moral sense making has drawn on Weick's work on organizational sensemaking in references 15 and 16.

[6] Situationist research in experimental social psychology has provoked some ethicists to challenge the importance that character has assumed in virtue ethics and popular thought. I am persuaded that specific situations tend to elicit specific responses, whatever the character of the respondent. But it is freely observable that in everyday life, similar situations evoke very different responses. Not every passenger leaps to offer their seat to pregnant, old or disabled travellers on the London Underground. In fact it is often me, while other passengers pretend to be engrossed in whatever they are reading on their Kindle. For a very readable introduction to situationist ethics see JM Doris's book listed in the further reading section at the end of this chapter.

That action determines the future: whether what we believed was true, or whether it was not. So whatever might be the underlying cause of moral trouble, what moral leaders think it is will shape their world. Sense, once made, has consequences.

Moral leadership begins, then, with sense-making bringing an event to attention. We are all making sense every moment of the day, ordering events into categories of the expected, the normal, the desirable; or perhaps the unexpected, the abnormal, the undesirable. Those who work in medicine inhabit a world where expected and unexpected complications and expected and unexpected deaths are part of the daily grind. This can make it a more than usually difficult place to detect that something is out of the ordinary.

Dr. Lister's moral attention was arrested by mortality data that those around him believed to be unexceptional. Taking on a new role in Trust-wide clinical governance processes he began to see figures that suggested what appeared to him to be an alarmingly high rate of complications and deaths in one particular department.

> Every month we were sitting looking at clinical incidents and complaints, and every month there was a serious incident or a death [in this department]. And I could never get anybody to tell me how many of these incidents we might expect in a unit of our size with this case mix. It was obvious that the key people from the [X] department weren't involved; they were not attending the meetings, couldn't give answers.

I asked Dr. Lister what had prompted his unease, when those around him viewed the data as unexceptional.

> It seemed obvious to me, so why nobody else had taken that action, I'm not sure .... Now the people within [crisis department] must have known. I still to this day don't know why they tried to look at each case as if it was an individual thing, and find excuses for what happened. It seemed that the trend was just so obvious to me, and I don't know why it seemed so obvious to me. And what did worry me was when I asked the questions, 'How many complications should we be seeing?', 'How many would you see in another unit?' nobody could answer that and nobody seemed willing to find the answers. But it seemed to me extraordinary. I suppose one thing that uncovered it was, I didn't know much about [specialty] .... And I was a bit astonished that it was actually so complicated, that there were so many high-risk cases, so many this that and the other. So alarm bells were already ringing. I was wondering, 'Is this the way it should be? I thought it was a safe thing. Is this the way it should be?' And it was only when I tried to find that out and realized that they either couldn't or wouldn't tell me that I thought there might be something wrong. And then I started to think about it and it was obvious there were serious things wrong. Even if the numbers weren't disproportionate, the way they were being looked at was not sufficiently rigorous .... Everybody kept just doing the routine, reporting these patient deaths, reporting the serious incidents, and nobody took any action to stop it happening.

Lister's description of how his moral leadership started introduces us to two important features of moral sense-making. First, moral sense is made in groups, and emerges from the activity of different people endeavouring to make sense of the world around them. Second, we make moral sense by setting standards for ourselves about how people ought to do certain things, or how things ought to turn out; and then we experience strong reactions when they don't.

Moral sense is made in groups

Looking back, Dr. Lister recalled having been somewhat at odds with colleagues. He remembered them treating each poor episode of care as a separate incident, and refusing to see them as a series suggestive of serious underlying problems. Sense-making seemed to create a gulf of understanding that separated him from his peers.

But the process of sense-making that Dr. Lister described was, from start to finish, one in which many people had a hand. Certainly Lister himself noted and framed important clues, pressed for an account and formulated his own alarming interpretation. However, he was a participant in organizational processes that generated certain types of information and determined who would have access to what. Information was identified, assembled, reported, filtered and interpreted by his colleagues. Different people could choose to circulate it, contain it, explain it away or suppress it. So the way this particular issue emerged out of the stream of day-to-day hospital activity reflected the different sense that different people made of it, and the different responsibilities that each felt they owed.

Comparing Ursula Usborne's description of becoming aware with Luke Lister's is illuminating. Usborne's account of her experience makes much more apparent the way that collective efforts, organized around different kinds of expertise, different role responsibilities and different responses to clues in the organizational environment, can pull moral trouble into focus. Lister experienced the discomfort of being a dissenter when he started to ask difficult questions about injuries and deaths recorded in the data. Although Lister felt he was on his own, colleagues making sense of events in ways he could either share or reject surrounded him. He was not starting from nowhere. When I asked Dr. Usborne how she had found out about the doctors whose practice might be cause for concern, her explanation highlighted group, or collaborative, cognition.

> There were [lay] managers who had lists of concerns, but that was all. And things had been being done, things had started to be addressed by the [organization] that pre-dated the PCT. But I think these were often managers who didn't have a medical colleague that they could turn to as an expert . . . .[7] So, my [professional medical] experience, alongside the [lay] managers' local knowledge, then started to say, 'This is acceptable, this is not acceptable, and this is what we can do about it'. So we fairly rapidly escalated some cases. . . .

We should notice the rather striking way Usborne described the process: 'my experience, alongside the [lay] managers' local knowledge, then started to say . . . .' This is not, it seems to me, a mere accident of expression. It is a very revealing use of words. What 'spoke' was the combined experience of the group, not just the individuals who contributed its constituent parts. The Primary Care Trust managers needed Dr. Usborne's clinical judgement, and what she self-deprecatingly described as her 'geeky' mastery of regulatory requirements, in order to make moral sense of the performance of local GPs. But equally, Dr. Usborne relied upon lay managers' understanding of patient complaints, practitioner reputations and their local community to do the same. Once these two intelligences were brought together within a 'knowledge network', it became possible for every member of the 'network' to state with confidence that certain activities failed to meet reasonable expectations: 'this is acceptable, this is not acceptable'. Each member of the group was now a participant in a narrative shared by all.

In Lister's case, the attempt to combine different intelligences was a process marked by a high level of disagreement. Lister brought to his colleagues' deliberations some bracing

---

[7] An additional reason is that the Performer's List Regulations upon which Usborne relied were only introduced with the Health and Social Care Act in 2001, so there were fewer ways of dealing with the situation prior to this.

expectations about how things ought to turn out for patients. His surprise at the level of risk tolerated by those around him was what prompted them to look again at what might reasonably be expected. So the group certainly assisted one another to make sense of what was going on. But whether Dr. Lister's group achieved the same level of collective cognition as Dr. Usborne's is doubtful. We shall see as the story progresses that Lister continued to interpret events differently from some key colleagues, remaining more isolated as a moral leader than Usborne may have done [17–21].[8]

Is moral expertise as much a quality of groups as individuals?

Research suggests that in groups which have made sustained collaborative efforts to solve problems and build knowledge, we can observe a form of expertise emerging that transcends individual limitations: 'networked expertise' [22–24]. Networked expertise is a form of higher-level cognitive competency that arises when people coordinate their actions effectively, bringing together their differing perceptions, skills, knowledges, role responsibilities and emotional orientations. Dr. Usborne's description of medico-moral sense-making directs our attention to the possibility that moral expertise may, sometimes at least, extend beyond individual capability to become a form of networked expertise.

It will become very apparent throughout forthcoming chapters that the process of enacting ethics rests upon people pooling, combining and coordinating their individual moral competencies and other social skills. We might perhaps achieve greater insight into the nature of practical moral expertise were we to conceptualize it as a quality possessed by a group of people, rather than the expression of individual character or skill alone.

On this account moral expertise is analogous to musical expertise, where a significant component is the capacity to work in harmony with others. Solos aside, the quality of a musical performance owes as much to the orientation of musicians towards one another, as it does to each musician's individual skill on an instrument. Over time, musicians who play together develop a collective musical character. Similarly, the quality of moral action may owe as much to the orientation of members of a group towards each other and their common values and goals as it owes to each individual member's capacity for moral reason or action. And over time, moral actors who work together develop a collective moral character. My argument here is not that individual ethical expertise is unimportant. Every member of an orchestra has to know how to play their instrument; but they also have to know how to play in concert with others. If the analogy is correct, ethical expertise consists of both individual moral know-how and collective moral know-how.

Thinking about enacted ethics as a group property, as well as an individual project, raises some important questions. If enacted ethics is a group property, moral leaders need to ask how those they lead will learn, assist and support one another when they face moral troubles either as individuals or as a group. Furthermore, it could prove fruitful to focus more of our effort on developing the moral expertise and moral resourcefulness of groups. At present we characteristically approach moral development as an individual concern,

---

[8] There is now a substantial body of research examining how members of healthcare teams work together and what factors may inhibit individual members from voicing anxieties or warnings about potential harm to patients. Although this literature deals with preventing harm to patients its arguments and supporting data are presented as being concerned with mechanisms of patient safety, rather than mechanisms of moral action. There are however obvious parallels. See references 17–21 for examples.

assuming we need to teach individuals how to reason and how to develop their own moral fibre. This approach remains important but, arguably, insufficient.

Sense-making builds on morally significant expectations

Events may sometimes suffice to draw attention to moral trouble. But it would be wrong to think that moral leaders wait for morally significant incidents to present themselves, or for the moral dimension of events to be evident. Something prompted Usborne and Lister to look further into situations they could as easily have ignored. Each, however, had the feeling that a gap was opening up in the moral order of things. That feeling was a response to unmet expectations: specifically it was a 'reactive attitude' shaped by 'normative expectations'.

Normative expectations are discussed in depth in Chapter 3, where the idea is explored alongside several examples of normative expectations in operation [2,25–27].[9] We need to consider them here, however, as part of the overall picture of moral sense-making.

Normative expectations are concerned with 'norms' in the sense that moral theorists use that word, referring to morally significant standards for behaviour. 'Respect patient autonomy' is a norm familiar to doctors. The existence of norms elicits expectations from those with an interest in them. So 'respect patient autonomy' elicits expectations from healthcare professionals, as well as from patients, carers, regulators and others. Such expectations are 'expectations' in two senses of that word. First we 'expect' others to adhere to certain standards, taking the view that they ought to respect these standards because the standards embody values important to us. Second we 'expect' that much of the time others will observe these standards, either because they have demonstrated a willingness to abide by them or because they have expressed sentiments suggesting they support them. So we expect (in a moral sense) doctors to respect patient autonomy, and we expect that (in a predictive sense) doctors will for the most part try to do so.

However, all of us live with the experience of disappointed expectations. We know that sometimes norms will be breached, for good reasons or bad. Knowing they will be breached does not immunize us, though, against reacting when they are. Quite the opposite. An important feature of normative expectations is that we feel strong 'reactive attitudes' – for example anger, disgust, shock or outrage – when they are violated. It may be the presence of just such a reaction that signals to us that an important normative expectation exists, and has been breached. Furthermore, knowing that a norm might be breached does not weaken the norm's moral authority. Knowing that some doctors fail to respect patient autonomy does not make respect for autonomy any less important. Indeed, it may make the norm itself even more compelling.

Significant moral habits and principles of medical professional conduct – for example, being candid with patients and colleagues when things go wrong – should be, and often are, held as normative expectations. Critically important to the moral quality of healthcare organizations are the normative expectations that come to prevail within professional groups. Equally important is the response that individuals or groups mobilize when a reactive attitude signals that their normative expectations have been breached. A reactive

---

[9] This discussion draws on Walker and Strawson; see references 25 and 26. For further discussion of Strawson's paper, see references 2 and 27.

attitude is a call to action. Ignoring, normalizing or excusing a breach in normative expectations may shape the future in ways that many will come to regret.

Care is required here, however. Normative expectations are not invariably morally sound. Some professional norms – medical paternalism, perhaps – may be open to question, and the normative expectations associated with them are then correspondingly problematic. Neither are reactive attitudes necessarily helpful. Anger or outrage may need to be tempered with a more considered response. Reactive attitudes are merely a signal that normative expectations have been breached. They invite consideration of events and of the expectations that surround them.

What inclines a medical leader to find clinical failure morally disturbing? In Chapter 5 we look in detail at the moral management of medical harm, and how medical leaders assign harm to categories of the blameless, the forgivable and the unforgivable. We are obliged to anticipate some of that discussion here, because a medical leader's awareness of actual moral trouble obviously rests on his or her assumptions about what is morally problematic. For current purposes, we should note that clinical failure is not necessarily a culpable failure. It might be wholly blameless; and if not blameless, then forgivable. Blameless and forgivable failures could still require moral repair – the restoration of patient and family trust in the clinical team, perhaps – but moral leadership within the team itself will often be sufficient to accomplish this. So what prompts medical moral leaders to suspect that something is afoot which may be neither blameless nor forgivable and calls for their intervention? In the following paragraphs, I note the comprehensive range of clinical, professional and role expectations that govern relationships between medical leaders and their colleagues. All of these are normative expectations that express important assumptions about what is proper care, and they thus afford a potentially powerful stimulus to ethical enactment.

Clinical normative expectations

Quite straightforwardly Usborne and Lister held a clear picture in mind of what constituted good care, coupled with a robust expectation that the clinicians accountable to them would provide it.

Lister believed that his colleagues experienced him as a supportive leader, but also one who had consistently high expectations:

> People feel good if they're encouraged .... But you have to deliver; you have to deliver as a clinician; you have to deliver as a manager .... One of the things which I think we as medical managers have to do, is show colleagues that *they* have to deliver .... The doctor has to be a professional, and what happens in that consultation environment is the critical thing. That's the sharp point; that's where it all happens. So doctors' professional standards have to be made the same; they have to be high.

We shall see later that Usborne, too, was very committed to supporting practitioners who she thought would benefit from help. But she also had high expectations, and was assured in her appraisal of standards. She recounted how an observer had charged her with being too severe in her judgement of one particular case, suggesting that it was a single instance of failure for which the practitioner could be excused. She had responded:

> where I felt justified was that [this single instance] was symptomatic of a systematic failure to take proper histories, to listen to patients, to value what you were being told, to listen to what was being presented, to even attempt to examine the patient, to try to formulate a hypothesis of what might

be going on, to share information with a patient, formulate a plan, to safety-net and keep informed, not just with that one case, with any case. There was no evidence of any critical thinking or compassion or kindness or professionalism or judgement at all, anywhere, in that doctor's clinical practice.

Few medical leaders will have any difficulty recognizing clinical excellence. But, axiomatically, excellence is not the norm. So the question arises how far from excellence it is permissible to fall. How do clinical leaders determine the proper threshold between 'good enough' clinical practice and 'not good enough'? This is a theme that will recur in later chapters, but it arises here for the first time because beliefs about what is 'good enough' practice are clinical normative expectations. Put another way, clinical normative expectations are embedded in and inseparable from practice knowledge.

To some extent clinical normative expectations are built on clinical and moral understandings that clinicians internalize during training, augmented or modified by what clinicians subsequently learn through experience. Increasingly, clinical standards can be measured by reference to clinical protocols. But settling the threshold of what is good enough is clearly a more complex matter than knowing what others do, or think they should do, or what protocols say. Some clinicians strive to improve upon the standards they observe in training or in practice, whilst others allow their own standards to lapse where they observe lower standards in others. Suffice it to say, for the present, that clinical standard setting is a *sine qua non* of medical leadership, and moral leaders will be those who fall into the first category of 'improvers' rather than the second category of 'laggards'. Commenting on the clinical unit he had developed, Lister was proud that

> We were really, really successful for twenty years .... Our unit was a leader ... and is still one of the best [specialist] units in [the region].

What he brought to his role as a medical director was an intense desire that others should strive to improve their services, together with a strong conviction that improvement was possible even in difficult circumstances.

> My objectives [on becoming medical director] were fairly clear cut, and they were to do with improving clinical care .... We had a lot of work to do to change the way people worked, to make the hospital more accessible, more welcoming, and more effective from the patient's point of view .... And I was very keen to get the clinicians involved; get them fired up and moving forward.

The assessment of clinical performance is a demanding art. There are legitimate differences in approach to a range of clinical procedures. Complicated clinical problems may confront the best clinicians with unexpected problems. Where performance is at the threshold of acceptability it may be a fine judgement whether it is 'good enough'. And a single instance of poor practice may be just that – a regrettable and forgivable single instance – or it may be early and important evidence of a larger, morally significant problem. Clinical normative expectations have to be sufficiently elastic to accommodate the complexity of clinical work, whilst remaining sufficiently stubborn to give direction.

Collegial normative expectations

Patients' first-hand experience of care, and data about patients' experience of care are of course critically important. But medical leaders also have access to their own first-hand data in respect of clinician performance, and it may be these data that supply the most compelling source of disquiet. These are the data relating to collegial normative expectations, expectations that bind clinical leaders and the clinicians they lead in relationships of trust.

Dr. Lister identified two 'unacceptables'. One was disquieting clinical data. The other was a disquieting degree of inaction by his consultant colleagues. It was his colleagues' attitudes to clinical governance data – their unwillingness to discuss it, their failure to answer to it, their refusal apparently to be disturbed by it – that signalled to Dr. Lister that the 'unfortunate' might be transmuting into the 'unethical'. What Lister remembered was that:

> it was only when I tried to find that out and realized that they either couldn't or wouldn't tell me that I thought there might be something wrong. And then I started to think about it and it was obvious there were serious things wrong. Even if the numbers weren't disproportionate, the way they were being looked at was not sufficiently rigorous .... Everybody kept just doing the routine, reporting these patient deaths, reporting the serious incidents, and nobody took any action to stop it happening.

Lister reiterated three times over how he had sought answers, and eventually concluded there was something amiss because people 'couldn't or wouldn't tell'. An apparent technical failure became morally culpable because those with an obligation to narrate an account of events assiduously avoided doing so. Had patients indeed suffered unintended harm, it would have constituted a serious, but probably forgivable, medical error. The same unintended harm became a culpable moral failure because the doctors who should have admitted to it both said, and did, nothing. This jeopardized the interpersonal bond between Dr. Lister and his colleagues as well as placing patients at risk [28–33].[10]

Dr. Lister was himself obligated to narrate an account of what was going on to his own bosses. One of his first actions was to report his concerns to the Long River Hospital Trust Board. Dr. Lister's recollection of the story he told at the time demonstrates the first stage in moral leadership moving into the second. From seeking to make initial sense of the situation, he set out to enlarge the circle of concern, involving others in further attempts to make moral sense of the situation.

> Eventually ... it became apparent that I couldn't assure the Board or the Clinical Governance Committee that this number of incidents was appropriate, that it was being managed, that steps were being taken to manage the risk. And we had to tell the Board I thought there was a real problem.

> I said to them I thought we were heading for another Bristol. 'I think we're having a large number of deaths and serious incidents; and we cannot explain them; and sooner or later this is going to get to the public domain. And I think it's as bad as Bristol. We've got to do something.'

Lister's description of the situation as 'heading for another Bristol' was intended to have a galvanizing effect on the Trust Board. It succeeded. Events at Long River had taken place after a determined whistleblower had finally drawn attention to serious failures in paediatric cardiac surgery at the Bristol Royal Infirmary. Their revelations had prompted an

---

[10] My account of how medical leaders distinguish between technical and moral failure parallels that of Bosk (see reference 28). For a review of Bosk, see references 29 and 30. Bosk noted in his preface that the terms 'normative error' and 'quasi-normative error' have been misinterpreted and used wrongly. They have now also achieved a currency within the literature. See references 31–33, where some of the most recent or influential articles have been included.

exhaustive public inquiry. The bruising nature of that inquiry, as well as its observations on the moral responsibilities of medical leaders, were a stark warning to hospital leaders, including Lister's colleagues [34–44].[11]

> I think Bristol scared everybody. I mean nobody had really appreciated . . . the failure to provide a safe environment until that problem; and people were really shocked at Bristol. They were shocked about the fact that the doctors could allow things to drift like that. And they were shocked at the degree of censure that applied to them.

Role-related normative expectations

Whether people notice what they ought morally to notice, and respond as they should respond, depends in part on their place within a network or community. Role responsibilities do not guarantee that people will become aware of matters they ought to take notice of, nor that they will do the right thing having becoming aware. But role-related normative expectations contribute to sense-making by 'priming' people to select out certain features in their experience and accord them a particular significance.

Dr. Lister gained access to data about what was happening at Long River Hospital because he assumed a particular role. But more to the point, he assumed an active attitude of responsibility in that role. This attitude alerted him to the presence of clinical risk, and pointed clearly to his duty to limit it. Ursula Usborne shared that active attitude of responsibility. Usborne occupied a newly created medical director role, and she felt keenly the normative expectations and accountabilities that went with it. They supplied, in her view, a mandate for robust moral leadership. Previous local medical leaders had been practitioners who retained their full-time clinical practice in the locality, and fulfilled more of an advisory than a managerial function. As Usborne pointed out,

> It is very difficult [to take action against other practitioners] if you're working in a community alongside colleagues as peers, and you're sharing the same out of hours, on-call service, and you're sharing the same referral pathways — [By way of contrast] I'm directly accountable to the Chief Executive for quality and I can be sacked.

Usborne's comments raise important questions about how quality and performance will be maintained in the doctor-led commissioning consortia to which PCTs have given way. In Usborne and Lister's cases, role-related normative expectations appear to have supported the practice of responsibility. But the normative expectations that accompany roles, particularly roles of authority, are not invariably sound ones. For example, normative expectations surrounding deference to clinical authority – expectations mobilized by doctors in either the senior or the junior position – can suppress moral initiative or legitimate dissent. In celebrated experiments Stanley Milgram demonstrated what history should already have taught us: that ordinary people willingly inflict suffering upon others when their role allows it, and authority instructs them to. (Milgram's experimental subjects were prepared to administer what they thought were life-threatening electrical shocks to strangers, because they believed it was a scientific experiment and received instructions to do so from a man in a white coat [45,46].) The normative expectations that accompany social roles may give rise to viciousness as well as virtue, and so they demand careful scrutiny.

---

[11] See reference 34 for the Bristol inquiry, references 35–39 for analyses, and references 40–44 for other inquiries into dangerous doctors.

Sense-making is cyclical

Hindsight is a familiar accompaniment to moral sense-making, which unfortunately does not progress reliably from suppositions to true facts. Moral leadership and enacted ethics are founded in what we believe to be true at the time that we act. Not infrequently, what we believe has to be revised when further information comes to light or when further reasoning brings us fresh insight. Moral sense can be affected by revisions of fact (we infrequently know all the facts, and often mistake the facts) and revised interpretations (we review the inferences that we draw from the facts).

Importantly, it may only become possible with hindsight to see how an instance of medical harm was one in a series and not an isolated incident. Lister was among the first to notice that a string of single instances could be an ominous trend, an insight that arrived in a moment of 'gestalt':

> It seemed that the trend was just so obvious to me, and I don't know why it seemed so obvious to me.

Although the first intimations of trouble came from the moment that he spotted the trend he could not, at that stage, be certain that he was right. In fact, what made him certain was not a careful suturing together of scraps of clinical data but the breach of normative expectations surrounding clinical accountability and clinical governance:

> So alarm bells were already ringing . . . . And it was only when I tried to find that out and realized that they either couldn't or wouldn't tell me that I thought there might be something wrong.

His revised view of the data, a view shaped by growing distrust of the clinicians involved, reinforced his initial anxious interpretation. It was an interpretation that appeared valid throughout the process and at its conclusion. However, the grounds of moral sense are constantly shifting beneath moral leaders' feet. The action that Lister was taking in response to events appeared at the time to be well founded. Later he reflected ruefully that some of what he had done had made the situation worse. But it was only when the process had wound its way towards its conclusion that it was possible to look back and declare the sense of it all. The internal inquiry that he instigated, for example,

> revealed some problems not only in practices leading to some of the events, but also in the way we were actually managing it at the time. This only became really obvious in retrospect.

As we continue to look at how moral leadership works, we will continue to encounter the constant remaking of moral sense and the disorientating effects of moral sense-making in time. Interpretations of reality that supply the moral justification for certain actions sometimes turn out to have been ill founded. There is no getting around this. I noted above how we are shaping the world even while we are still making sense of it. Inaction is not an option; or rather, inaction is an option but it has as much of an effect as action. To overlook or ignore a clue that patients are facing unacceptable risk affects the world; so too does spotting a clue and doing something about it; so too does acting on a suspicion of clinical risk even when there is none.

The cycle continues: moral leaders involve others in making deeper moral sense of the situation

We now move on to consider the second stage of the process by which moral leaders catalyse enactment of ethics. In the first stage the central task is becoming aware of potential concerns and beginning to make sense of situations. In the second stage, work moves on to assembling and testing a coherent narrative of what has happened and what must be done.

The business of moral leadership begins with signals, hints and warnings that emerge from the messy data of experience. Something potentially harmful to what the moral leader cares about, or has responsibility for, is thought to be happening 'out there'. What is 'out there' and ethically relevant is people's past, current and future actions towards others. Most often, what is 'out there' at the beginning is still very uncertain. The chief means of resolving uncertainty is to seek further information.

But to take notice of moral signals, hints or warnings implies that some kind of human reasoning is also going on, 'in here' so to speak. What is 'in here' is an orientation towards making a moral assessment of actions and situations. The grounds for a moral assessment may sometimes be clear, but as often as not the moral substance in 'troubling' situations turns out to be equivocal. Although normative expectations provide a basis for moral understanding, many situations are open to different moral interpretations and assessments. When a consultant loses her temper with a junior she may be a bully, she may be a stickler for high standards in surgery, or she may be both. How are her actions to be judged? Whereas *uncertainty* can often be resolved (at least partially) by seeking information, *equivocality* yields primarily to normative reasoning and normative judgement [16(p95–9)].

That is what can make it discomfiting.

To contend with uncertainty, moral leaders work towards creating a believable narrative: an account of the past, the present and the likely future that will help to guide action. To contend with equivocality, leaders need a narrative that is morally compelling, as well as believable. The narrative that emerges has to tie what is going on 'out there' to moral beliefs 'in here', and lead towards a solution. So over the course of moral leadership, what is 'out there' becomes better known and less uncertain; whilst what is 'in here' becomes better understood and less equivocal.

Sense-making involves resolution of the uncertain and the equivocal

It is a commonplace observation that medicine is an uncertain art. Paul Atkinson observed that sociological inquiry into medicine had too often relied on uncertainty 'as a catch-all term', so that sociological analysis of medical reasoning remained imprecise [47–56].[12] Ethicist Richard Ashcroft has noted, on the other hand, that medical ethical commentary tends to acknowledge three sources of ambiguity or indecision. First, moral norms themselves do not readily supply answers to difficult problems, so reference to norms frequently does not settle the matter. Additionally, information may be incomplete, in which case it is not clear to what facts relevant norms should be applied. Finally, values and principles do not generate practical plans for action, so something other than moral reasoning is required to fill the gap between awareness of a moral problem and implementation of a moral solution [57].[13]

---

[12] However, more work has been done to refine the concept of uncertainty in medicine by sociologists since Atkinson wrote this in 1995; see references 48–56 for further analysis.

[13] Also, medical ethics assumes that resolving these will result in good outcomes.

The accounts that medical leaders supplied of moral leadership suggest that Ashcroft's three classes of doubt can usefully be more closely specified. Medical leaders in my study worked towards ethical enactment by constructing a moral narrative around six areas of concern:

(i)   what moral norms apply (normative concerns);
(ii)   what actually happened (empirical concerns);
(iii) what might happen next (predictive concerns);
(iv)   how what happened and what might happen can be known (epistemological concerns);
(v)   what can be done about it (tactical concerns);
(vi)   what they personally feel to be right or wrong (virtue concerns).

These different varieties of doubt call for different responses. We noted earlier the distinction between uncertainty and equivocality: matters that are uncertain may be clarified (but not necessarily resolved) by seeking further data, while matters that are equivocal call forth the exercise of judgement. Thus empirical, predictive and tactical concerns present the problem of uncertainty; while normative, epistemological and value concerns are equivocal.

Normative equivocality

Looking back, neither Dr. Usborne nor Dr. Lister remembered feeling much doubt about the broad moral principles that applied to their situation. The primacy of patients' interests was an unequivocal commitment, the foundation stone of the moral narrative that each pursued. Ursula Usborne regretted the historical injustices that had brought some of her failing doctors to Churchland, but she was clear that patients had first claim on the Primary Care Trust's beneficence.

> There are issues about the history of these doctors. They were brought here, quite deliberately, by the NHS, given the impression that the streets were paved with gold. They were often treated very badly. They were not promoted as fairly. They were put into jobs that were unattractive. They may well have been victims of discrimination years ago. Many of them have been abused in employment relationships in General Practice, been promised things that never happened – you know, become [an employee in the partnership] with a view to [becoming a partner] – that never materialized — But you can't excuse unacceptable patient care. Even taking all of those things into account . . . .

Dr. Lister had countenanced three different domains of harm. One was harm to patients resulting from failure to manage clinical risk in the problem department; another was the more remote harm associated with loss of public trust in Long River Hospital in the wake of poor publicity; a third was the impact on colleagues. It was plain to Dr. Lister that protecting patients from the heightened risk of medical error had to take precedence over preserving the hospital's reputation. Equally plainly, patients' interests should prevail over the interests of doctors and their families.

> There were several areas there, which I thought were very difficult. One, the duty to open this all up in the first place. Knowing what a problem it was going to create, and expose us to all that publicity . . . . The actions that we were going to have to take were going to have really serious impact on peoples' livelihoods . . . family relationships, and everything else. But realizing you couldn't do it – and make life safe for the patients – in any other way.

However, knowing the nature of one's moral responsibilities does not, without more, generate a solution. If the problems Lister and Usborne identified had to do with the competence of individual doctors – poor clinical decisions, lack of skill, bad management or inappropriate behaviour – then close supervision, training, retraining or dismissal might be appropriate. On the other hand, if the problems were institutional in origin – malfunctioning systems, insufficient trained staff, excessive workload or a lack of resources – then retraining, disciplining or dismissing doctors would not solve them. It is hard enough to identify all the contributory factors, and close to impossible to ascribe due weight to each. Dr. Lister had disciplined staff, and he still harboured lingering doubts that he had done, in the circumstances, the right thing.

> And [I was] always asking myself 'Well do we really need to do it this way? Are we being really honest? Are we victimizing people? Are we right?' And I still don't know the answer to that question.

Dr. Lister's continuing questions about what he had done, about how it was done, about his conscientiousness and about his moral perspicacity, are telling. Doubts like these are the doubts of those who must do more than merely think about the issue. They are the doubts of those who have to act. In much of the literature of medical ethics, the central issue is normative ambiguity. In enacted ethics, normative ambiguity may well be present, but it is often not the most taxing problem. This is because moral leadership is about creating the world, when what the world is, and what the world will become as a result of what leaders do, can never be fully known.

Empirical and predictive uncertainty

Living in real time, what drains ethical determination is empirical, predictive and tactical uncertainty alongside personal doubt. Moral leaders face uncertainty about what actually happened; about whether a person did what others say they did; about whether if they did do it, they acted in error or carelessness or malice; about what might happen if the moral leader acts or if they don't act, or if they act this way or if they act the other way. We add to this empirical, predictive and tactical uncertainty a degree of ambivalence. We are not sure about the grounds on which we can decide any of these things; and we wonder whether, when we did act, we enacted our values or merely succumbed to expedience.

One way of managing the problem of empirical uncertainty, and the predictive uncertainty that is associated with it, is to pay attention to procedural fairness. Even if we cannot be absolutely sure that we have found the right facts, we can at least be certain that we have gone about finding them the right way.

Ursula Usborne spoke assuredly about her experience of dealing with doctors whose performance gave her cause for concern. She seemed to me resilient, sure, and admirably able to carry the moral weight of what she does. So I was surprised by her answer to my question whether she had ever doubted that she had been right to act as she had.

> I'm plagued with doubts all the time. I do worry tremendously. About, am I being unfair? Are my standards too high? Is this . . .?
>
> —
>
> [In one of the practices where I worked as I GP I witnessed the effect of] a complaint that I thought was quite unjustified. That was a terribly conscientious doctor. Now he killed himself. He committed suicide. And it traumatized not only his family, the partnership, the practice team, but

the whole community. All of his patients felt guilty – that this wonderful man had died over this wretched complaint, that was ill founded.

That experience has really made me think. When we do discipline somebody, they have to have help. They have to have support. We could be wrong. It's been painted this way but there's another side to the story. We have to be terribly careful, because I don't want . . . I don't want another doctor's death on my conscience through mishandling a disciplinary process.

Dr. Usborne managed these anxieties about the outcomes of her action by adhering faithfully to principles of justice and fairness, particularly giving a proper hearing to both sides of a story. She contended with empirical and predictive uncertainty, and her own conscience, by paying careful attention to the ethical dimension of fact-finding as a procedure.

Of course, there are sound practical reasons to attend to procedural fairness. Disciplinary processes impose their own quasi-legal requirements. Where events could lead to proceedings with serious penalties (such as losing the right to provide care to NHS patients, or losing the right to practise altogether)[14] a legalistic approach is essential. But this is not the story Usborne chose to tell, and nor does this supply the reasons that are to her morally compelling. The reason Usborne needs to hear the other side is that she has witnessed the tragic effects of being wrong. She needs the moral narrative that she enacts to be, as far as it can be, true and for blame to fall only where it is justified.

Moral narratives assign what may be weighty and long-lived moral judgements. Veracity is therefore of the essence. The most significant difference between an ordinary story and a moral narrative is that the value of an ordinary story does not rest on how well it represents the facts as others understand them to be [58]. Moral narratives, however, have to allocate responsibility consistent with the believable facts of the matter if justice is to result.

Usborne had to be as certain as she could be that her narrative was a credible version of what happened, and who was responsible. Procedural fairness offered the most reliable route to narrative credibility. It was what enabled her, in good conscience, to hold doctors morally responsible for what happened to their patients. The requirement for veracity in moral narrative leads us into a further difficulty with which moral leaders must contend. How is the truth to be known?

Epistemological equivocality

Moral narratives require a plausible account of cause if they are to be convincing as well as just. But a sound explanation may not be easy to formulate, and generating a causal account raises considerable epistemological anxiety. Moral leaders may harbour genuine doubts about their understanding of what is going on. They may question whether (to recall to the traditional analysis of knowledge in Western philosophy) they have a justified true belief about the causes of their moral trouble.

---

[14] Doctors are granted their licence to practise by the General Medical Council and may be deprived of their licence to practise, or have conditions placed on their practice, through the General Medical Council's fitness to practise procedures. Separately from this, General Practitioners must be on a 'Performers List', hitherto maintained by Primary Care Trusts, if they wish to be reimbursed for providing care through the NHS. They can be removed from the Performer's List on grounds of performance or probity, so it operates as an additional tier of local control. GPs who are not on the Performers List may provide primary care privately, so long as they are still registered with the General Medical Council.

It is important to note here how different approaches to attributing cause are capable of generating very different moral narratives. Lister and his colleagues at Long River Hospital divided over two conflicting narratives derived from the same clinical data. Lister described the first of these with disdain as a 'medico-legal' narrative, a story of individual acts and omissions. Lister's preferred narrative was a narrative of related actions and omissions. The failure to relate actions and omissions to one another was, in Lister's eyes, both a reason for their continuing occurrence and grounds for assigning moral blame.

[During the internal inquiry, the consultant who was responsible for managing clinical risk was able] to stand there and give evidence in this medico-legal way without looking at systems. And that was immediately apparent to me. It was immediately apparent to me during the investigation what he was doing. And the fact that he wasn't being called to account for that. The major gaps between the professions [working together in the department] were apparent. There was no systematic analysis of risk. There was no systematic getting together of the professions to look at it, to look at practice, and change things.

[In a medico-legal approach] somebody looks at the facts and says 'Was there an adverse outcome? Is there any evidence of individual performance failure?' And the answer is, 'No.' And then that's put to one side, and you look at the next one. Instead of looking at all of them, and looking for common factors. The aims seem to be merely to exonerate individuals, or a unit, from any blame, and not to look at underlying practices and systems. It's as if you were being sued and you just want to create your defence.

The medico-legal paradigm protects innocent doctors from false allegations and faulty logic. It proceeds from a presumption of innocence and treats every event as a single instance. Evidence that a doctor caused harm on one occasion is not evidence that they have caused harm on a different occasion. Suspicions that a doctor might have caused harm once-upon-a-time cannot ground suspicions that they have caused harm in the here-and-now. Its antithesis is the preventive paradigm. This aims to safeguard innocent patients from potentially dangerous doctors and dysfunctional systems [59].[15] It proceeds from a presumption of protection and treats every event as an instance potentially causally connected to others. All harmful events should be investigated for the possibility that they share the same origin. Hitherto unseen patterns are sought and weak hypotheses formulated. All findings of past harm are potentially relevant to the prediction of future risk.

Just institutions – and ethical healthcare organizations strive to be just – have to find an acceptable balance between wrongful blame and wrongful exoneration. The moral hazard of mistakenly blaming a doctor has to be weighed against the moral hazard of exposing patients to harm because they have unjustly avoided blame. When the medico-legal paradigm is used to promote fair procedures, it is morally defensible. When it is used to shield doctors from reasonable accountability, however, it becomes morally offensive. Equally, the preventive paradigm is morally defensible when it used to protect patients. It is morally offensive when it is used as a justification for punishing individual practitioners in order to be seen to be doing something.

The medico-legal and preventive paradigms are a response to empirical and predictive uncertainty, to past and future unknowns. Each is based in its own epistemology. Each seeks to avert the harm that follows from making the wrong sort of sense, deriving the

---

[15] The preventive paradigm is comparable to Holm's concept of protective responsibility.

wrong narrative, from difficult settings and circumstances. Conversely, used cynically, each paradigm is capable of producing harm precisely by making the wrong sense, and procuring the wrong narrative.

Tactical uncertainty

Making sense and deciding what to do are iterative processes. Each informs the other. It will be recalled that one of Dr. Lister's first narrative acts was to report up to his superiors.

> I think it's as bad as Bristol. We've got to do something . . . .

The way forward was an internal investigation, a tactic that resolved one uncertainty, only to open up a host more.

> I had no doubts about what I had to do at that time, but I was so ignorant – I didn't know what we had to do! I knew we had to do something, but I'd got no idea really about how to construct an investigation, how to draw conclusions, how to make an action plan and deliver it.

The initial decision to hold an internal inquiry led more or less directly to the emergence of the two diametrically opposed moral narratives we examined above. And thus arose a new normative dilemma: how to resolve the incommensurable moral judgements in which each narrative concluded.

By the time Dr. Usborne joined Churchland Primary Care Trust, she knew enough not to have to contend with such a high degree of tactical uncertainty.

> I'm a bit of a geek about regulations and powers and where certain things have come from . . . .
> I was an advisor to [various working groups], I've a fairly encyclopaedic knowledge, a lot of experience hands on.

Knowledge and experience reduced the scale and scope of ambiguities. There were fewer novel tactical choices. Because Usborne could anticipate future events, she could calculate the likely effects of intervening in them, and build in protective manoeuvres. Knowing what to do, however, does not make moral leadership exactly easy.

> I wasn't afraid of it because I'd done it before, and I'd had experience of other people, going down this road . . . . And because I'd been involved in some quite serious cases in the past, I was able to approach people like Professor [. . .] and say, 'Look here's a report, what do you think?' and get that external validation of what we were doing. Because at every stage you're vulnerable to challenge, either through the defence societies or through judicial review, or in the High Court. So there have been times when it's been really quite draining. So again, having got networks nationally, that helps resilience because you can talk to chums who are in a similar position. But it can get depressing. This hasn't been done without an impact on my personal health; it's affected my mental and emotional health . . . .

Virtue concerns

As Lister and Usborne pursued the development of a moral narrative appropriate to the circumstances they found themselves in, they had concerns both for their own moral identity, and for the moral reputation of their organization. Neither wished to be associated with an organizational culture that was uncaring, bullying or unjust, but neither were they inclined to tolerate unacceptable clinical risk. Both described expressive virtues – kindness, humility and candour for example – as morally important.

I noted earlier that Ursula Usborne attempted to contain the pervasive doubt that accompanies the enactment of ethics by adhering strictly to her conception of core principles of justice. In a similar way, she managed her doubts about where to draw the line between acceptable and unacceptable care by balancing her commitment to robust performance management with an equal commitment to practical support and compassion.

> There is a danger of, you get a medical director who's a complete bully, who has impossibly high standards, who throws the book at everybody. But I'd like to think that we do take a formative approach at first. We understand nobody's perfect. We're all human, nobody's error free, one case doesn't mean 'end of career', or at least, it shouldn't . . . . We do a lot of support for doctors in trouble. So doctors who have illnesses get support. Quite a number of doctors who've been in trouble one way or another, we've offered psychological support to, behavioural counselling, mentoring, peer support. It has to be by its very nature invisible and confidential. The disciplinary cases are highly visible because everyone knows about them and they're all in the public domain. But the support is all hidden so people don't see that bit. But I'm equally proud of that stuff, because I know that we've prevented doctors going under.

Lister was agreeably surprised to discover it was possible to develop a moral narrative on behalf of the organization that remained consistent with personal values he had defended throughout his professional life. He recalled how he looked for some concordance between his personal narrative of value – a sense of his own integrity – and his public acts of moral leadership [60].[16]

> You know, clinicians are used to pressure. But I felt a sort of pressure through that process that I never experienced as a clinician — I went through a process of coaching, which I found really, really helpful . . . . Sorting out what my values were, and what [values] I was going to apply to this . . . I think what really came of it was that one's values are all right. There's a sense that when you come into a job like this, you have to behave in a corporate way [and set aside personal virtues such as kindness and honesty]. (Dr. Lister, Long River Hospital NHS Trust)

How do moral leaders know they are doing the right thing?

To be a moral leader means to commit to action, despite persisting equivocality or uncertainty. How do moral medical leaders judge whether they are doing more good than harm? In moral theory, where moral reasoning proceeds on more certain grounds than generally obtain in reality, determining what is right is hard enough. Enacting ethics is even harder.

From a pragmatic perspective, the most and least that can be asked of people is to enact what they believe to be best in the circumstances. Moral leaders have to satisfy themselves that the moral narrative they are orchestrating is the best, or at least 'good enough'. They appear to do this by looking for 'fit'. Moral narratives may be thought of as 'fit' in three senses.

First, a moral narrative is 'fit' in a vaguely ecological sense if it survives. A 'fit' moral narrative in this sense is not necessarily objectively the best, or the one that will achieve the most good. It is simply the one that prevails. It is the one that has been adopted, for good or bad reasons, by an influential proportion of the members of a group. Moral leaders have to give consideration to what a group currently believes to be good or right, if only to decide whether they will challenge it.

---

[16] Cf. Storr.

Second, a moral narrative stands a better chance of being compelling if it 'fits with' the ethical concerns, moral customs and existing moral narratives of a particular community. But shaping a narrative that 'fits with' a community's concerns is no easy task. One difficulty is that most people belong to, and feel loyalty to, several different moral communities. A doctor's moral communities may include her department, her specialty, her patients, her employing organization, the larger professional community that licenses her practice, her family, her social circle or her neighbourhood. Each of these communities has its own 'local' moral narratives and normative expectations, and each is keenly interested in what moral responsibilities are owed to them. A doctor's patients and her colleagues may – for example – hold very different views on what is morally fitting when a patient has suffered a medical injury. Individuals may therefore feel torn between the needs of different moral communities and the moral solutions they each favour.

Finally, for a moral narrative to stand a reasonable chance of prevailing for any extended period of time, it has to be 'fitting' in the sense of reflecting deeper moral values. A narrative's 'fit with' the norms of one's close moral community is no guarantee that it is 'fitting' in the eyes of others more removed. George Bernard Shaw famously accused the medical profession of conducting a 'conspiracy against the laity', protesting that it served its own interests better than it served the interests of patients [61]. Others have echoed him, portraying the community of doctors as, at times at least, a somewhat immoral community [62–68].[17] If the moral narratives created within the medical community are to be seen as instances of ethics enacted, such narratives must reasonably reflect the moral perspectives of outsiders.

Fitness in all three senses requires leaders to orientate themselves to their own moral communities, whilst retaining a degree of ethical independence. As moral narrative begins to emerge from doubt and ambiguity, astute moral leaders begin to test it for 'fit'.

In common with all of the medical leaders in the study, Usborne had recourse to her own informal networks in order to test her narrative for fit.

> Because it's a pretty lonely furrow to plough, we do tend to ring each other up or email each other, just chat things through as a sounding board. Just to take the temperature of, 'Where do you think this is going? Am I completely off beam here? Or what do you think?' And that's useful. There is a need for ... some kind of validation of your actions, [to] act as a damper on excessive zeal on the one hand, or as a spur to being too tolerant at the other extreme.

How can a person who needs to seek moral advice judge the ethical expertise of those who dispense it? This is the so-called 'credentials' problem, a logical conundrum that has taxed philosophers since Socrates [69]. Medical leaders were quick to acknowledge the importance of using peers and colleagues as sounding boards. But several had found themselves ruing their choice of advisor. Luke Lister reflected that he had lacked a steadfast moral confidant, someone on whom he could rely to test his emerging views as the situation unfolded. The colleague with whom Lister worked most closely at the beginning turned out to be a poor choice. Lister felt his colleague's ethical perception had been coloured by a concern to protect his own position and to defend other professionals involved in the case. We noted earlier in this discussion the moral importance of 'reporting up': when Dr. Lister

---

[17] Freidson is one of the best known critics of self-serving professionalism. See references 63–68 for updated critiques.

found his ally slow to report up, his trust in him began to drain away. Not reporting up was the first worrying signal of a lack of ethical expertise in his ally.

> He had quite a lot of individual expertise in clinical risk ... and he'd come to enjoy being an expert ... I think he was frightened that if he did refer things upwards, his role might be undermined, his status might be undermined. And in another way I think he felt that if he did put things upwards, then that would be a personal failure for him .... At that time [the person] I would regard as my key ally was actually the last person I should have been relying on.

The ostensible purpose of many formal meetings in organizations is to make decisions. They might be better understood, however, as arenas for testing and determining organizational narratives. Committees and boards do decide, sometimes. But perhaps more importantly, they work to secure consensus; to settle the question of 'whose say goes' when consensus cannot be achieved; and to make a record of organizational narratives. Dr. Usborne described how one, the 'Performance Committee' of the Churchland Primary Care Trust, operated:

> we have the formal performance committee where I take cases. And it's very important that we have representatives from other professions, so we have nurses and pharmacists and dentists and managers and also a GP representative as an observer. Their task is to make sure that the PCT is observing natural justice. We have a wonderful member, a doctor in one of our practices, for whom I have the utmost respect. If that doctor says, 'Sorry Ursula, that's over the mark', well that's important. I will pay attention to that.

> *If you were anxious about a certain case, might you chew it through with that particular person?*

> No, it's different. It is different. This person's there as a representative, almost as the trade union. They know the regulations probably about as well as I do. So I would want to be confident of my case before I even shared it with them. I would cross check before that, because I know that this doctor would challenge me and I don't want to be caught wanting in front of them.

The performance committee as Ursula Usborne described it provided two important points of comparison. It was a forum for testing her moral narrative against the views of professionals from different moral communities. It also allowed her to test it against the views of members of her own moral community of General Practitioners.

The cycle matures: moral leaders elicit the commitment of others who enact a shared vision

We have now reached a third phase in the leadership process, during which a plausible and fitting moral narrative is used to coordinate action throughout an ever widening circle of confederates. We saw in the first section of this chapter how moral leadership starts in awareness of possible harm, and preliminary sense-making. We then saw in the second section how a moral narrative begins to take shape as a result of concerted efforts to resolve uncertain facts and equivocal values. Next, the leader's task is to secure the commitment of those around her to agreeing and acting out appropriate solutions.

We shall continue to follow Dr. Usborne's story, but for reasons of confidentiality we have to set aside Dr. Lister's tale for now. We return to Usborne's account of moral leadership to consider one case in particular. When she took up her role as medical director at Churchland Primary Care Trust, Usborne became accountable for local oversight of the area's General Practitioners. Shortly after she arrived, she was informed that a patient had died in what, in Usborne's view, were 'appalling circumstances'. When she investigated the surgery that was responsible for looking after the patient, Dr. Usborne found a practice that was

> devoid of any kind of [clinical] governance systems at all, for which the partners were jointly responsible. And all of [them] had abdicated any kind of responsibility for quality. [They] were just overwhelmed by the challenge of caring for this very demanding and very difficult population . . . .

Over the next two or so years, Dr. Usborne led the PCT through a labyrinthine and very expensive process aimed at calling the practitioners to account, and protecting other patients from harm. This eventually resulted in several doctors in the practice being removed from the list of General Practitioners eligible to receive payment from the NHS (the 'Performers List'). Some doctors were stripped of their licence to practice and removed from the GMC's Medical Register. This is part of Dr. Usborne's explanation of how this was done.

> We were doing three things simultaneously.

> On the one hand we were trying to develop these doctors, and demonstrating that they were just not able to develop. We used the National Clinical Assessment Service . . . . The [doctors] were found to be just not competent at all, not remediable. The marker . . . was that they had absolutely no insight into there being anything wrong. There was almost a thing of, 'Well I've qualified as a doctor, why would I need to do anything more once I've qualified?' But their qualifications were so old and out of date, and they'd not kept abreast of things. So it was very difficult. Having to sit across the table from somebody and say, 'Look, yes you're a doctor. Yes, you've got the qualification but actually no, you're not fit to practice'. It's not nice.

> We were also using our own powers deriving from the Health and Social Care Act 2001 and so-called Performers List Regulations. The GMC was a parallel process because the findings on the doctors were so bad that we were able to say, 'We're removing you from our lists, but also we think that you should not be fit to practice as a doctor at all.'

> We proved [a number of] different charges [where] the GMC failed to impose a sanction. They said, 'You're guilty of all these charges but that doesn't constitute serious professional misconduct'. We then appealed that [through further regulatory and legal forums].

What are we to make of this account? From one perspective, Dr. Usborne is simply relating the tortuous process through which incompetent doctors are deprived of the privileges of practice. From a different perspective, however, she is describing how a moral narrative extends beyond a leader and their confederates to engage a wider circle of 'enactors'. In this case, her moral leadership resulted in several different groups adopting an understanding of events that permitted them to redefine the moral and professional status of the doctors involved.

Both of these two perspectives help us to understand the task of moral leadership. First, Usborne's own perspective draws our attention to a critical factor in ethical enactment: context. What can be done about a potential moral harm depends entirely upon what practical action the context permits. What this implies, in turn, is that a sound working knowledge of the institutional, organizational and policy landscape is just as important to moral leadership as more obviously 'moral' knowledge. Next, thinking about moral leadership as a narrative activity, we see Usborne's moral narrative being enacted through institutions (e.g. NCAS), through institutional practices (e.g. the NCAS assessment) and through 'micro-practices' of responsibility (e.g. explaining to a doctor that they are not fit to practise). The more a moral leader knows about institutions, their practices, and their cultures, the greater is the likelihood of formulating and implementing a sound narrative response to moral trouble.

Institutions, practices and micro-practices of responsibility

Much of this chapter has already been taken up with practices of responsibility: specifically the practices of responsibility that are engaged when people set out to make sense of morally troubling events. I now move on to consider the practices of responsibility that are engaged when sense has largely been made and a moral narrative is becoming social reality. What we will see is that although institutions, practices and micro-practices are extraordinarily varied, the strategies available to us to manage moral trouble are rather limited. We should start by noticing, though, the rich array of institutions and practices surrounding medicine and through which moral narratives may be constituted.

Institutions include the courts; the professional associations such as the medical Royal Colleges, the British Medical Association, the Medical Defence Union and the Medical Protection Society; the regulatory bodies including the General Medical Council, the Council for Healthcare Regulatory Excellence, and the Care Quality Commission; the advisory agencies such as the National Institute for Health and Clinical Excellence, the National Clinical Assessment Service, the National Patient Safety Agency, and other organizations with a specific remit such as the NHS Litigation Authority; the commissioning bodies such as Primary Care Trusts; and of course, the healthcare provider organizations themselves, whether public or private, tertiary, secondary or primary care.[18] (At the time of writing, the regulatory and advisory landscape is changing and the functions of several of these bodies will eventually be carried out by different agencies.)

Within these institutions, responsibilities are defined and practised through such avenues as: primary and secondary legislation; the conditions of membership, ethical codes, disciplinary procedures, review processes, collegial networks, and educational resources in professional associations; the Department of Health operating frameworks; the quasi-legal guidance emanating from advisory organizations; the licensing and registration requirements of regulators; high-level inquiries into medical wrongdoing; protocols, committees, reports of working parties; contracts and performance standards governing primary and secondary care; and role hierarchy, appraisal processes, contractual terms, disciplinary codes and legal rights and responsibilities in medical employment.

And of course micro-practices of responsibility are even more extensive. Micro-practices are the myriad intricate operations that sustain moral relations minute-by-minute in healthcare organizations [70,71]. They are ways of taking care of the well-being of patients, families and colleagues, practices which run the gamut from A to W, if not quite to Z: for example apologizing, blaming, conciliating, demanding and excusing; through praising, questioning, reprimanding and soothing; to voicing values and to whistleblowing [72].[19]

These lists of institutions, practices and micro-practices above do not even begin to be comprehensive. However, they suffice to illustrate the profusion of ways in which moral narratives come to be expressed. In striking contrast to the profusion of local tactics, however, the strategies through which responsibility and accountability are elicited and enforced can

---

[18] See Appendix 2. [19] The term 'voicing values' is MC Gentile's.

be quite succinctly stated. In this study a total of six strategies became apparent: scrutiny; moral suasion; moral bargaining; gate-keeping; exclusion; and making reparation.

Each one of these strategies endeavours to determine an individuals' place in relation to their a community. They seek to enforce responsibility and accountability first by drawing members closer into the community and its norms (scrutiny, moral suasion); then by making inclusion in the community conditional (moral bargaining, gate-keeping); and finally by distancing members from the community (exclusion). Making reparation is a special case. Rather than being about inclusion or exclusion, moral repair is about reordering moral relations, adjusting victims' and offenders' standing vis-à-vis one another. Moral leadership is, thus, about nothing if not defining an individual's standing in the community.

Drawing members into community

Scrutiny and persuasion are deployed to maintain and reinforce community norms on a day-to-day basis, and to bolster their authority when they are at risk of being breached. Scrutiny may come in the form of direct supervision, or through familiar organizational devices such as mortality and morbidity data, clinical audit and accreditation of services. Persuasion might come in the form of rhetorical address, written communications, policies and protocols, one-to-one moral suasion and, when norms have been breached, various forms of reprimand.

When she found herself confronted by the egregious breach of normative expectations described earlier, Usborne started out with a strategy of enhanced scrutiny. In the early stages of this affair, there was the prospect (albeit increasingly remote) of rehabilitating doctors who were thought to lack competence. Her first steps were supervision and assessment of colleagues to ascertain the cause of their difficulties, as well as to contain the possibility of future harm being done to patients.

Scrutinizing the performance of the individuals concerned was not the only action to be initiated in the early phases. Moral leadership of colleagues was mandated too. When the problems first arose, one of the difficulties Dr. Usborne faced was a perception among colleagues that when patients came to harm because their doctors failed to monitor their health, this was less morally blameworthy than when patients came to harm through doctors' dangerous actions. The reasons for these different assessments of harm are complex, but the results familiar. The months of life a patient might lose through, say, physician-assisted dying capture the moral imagination more readily than the years of life a patient loses through passive neglect of a chronic condition such as diabetes. Usborne's rhetorical solution was to recast what many would tell as a story of passive neglect into a morally compelling tale of active harm. She did so in a single powerful phrase that spelled out the moral parity between medical neglectfulness and killing, and reformulated colleagues' moral understanding.

> One of the phrases we used when we were discussing this with colleagues, we said, 'This practice is supervising the premature death of hundreds of people'. There wasn't a Shipman [73][20] there ... but these doctors, through indolence and just despair, were neglecting the care of patients; who were suffering in consequence.

---

[20] The name Harold Shipman may not resonate internationally quite as it does with UK readers. Harold Shipman was a General Practitioner who was also a prolific serial killer. In 2000 he was convicted of the murder of 15 of his patients, and a subsequent inquiry attributed a further 218 premature patient deaths to his actions.

Negotiating conditions for community membership

It is a trite observation that humans are social animals. It is less trite, perhaps, to observe that promises of fellowship or threats of ostracism are powerful modes of moral influence. Where conditions for community membership are stringent – as they are in medicine – continuing membership becomes all the more desirable and the prospect of exclusion becomes an even more effective threat. Total exclusion from the community of medicine means, of course, to be denied the privileges of practice as well as to be disgraced in the eyes of peers and public.

Here I consider how the several steps leading up to exclusion allow for a degree of negotiation between the parties. One effect of such negotiations is to classify the practitioner either as a person deserving of support, whose moral standing remains intact; or as a person fit for exclusion, whose moral standing may properly be degraded in ensuing processes and procedures.

Moral bargaining seeks to elicit reformed behaviour through the threat of sanctions or the offer of inducements. It can take the form of deferring disciplinary or other action in exchange for an agreement to modify behaviour, or to undertake or to cease certain activities voluntarily; it can be a warning that proceedings will be instigated if behaviour does not change; it may be a promise to provide benefits such as additional training or different duties, in exchange for concessions from the practitioner. Used beneficently, this strategy is rightly described as moral bargaining. Used cynically, or used in circumstances where there is real inequality of bargaining power, the strategy might be more accurately described as moral blackmail.

Early in her dealings with them, Usborne quite properly referred her doctors to the National Clinical Assessment Service (NCAS) before taking any further steps. Although Usborne may not have perceived it as moral bargaining, referral to NCAS is an informative example of the strategy. NCAS is a national body that assesses the competence and professional behaviour of doctors referred to it and advises, where appropriate, on remediation. NHS organizations wishing to suspend a doctor from NHS employment must refer to them to NCAS, but in all other cases referral is voluntary. NCAS is an advisory body so it cannot compel doctors or their organizations to follow their recommendations and it will only carry out an assessment if the doctor concerned agrees to it. As organizations can choose whether to refer a practitioner to NCAS, and as practitioners can elect whether to be assessed, referral to NCAS can be used as a form of moral bargaining. What is the nature of this exchange?

NCAS differentiates between what it deems incompetence on the one hand and moral turpitude on the other, restricting its sphere of activity to dealing with technical incompetence. Cases involving matters of probity, such as dishonesty or inappropriate relationships with patients, are referred directly to the regulator. By resolutely distinguishing 'technical' matters from 'moral' infractions NCAS maintains the moral standing of doctors undergoing assessment. Furthermore, NCAS views its assessment processes as developmental. It takes pride in the number of doctors who return to work – with remediation where necessary – following an assessment [74–77].[21]

---

[21] See references 74–76 for a list of NCAS publications, and 77 for a study done at King's College London about assessment and remediation of doctors in difficulty.

NCAS describes its review processes in noticeably neutral, almost soothing tones, emphasizing its reasoned, supportive, evidence-based approach. Doctors referred to NCAS participate in a thorough review of their health, clinical skills and character. References to moral character are limited to the qualities required of a good doctor: that is, empathy, sensitivity, self-awareness, ability to learn, and so on. A core requirement (the one most widely cited by medical directors) is that doctors exhibit 'insight'. 'Insight' serves as a marker for the practitioner's capacity to understand his limitations and learn from his mistakes. Having 'insight' implies that the practitioner defers to the judgement of those who consider that his behaviour is at fault. To contest this judgement may be evidence that the practitioner is unable to see himself as others see him, and is therefore incapable of change.

Two further features of NCAS processes are worthy of comment. The first feature is that NCAS resists categories of blame and moral judgement, preferring to classify practitioners' behaviour as either remediable or irremediable. The clearest example of how this cuts across commonly conceived moral categories is in the case of drug misuse. By classifying this as (at least in principle) an illness capable of cure, and a behaviour that is remediable, NCAS protects the practitioner from the moral stigma associated with criminal activity or lapses of probity. The second feature is that NCAS assessment is one of few ways for practitioners to contest the perspective from which an organizational moral narrative is organized. NCAS allows for the possibility that what has been perceived as a problem with the practitioner's performance may turn out to be problem with the organizational setting in which a practitioner performs. Seen from another perspective, what looks like incompetence may really be excessive workload, prejudicial judgements by colleagues, dysfunctional teams, unrealistic expectations, and so on. NCAS encourages the parties to consider both how a practitioner's behaviour has been construed, and also what organizational factors may be driving it.

On the surface of it, this is a rational-technical appraisal of clinical performance. Stripped to its narrative essentials however, NCAS assessment looks oddly familiar. In return for submitting themselves to NCAS procedures, doctors get a shot at redemption. Some will confess to mistakes in the hope that suitable penitence will open the door to remediation. Others will hope to demonstrate that a negative judgement of their ability, behaviour or character is wrong. In the latter case, NCAS procedures hold out the promise of restitution, restoring the doctor to their former moral standing as a trustworthy member of the community of practitioners; but non-compliance or an unsuccessful assessment carries the ultimate threat of excommunication, expulsion from the community of practice.

So one way of understanding NCAS processes is to view them as a redemption narrative. NCAS procedures are private and confidential. The agency avoids the language of blame and fault, emphasizing that its role is to understand apparent performance difficulties. It endeavours to maintain the social status of the participant by supporting and, where possible, rehabilitating the individual. This redemptive narrative is quite different from the fault and blame narrative associated with referral to the General Medical Council under the 'fitness to practice' procedures. The disciplinary measures of the medical regulator represent the punitive face of medical professional morality. The regulator's processes are public and open. As such, they inevitably degrade the social status of the practitioner. Whatever the outcome, the practitioner will bear the stigma of having been the subject of proceedings that have the power to sanction or exclude them from the community [78].

We noted earlier that justice lies in finding the right balance between the medico-legal and the preventive approaches to making sense of medical harm. So too, justice for patients and practitioners lies in finding the right balance between redemption and degradation narratives.

Distancing members from community

As the last part of Usborne's tale suggests, the most draconian strategy in the armoury of moral leadership is to seek excommunication of a moral offender. It is easy to see how a moral judgement is made when a practitioner's personal behaviour or probity has been called into question. Is it also moral judgement where the grounds for exclusion are purely those of technical competence? Undoubtedly so. Expelling a doctor from the professional community by suspending or withdrawing their licence to practice results in a profound change to an individual's moral standing, both within the professional community and in a wider social circle. A doctor 'excommunicated' for reasons of technical incompetence experiences both professional and personal disgrace.

It should be no surprise to any observer of medicine that assessing the technical ability of qualified practitioners is an activity accompanied by significant moral unease, however well justified the final judgement. The implementation of revalidation – the process by which UK doctors will from 2012 be required to renew their license to practise on a quinquennial basis – will no doubt be a significant source of moral anxiety in forthcoming years [79,80].[22]

Conclusion

Thinking and writing about moral narrative leaves one with an appreciation of the importance of having the last word. Final words resonate. It is in the epilogue, the obituary, the official minutes, the last will and testament, the final report, that a claim to definitive meanings is staked. He who speaks the final words has the best chance to assert that his reality is the reality. So assigning the last word is a profoundly moral decision. For this reason, I want to leave the last words of this chapter to Dr. Lister and Dr. Usborne. But before I can do so, I should summarize the argument that I have presented here.

Moral leadership becomes apparent in three linked processes. First, moral sensibilities are provoked by something in the data of everyday experience, and moral sense-making begins. Then, leaders involve those around them in making moral sense out of the heady confusion of information, predictions, perspectives and values that surround them. Finally associates are engaged in implementing the moral narrative that best expresses a fitting way forward.

I identified seven features characteristic of moral leadership. First, it reflects the collaborative nature of moral expertise. Second, it is grounded in the normative expectations that accompany specific social relations and social knowledge. Third, moral sense-making takes place through time, and is in some significant respects retrospective. Fourth, credible moral narrative emerges out of action to resolve normative, empirical, epistemological, predictive, tactical and virtue concerns. Fifth, moral narratives make sense to and within moral

---

[22] For a comparative account of American, Canadian and UK policy on recertification and revalidation, see reference 80.

community. Sixth, the potential to actuate moral narrative is supplied by practices of responsibility significantly embedded in social structures. Seventh, moral narrative is implemented through a range of strategies that define the relationship between individuals and their communities.

In the final section I present evidence for my eighth and final argument. To enact ethics is not only to reason, but also to perform the value commitments that make us who we are and worthy in our own eyes. We have to commit to making a moral narrative, even when we are uncertain what good will come of it, even when we cannot be sure how others will judge us, and even when we wonder whether we are good ourselves. So now the final words.

Final words . . .

Dr. Luke Lister, Long River Hospital NHS Trust:

> I'm talking more than I thought I would . . . I suddenly wondered why I was doing it, you know! I sense that my speech was fairly upbeat, and it almost sounded to me as though there was brio there. [Doing what I did] is not something I'm particularly – I am proud of it, in a way, as having done it and learnt a lot and seen it through – but I'm not boasting about having sacked people and created chaos in their lives. And then suddenly hearing my own tone of voice – I'd be very sad if that came over.

Dr. Ursula Usborne, Churchland Primary Care Trust:

> I know exactly what you mean when you say, 'dig deep'. And I recognize that as, as shut your eyes, take a deep breath, and focus. I have to do that from time to time. Earlier on I referred to the 'grasping the nettle moment' where the pain kicks in and you have to just get through it. One of those situations was where I had to say to somebody, 'You are resigning. But I'm going to have to tell you either you should give up work completely and not work as a doctor any more, or I'm going to have to take it further and pursue this matter'. . . .

> What happens in that moment of focus? I suppose it's almost like checking off a rosary. It's the right thing, it's correct, it's based on this, it's based on that, it's rational. It's going to feel unkind. You don't have any choice. But you can offer this, that, and the other safety netting. That's it, and it has to be faced.

> The moment's now.

Further reading

Weick KE. *Making Sense of the Organization.* Oxford: Blackwell; 2001.

Bosk CL. *Forgive and Remember: Managing Medical Failure.* 2nd edn. Chicago: University of Chicago Press; 2003.

Walker MU. *Moral Understandings: A Feminist Study in Ethics.* 2nd edn. New York: Oxford University Press; 2007.

Hunter KM. *Doctors' Stories: The Narrative Structure of Medical Knowledge.* Princeton: Princeton University Press; 1991.

Klein G. *Sources of Power: How People Make Decisions.* Cambridge, MA: MIT Press; 1999.

Doris JM. *Lack of Character: Personality and Moral Behaviour.* New York: Cambridge University Press; 2002.

References

1. Morgan G. *Images of Organization.* London: Sage; 1997.

2. Walker MU. *Moral Understandings: A Feminist Study in Ethics.* 2nd edn. New York: Oxford University Press; 2007.

3. MacIntyre A. *After Virtue.* 3rd edn. London: Duckworth; 2007.

4. Maines DR. Narrative's moment and sociology's phenomena: toward a narrative sociology. *Sociological Quarterly*. 1993;**34**(1):17–38.

5. Maines DR. *The Faultline of Consciousness*. New York: Aldine de Gruyter; 2001.

6. Boseley S. Doctors failing 3m patients: call for tight checks to improve service. *The Guardian*. 2004: Available from: http://www.guardian.co.uk/society/2004/dec/18/medicineandhealth.lifeandhealth?INTCMP=SRCH.

7. Donaldson LJ. Doctors with problems in an NHS workforce. *BMJ*. 1994;**308**(6939):1277–82.

8. Donaldson LJ. Facing up to the problem of the poorly performing doctor. *Student BMJ*. 1996;**4**:276–7.

9. Scally G. Dealing with duffers. *The Lancet*. 1995;**346**(8977):720–.

10. Smith R. All doctors are problem doctors. *BMJ*. 1997;**314**(7084):841.

11. Mayberry JF. The management of poor performance. *Postgraduate Medical Journal*. 2007;**83**(976):105–8.

12. Smith R. Managing the clinical performance of doctors. *BMJ*. 1999;**319**(7221):1314–5.

13. Firth-Cozens J. Doctors with difficulties: why so few women? *Postgraduate Medical Journal*. 2008;**84**(992):318–20.

14. Kohn LT, et al., eds. *To Err is Human: Building a Safer Health System*. Washington DC: Institute of Medicine: National Academy Press; 2000.

15. Weick KE. *Making Sense of the Organization*. Oxford: Blackwell; 2001.

16. Weick KE. *Sensemaking in Organizations*. London: Sage; 1995.

17. Waring JJ. Beyond blame: cultural barriers to medical incident reporting. *Social Science & Medicine*. 2005;**60**:1927–35.

18. West E. Organisational sources of safety and danger: sociological contributions to the study of adverse events. *Quality & Safety in Health Care*. 2000;**9**(2):120–6.

19. Lawton R, Parker D. Barriers to incident reporting in a healthcare system. *Quality and Safety in Health Care*. 2002;**11**(1):15–8.

20. Vincent C, Stanhope N, Crowley-Murphy M. Reasons for not reporting adverse incidents: an empirical study. *Journal of Evaluation in Clinical Practice*. 1999;**5**(1):13–21.

21. Reason J. Understanding adverse events: human factors. *Quality in Health Care*. 1995;**4**(2):80–9.

22. Hakkarainen KPJ, Palonen T, Paavola S, Lehtinen E. *Communities of Networked Expertise: Professional and Educational Perspectives*. Amsterdam: Elsevier/EARLI; 2004.

23. Paavola S, Hakkarainen K. The knowledge creation metaphor – an emergent epistemological approach to learning. *Science & Education*. 2005;**14**(6):535–57.

24. West R, Graham C, Hakkarainen K, Palonen T, Paavola S, Lehtinen E. Communities of networked expertise: professional and educational perspectives. *Educational Technology Research and Development*. 2007;**55**(4):391–3.

25. Strawson PF. Freedom and resentment. In: Strawson PF, ed. *Studies in the Philosophy of Thought and Action*. New York: Oxford University Press; 1968.

26. Pears D. Strawson on freedom and resentment. In: Hahn LE, ed. *The Philosophy of P.F. Strawson: The Library of Living Philosophers*, vol. **XXVI**. Chicago: Open Court; 1998, pp. 245–58.

27. Strawson PF. Reply to David Pears. In: Hahn LE, ed. *The Philosophy of P.F. Strawson: The Library of Living Philosophers*, vol. **XXVI**. Chicago: Open Court; 1998, pp. 259–62.

28. Bosk CL. *Forgive and Remember: Managing Medical Failure*. 2nd edn. Chicago: University of Chicago Press; 2003.

29. Anderson JG. Forgive and remember: managing medical failure. *JAMA*. 2004;**291**(14):1775–6.

30. Conrad P. Forgive and remember: managing medical failure (review). *Social Forces*. 2004;**83**(1):426–8.

31. Rosen P, Markovchick V, Dracon D. Normative and technical error in the emergency department. *Journal of Emergency Medicine.* 1983;**1**(2): 155–60.

32. Cassell J. Technical and moral error in medicine and fieldwork. *Human Organization.* 1981;**40**(2):160–8.

33. Holtman MC. Paradoxes of professionalism and error in complex systems. *Journal of Biomedical Informatics.* 2011;**44**(3)95–401.

34. Learning from Bristol: The Report of the Public Inquiry into Children's Heart Surgery at the Bristol Royal Infirmary. *Cm 5207;* 2001.

35. Smith R. All changed, changed utterly: British medicine will be transformed by the Bristol case. *BMJ.* 1998;**316**: 1917–18.

36. Davies HTO, Shields AV. Discussion paper: Public trust and accountability for clinical performance: lessons from the national press reportage of the Bristol hearing. *Journal of Evaluation in Clinical Practice.* 1999;**5**(3):335–42.

37. Horton R. How should doctors respond to the GMC's judgments on Bristol? *The Lancet.* 1998;**351**(9120):1900–1.

38. Smith R. Regulation of doctors and the Bristol inquiry. *BMJ.* 1998;**317** (7172):1539–40.

39. Willis JAR. The aftermath of the Bristol case. *BMJ.* 1998;**317**(7161):811.

40. *An inquiry into quality and practice within the National Health Service arising from the actions of Rodney Ledward.* Department of Health; 2000.

41. Independent investigation into how the NHS handled allegations about the conduct of Richard Neale. *Cm 6315;* 2004.

42. Independent investigation into how the NHS handled allegations about the conduct of Clifford Ayling. *Cm 6298;* 2004.

43. Independent investigation into how the NHS handled allegations about the conduct of William Kerr and Michael Haslam. *Cm 6640* 2005.

44. Shipman Inquiry. Safeguarding patients: lessons from the past – proposals for the future. *Cm 6394;* 2004.

45. Milgram S. Behavioural studies of obedience. *Journal of Abnormal and Social Psychology.* 1963;**67**:371–8.

46. Milgram S. *Obedience to Authority: An Experimental View.* London: Tavistock; 1974.

47. Atkinson P. *Medical Talk and Medical Work: The Liturgy of the Clinic.* Thousand Oaks, CA: Sage; 1995, p. 110.

48. Geoffrey HG, Sandra KJ, Jennifer B. Physician expressions of uncertainty during patient encounters. *Patient Education and Counseling.* 2000;**40** (1):59–65.

49. Timmermans S, Angell A. Evidence-based medicine, clinical uncertainty, and learning to doctor. *Journal of Health and Social Behavior.* 2001;**42**(4):342–59.

50. Parascandola M, Hawkins JS, Danis M. Patient autonomy and the challenge of clinical uncertainty *Kennedy Institute of Ethics Journal.* 2002;**12**(3):245–64.

51. Ogden J, Fuks K, Gardner M, Johnson S, McLean M, Martin P, *et al.* Doctors expressions of uncertainty and patient confidence. *Patient Education and Counseling.* 2002;**48**(2):171–6.

52. Lingard L, Garwood K, Schryer CF, Spafford MM. A certain art of uncertainty: case presentation and the development of professional identity. *Social Science & Medicine.* 2003 Feb;**56**(3):603–16.

53. Williams SJ. Parsons revisited: from the sick role to...? *Health (London).* 2005;**9** (2):123–44.

54. Pilnick A, Hindmarsh J, Gill VT. Beyond 'doctor and patient': developments in the study of healthcare interactions. *Sociology of Health & Illness.* 2009;**31** (6):787–802.

55. Spafford MM, Schryer CF, Campbell SL, Lingard L. Towards embracing clinical uncertainty. *Journal of Social Work.* 2007;**7** (2):155–78.

56. Fox R. Medical uncertainty revisited. In: Gary L. Albrecht RF, Susan Scrimshaw,

eds. *Handbook of Social Studies in Health And Medicine*. London: Sage; 2000, pp. 409–25.

57. Ashcroft R. 'Power, corruption and lies': ethics and power. In: Ashcroft R, Lucassen A, Parker M, Verkerk M, Widdershoven G, eds. *Case Analysis in Clinical Ethics*. Cambridge: Cambridge University Press; 2005, pp. 77–94.

58. Gabriel Y. *Storytelling in Organizations: Facts, Fictions, and Fantasies*. Oxford: Oxford University Press; 2000, p. 28

59. Holm S. *Ethical Problems in Clinical Practice: The Ethical Reasoning of Healthcare Professionals*. Manchester: Manchester University Press; 1997, p. 126.

60. Storr L. Leading with integrity: a qualitative research study. *Journal of Health Organization and Management*. 2004;**18**(6):415–34.

61. Shaw GB. *The Doctor's Dilemma*. London: Constable; 1911, pp. xxii, Act 1: pp. 28,47,48,49,50,51,52,53,54.

62. Freidson E. *Profession of Medicine: A Study in the Sociology of Applied Knowledge*. Chicago: University of Chicago Press; 1970.

63. Brennan T. Medical professionalism in the new millennium: a physician charter (project of the A.B.I.M Foundation, A.C.P–A.S.I.M Foundation, and European Federation of Internal Medicine). *Annals of Internal Medicine*. 2002;**136**:243–6.

64. Blank L, Kimball H, McDonald W, Merino J, for the ABIM Foundation AF, EFoIM. Medical professionalism in the new millennium: a physician charter 15 months later. *Annals of Internal Medicine*. 2003;**138**(10):839–41.

65. Wear D, Aultman JM. *Professionalism in Medicine: Critical Perspectives*. New York: Springer: 2006.

66. Davies M. *Medical Self-Regulation: Crisis and Change*. Aldershot: Ashgate; 2007.

67. Cruess RL, Cruess SR, Johnston SE. Professionalism: an ideal to be sustained. *The Lancet*. 2000;**356**(9224):156–9.

68. Emanuel L, Cruess R, Cruess S, Hauser J. Old values, new challenges: what is a professional to do? *International Journal For Quality in Health Care*. 2002;**14**(5):349–51.

69. Cholbi M. Moral expertise and the credentials problem. *Ethical Theory & Moral Practice*. 2007;**10**:323–34.

70. Nikku N, Eriksson BE. Microethics in action 1. *Bioethics*. 2006;**20**(4):169–79.

71. Reiter-Theil S AG. Research on clinical ethics and consultation. Introduction to the theme. *Medicine, Health Care and Philosophy*. 2007;**11**(1):3–5.

72. Gentile MC. *Giving Voice to Values: How to Speak Your Mind When You Know What's Right*. New Haven: Yale University Press; 2010.

73. Field R, Scotland A. Medicine in the UK after Shipman: has 'all changed, changed utterly'? *The Lancet*. 2004;**364**(Supplement 1):40–1.

74. NCAS. *Back on Track: Restoring Doctors and Dentists to Safe Professional Practice*. 2006.

75. NCAS. *Handling Concerns about the Performance of Health Professionals*. 2006.

76. NCAS. *Understanding Performance Difficulties in Doctors*. 2004.

77. Humphrey C, Locke R. *Provision of assessment and remediation for physicians about whom concerns have been expressed: an international survey*. London: King's College; 2008.

78. Garfinkel H. Conditions of successful degradation ceremonies. *American Journal of Sociology*. 1956;**61**:420–4.

79. Shaw K, MacKillop L, Armitage M. Revalidation, appraisal and clinical governance. *Clinical Governance: An International Journal*. 2007;**12**(3):170–7.

80. Shaw K, Cassel CK, Black C, Levinson W. Shared medical regulation in a time of increasing calls for accountability and transparency. *JAMA*. 2009;**302**(18):2008–14.

Understanding normative expectations in medical moral leadership

The purpose of this chapter is to understand the nature of normative expectations; to observe how they differ from, and how they interact with, other elements in our moral life; and to consider their expression in narratives of medical moral leadership.

The concept of normative expectations, and the associated concept of reactive attitudes, were both introduced for the first time in Chapter 2. Normative expectations reflect our understanding of the responsibilities that we each owe to one another, and our views on how these responsibilities ought to be discharged. Normative expectations give rise to a keen sense that we 'have a right' to demand certain actions of others. Normative expectations are also frequently accompanied by strongly felt 'reactive attitudes' of anger, outrage, resentment, disgust, dismay and the like. These emotions arise when we perceive that we have been let down, particularly when we have been let down in relation to something to which we felt entitled.

In this chapter, I analyse five examples of moral leadership. We will explore the way in which normative expectations and reactive attitudes inform and shape medical leaders' action, and also consider their interplay with other components of moral life. The examples are not just of interest as examples of normative expectation. They also illustrate something of the range of 'moral troubles' with which medical leaders in the study were concerned.

Normative expectations and reactive attitudes explained

Philosopher Margaret Walker begins her account of normative expectations by noting 'a sensibility attuned to norms is a basic part of human social functioning' [1(p24)]. I noted in Chapter 1 that bioethical debate is made more difficult where different disciplines use the same words in different ways. 'Norms' is one of those words. So what sorts of norms are we referring to when we use the term 'normative expectations'?

The 'norm' element in normative expectations refers primarily to 'norms' in the sense that moral theorists use the word. 'Norms' either signify behaviours that are more or less prescribed and desirable, in which case we consider the norm something we 'ought' to do; or they signify behaviour that is more or less prohibited and undesirable, in which case we consider it something we 'ought not' to do. 'Norms' in this usage are standards for conduct, standards that we appraise from a moral point of view. Adopting a moral point of view we might ask, for example, whether reason commands us to treat the norm as a universal law, as Kantian ethics invites us to do; or we might ask whether the conduct it commends will have good consequences.

Social theorists are more inclined to use the term 'norm' in a statistical sense, referring to the frequency with which we observe certain patterns of behaviour. 'Norm' in the social theorists' lexicon by and large suggests conduct that falls within the usual range, the 'normal' way of going about things. For the social theorist, identifying behaviour as a 'norm' does not imply any evaluation of the behaviour, and the theorist may reserve judgement on whether the 'norm' is in any way desirable.

These two meanings of 'norm' are of course related, but philosophers have long cautioned against conflating the two. In a well-ordered society, consensus about 'how things ought to be done' will probably lead towards this becoming the 'normal' way of doing things. Normative expectations and reactive attitudes have a role to play here, as we shall see: when there is a belief that things ought to be done a certain way, people act and react in ways that aim to elicit the desired behaviour in others.

The association between statistical and moral norms works far less well the other way around, however. The 'normal' way of doing things *may* be desirable, but there is no guarantee that the statistical norm embodies the right or good. So moral norms cannot be read off from statistical norms. And indeed the 'normal' might be thought to be highly undesirable, thus generating moral and political debate and movements for change.

It is because 'a sensibility attuned to norms is a basic part of human social functioning' that norms come to be accompanied by 'expectations'. Like norms, 'expectations' concern both what we believe to be valuable and what we find predictable. Morally speaking we 'expect' others to adhere to certain standards, taking the view that they ought to comply with standards because the standards embody important values. Statistically speaking we 'expect' that much of the time others will observe these standards, either because they have already demonstrated a willingness to abide by them or because they have expressed sentiments suggesting they support them. Such expectations can be either general, concerning what we think groups of people or types of people should do; or specific, concerning what I think you or another particular person should do. My general expectation might be that people tell the truth. If I know that someone has a propensity to lie in difficult situations, I might accurately predict that they will lie to me in this one. But I still hope that they will not. Moreover, my doubting their truthfulness does not weaken the normative expectation of truth telling, which continues to apply to them as much as to others whom I trust more.

Normative expectations thus yoke together a demand to behave in a certain way and a degree of anticipation that this will be done. They are an expression of hope and trust that in the normal course of events people will behave as they should behave.

We may now revisit the example of respect for patient autonomy that I briefly considered in Chapter 2 to illustrate how normative expectations function. The requirement to respect patient autonomy is a moral norm familiar to doctors. The existence of this norm elicits expectations: from healthcare professionals and their regulators that professionals will comply with it; from managers that healthcare professionals will pursue it; from patients that doctors will respect their autonomous wishes, and from professionals that patients will wish to exercise autonomy; from patients and professionals that family carers will respect patient autonomy; and so on. These expectations are both moral expectations, a belief that these things ought to happen and that patients are entitled to them; and a predictive expectation, that patients will experience (in some degree at least) respect for autonomy [2-7].[1] Knowing that some doctors will fail to respect patient autonomy

---

[1] O'Neill has observed that in medical settings respect for autonomy has come to be seen as broadly synonymous with informed consent, see reference 2. Anspach (reference 3) was one of the first to write in detail about how 'informed consent' was produced in practice. See references 4-7.

when this is required does not make the general principle of respect for autonomy any less important. Indeed, it may make the norm itself even more compelling. And as normative expectations are both general and specific, patient expectations of doctors crystallize around tangible expectations of this doctor, who they anticipate will be particularly focussed on patient choice, or particularly paternalistic, perhaps; and doctors generally, of whom they hold more nebulous expectations.

Normative expectations create a sense of entitlement to what is normatively expected: to have autonomy respected, to be told the truth, to be treated kindly, to be granted privacy, to be kept clean and safe in hospital, to have our feelings taken into account. This sense of entitlement becomes most apparent in how we respond when normative expectations have been violated. We react with feelings such as resentment, anger, disgust, outrage, guilt, shame or remorse, feelings that the philosopher Peter Strawson described as 'reactive attitudes' [8]. These reactive attitudes bring to the level of bodily experience both our normative expectations and the sense of entitlement that accompanies them. Reactive attitudes are a visible expression of feelings of hurt, betrayal, sadness, embarrassment, disrespect and the rest, and they emanate from a normative judgement. Strawson pointed to how our strongly felt attitudes literally embody our interpretation of the moral status of actions.

> If someone treads on my hand accidentally, while trying to help me, the pain may be no less acute than if he treads on it in contemptuous disregard of my existence or with a malevolent wish to injure me. But I shall generally feel in the second case a kind and degree of resentment that I shall not feel in the first. If someone's actions help me to some benefit I desire, then I am benefited in any case; but if he intended them so to benefit me because of his general goodwill towards me, I shall reasonably feel a gratitude which I should not feel at all if the benefit was an incidental consequence, unintended or even regretted by him, of some plan of action with a different aim. [8(p5)]

If we are angry or vengeful, we regard it as justified, at least in principle, by the normative breach. If we are forgiving or mortified, we sense the 'rightness' in being so. Furthermore, we may feel that we ought to feel these ways, even when we do not; and others may expect us to express such feelings, even if we do not in fact own them.

The presence of a reactive attitude is a signal that something has disturbed our normative expectations. It may be obvious exactly what that is, or it may require some sense-making before the expectation that has been violated becomes apparent. I suggest that the moral quality of healthcare organizations rests upon the normative expectations that come to prevail within professional groups, and the response that individuals or groups mobilize when a reactive attitude signals that their normative expectations have been breached.

Because I expect you to act as you should act, I treat you as responsible for meeting my normative expectation, and as accountable to me if you do not. How I hold you accountable may depend upon my own 'reactive attitude'. If you let me down I may for instance scold you, demand an explanation or offer you forgiveness. Considerable care is required here. Normative expectations are not always morally sound. Some professional norms – medical paternalism, perhaps – may be open to question, and the normative expectations associated with them are then correspondingly problematic. Neither are reactive attitudes necessarily helpful. Anger or outrage may need to be tempered with a more considered response. Or I might suppress the signal that something is wrong and ignore, excuse or normalize your behaviour. Reactive attitudes are merely a sign that normative expectations have been threatened. They do not supply a reasoned response to the breach.

To summarize, normative expectations express expectations both of myself and of others that we will act in accordance with the shared moral understandings that are available to guide behaviour. Moreover, when one of us acts in a way that seems to violate such shared understandings, others are entitled to hold the putative offender responsible, to demand an account and, where appropriate, to receive some form of restitution. Whatever the nature of our emotional responses to lapses or violations, we are inclined to consider our feelings justified, a signal that moral understandings have been betrayed. As Walker concludes, normative expectations 'can only be explained as expressing a kind of presumption that is also an insistence that people live up to standards' [1(p68)]. Medicine is full of standards: standards for clinical care, standards for behaviour towards colleagues, standards for the performance of one's role, and so on. These standards are not ordinary moral norms, but the norms that are part of a particular practice. Normative expectations and the associated reactive attitudes are, then, the practised, enacted and embodied expression of a negotiated order of community norms and formal moral propositions [1(p68),9 (p186ff),10,11].[2]

How certain are our normative expectations?

We saw in Chapter 2 that moral leadership begins with, and proceeds through, making moral sense of the events that the leader confronts. Sense-making must address two sources of confusion. Some sources of confusion are matters that are equivocal. We are equivocal when we are not yet certain about what is right or good or otherwise ought to be thought; and equivocality can only be settled through reasoning, logic or commitment to certain values. Other sources of confusion are matters about which there is uncertainty. Uncertainty concerns what has happened, or what could happen, or what is practically possible; uncertainty can sometimes, but not always, be resolved by seeking further information.

What effects do equivocality and uncertainty have on normative expectations and reactive attitudes? Equivocality may weaken normative expectations, inviting questions about whether we are right to presume or insist on certain standards. Normative expectations may be far from settled, an ongoing subject of negotiation or a source of contention. Those who hold normative expectations may not know how they ought to think or feel, or they may think or feel in ways others believe are unjustified. Uncertainty in turn may weaken reactive attitudes, inviting questions about whether the standards that we insist upon have after all been broken, and if they have whether anything can in any event be done about it. Even if normative expectations are clear, and our reactive attitude legitimate, we may not know what we should do, or how to do what needs to be done, in order to vindicate them.

In the next part of this chapter, I examine five narratives that illustrate how normative expectations and reactive attitudes function to inform medical managerial experience. They show how normative expectations are prioritized; how they may elicit 'moral address'; how moral leaders may work to alter them; how they are negotiated when norms are

---

[2] Normative expectations are thus intrinsic to a practice in much the same way that MacIntyre proposed virtues were. See reference 9, pp. 186ff. Walker approves Hollis's observation that normative expectations 'hover uneasily between moral obligations and the local requirements of a particular society'. See references 1 (p. 68), 10 and 11.

equivocal; and how responsibility is accepted even when others' expectations are at odds with an individual's moral beliefs.

The narratives that follow were recounted in research interviews, but rather than reproduce the interviews verbatim the narratives have been extracted and reported in the third person. This is because my purpose at this point is not to analyse the narrative as an interview narrative, but to comment on the interplay of normative expectations and reactive attitudes in the events that interviewees reported. Some of the subjective language and tenor of the interviews remains, however, because it is strongly suggestive of how normative expectations and reactive attitudes prevailed at the time.

Example 1: normative expectations surrounding waiting times for treatment

The time a patient waits for treatment is a moral issue. Patients waiting for treatment are often in pain or anxious, their condition frequently deteriorates, and they may face higher health risks when they do eventually receive care. The time patients spend waiting for treatment is also a political issue. Time spent waiting is (superficially) easy for the electorate to understand and (superficially) easy to measure.[3] It is therefore an obvious object of political rhetoric. In the period from 1997 to 2010 a Labour administration sought to fulfil its promise to the electorate to reduce the amount of time that patients spent waiting for treatment; the Department of Health set and enforced stringent targets for hospitals to achieve. These were accompanied by financial incentives, publication of standards of performance, and penalties for failure. Those who suffered the greatest penalty for failure were probably 'lay' NHS managers, whose jobs and reputation often rested upon hospitals delivering services in compliance with central targets. But the prospect of their failure created tensions across the system, as they sought to manage the change.

One of the most high-profile of the targets for NHS hospitals has been the length of time that patients spend waiting for treatment in the emergency department (until recently, more frequently referred to as Accident & Emergency or A&E). The government foresaw clear benefits for patients; but those charged with implementing the changes on the ground confronted the practical and moral difficulty of meeting the targets while still providing acceptable care to all of their different patient populations. First, was it best to recognize the moral legitimacy of the targets and to endeavour to meet them, even at considerable cost? Striving to meet demanding targets could mean diverting limited organizational resources (time and money) from other equally important areas of health need, thus disadvantaging some groups of patients and distorting local healthcare priorities. But equally, failing to meet the targets could bring organizational penalties that reduced the hospital's capacity to serve their population (as well as damaging individual careers). Perhaps it would be better to protect the interests of the organization, and protect the interests of the wider patient population, by merely creating the impression of meeting the targets?

---

[3] The difficulty is – for example – determining what duration and kind of waiting time is relevant. Clearly it is unacceptable to leave a patient to suffer in anxiety and pain for a long period. Is it good enough care, though, if a patient is assessed and given pain relief but then spends another 12 hours waiting for further treatment or admission to hospital? Does this 12 hours become morally acceptable if several other patients with worse conditions are treated while the first patient waits?

Dr. Breedon believes that morals and management go together in medicine; if you think something's absolutely the wrong thing to do, then how can you manage it into place? He would find it very difficult to sell a management change he wasn't morally convinced of. He thinks that government targets for hospitals, the subject of a great deal of criticism, have been valuable. Some of the targets have been a bit too specific and too stringent, but – for example – the idea that patients shouldn't generally wait more than 4 hours in an emergency department seems to him entirely right.

Dr. Breedon has been a patient in A&E, and knows what it's like from that perspective. He's seen fights in the waiting room and people getting fractious, the staff getting abused. He knows that patients sometimes don't realize that what's going on is that one person's had a heart attack, while another's only got a cut finger, so the person with a heart attack goes before you. When the waiting time is reasonable and someone's being disruptive in the waiting room, then frustration is no excuse – you can legitimately get them escorted off the premises and say 'When you calm down come back, but we're not seeing you at the moment'.

The difficulty with the government targets is not the targets themselves, in his view: it's the 'Stalinist' response if hospitals and their managers don't make the targets. A punitive approach has been really unhelpful. It gets to people, who feel unfairly blamed when even their best efforts haven't been sufficient to solve an insoluble organizational problem.

He's much more interested in satisfying the moral intention underlying targets than with technically meeting the target itself. The technical fix that some hospitals applied to the A&E wait was to create an additional area behind the A&E department, and stipulate that it was not an A&E. At a time when Barton Dene Hospital was struggling to meet the 4-hour target, his A&E staff were invited to visit hospitals where the problem had been solved. So they went to a few places, and came back and said 'Well, there's one place they just painted a line across the corridor; and this side's A&E and that side's not A&E!' Breedon thought, 'That doesn't solve the problem at all! What's that for!'

They spent quite a lot of time arguing through the morality of the whole situation and his A&E colleagues were absolutely adamant they were not going to accept a technical fix. One came to say they'd heard a rumour that something was going to happen at Barton Dene by way of 'fixing' the target, and threatened to resign. Perhaps they went a bit too far on the moral high ground, but they weren't interested in technical compliance. They wanted to sort out what they did in A&E so that patients could be discharged promptly, and they wanted to engage with the physicians and the surgeons and others in the hospital to make sure patients could be admitted quickly when that was needed. The A&E staff were emphatic about meeting this target by changing the way the hospital worked, by mapping the process and seeing where the blocks were and unblocking the blocks and making sure that the process was smooth. They were absolutely adamant they wanted to do it that way.

Barton Dene got into some trouble in the early stages, because it appeared to be lagging in meeting the target. But now they have a solution that is sustainable. And they're going to take that a step further, and change the system yet again, to do something even better.

(Derived from interview with Dr. Breedon, Barton Dene Hospital)

Dr. Breedon's narrative renders several clusters of normative expectation and reactive attitude apparent. To start with Dr. Breedon himself, he holds the overarching normative expectation that medical management should have as its first concern organizing services to meet the needs and interests of patients. (Interestingly, this expectation seems to have been fortified by Dr. Breedon's experience of being a patient himself.) Added to this there is a normative expectation that colleagues should work collaboratively to promote the interests of the organization and its patients; together with the normative expectation that staff should be treated fairly when they have endeavoured to do their best. His reactive attitudes seep through his account of events. He resents that NHS staff have been penalized for failing to solve insoluble problems. He is also dismayed that some organizations and managers appear to have descended to gamesmanship over the targets, missing their moral core.

The emergency department staff clearly shared the normative expectation that medical management should focus on serving the interests of patients. Indeed, in Dr. Breedon's narrative there is a sense that the clarity of their convictions functioned so as to shore up his own. His colleague's threat of resignation evidences, I think, two normative expectations: that medical managers should make good clinical care their first concern, and that the medical director should support clinicians who are in difficult situations because of their determination to stand up for good clinical care. The threat to resign expresses a reactive attitude of outrage to what was thought to be a breach of these expectations. Reactive attitudes, we noted earlier, may be formulated with the intention of calling forth a response to a breach. In this case the expressive reaction was geared towards eliciting Dr. Breedon's support, and it appears to have fulfilled its aims.

Dr. Breedon also hints at the normative expectations of fair treatment that he believes patients hold. In his view, patients expect to receive equal consideration, each being cared for according to their needs. He assumes that patients will tolerate the waiting that goes along with allowing those most gravely ill to take priority, but, to be tolerant, patients need to know that meeting other more urgent needs is the reason for delay. Whether or not he is right about what patients think, his narrative expresses Dr. Breedon's own normative expectation that patients ought to tolerate reasonable waiting times. When waiting times are reasonable, he argues, patients can be expected to behave well and be excluded if they become disruptive.

Breedon's narrative presents what appears to be a rather simple choice between the moral good of taking time and resources to improve the emergency department and the moral vacuity of 'gaming' the targets. The situation is only simple once events have been clearly perceived, however, and when the choice is reviewed in retrospect.

In the period that Dr. Breedon was recalling, administrative pressure to comply with targets was considerable. However, their clinical and moral validity was heavily contested, with some clinicians arguing that a focus on targets distorted clinical decision-making and undermined care for patients [12–21].[4] The contestability of the targets made it possible to hypothesize that it might be more morally defensible to 'game' than it was to comply. Moreover, organizational reputations were at risk when targets were not met. It was feared that where the regulator[5] criticized non-compliant

---

[4] The objections were not without merit. When the 4-hour target for A&E was first introduced, 100% compliance was required. This led to the situation reported by more than one medical director in this study: clinicians or managers requesting permission to breach the target on grounds of clinical need, where a seriously ill or badly injured patient was best cared for in the emergency department. The most egregious and well-known case in which an unbalanced focus on financial and clinical targets distorted clinical care occurred at the Mid-Staffordshire Hospital, subsequently the subject of a high-profile inquiry (see reference 12). In December 2010 the targets for emergency care were replaced by a set of indicators that are not, for the most part, mandatory (see reference 14). The aim to treat all patients within 4 hours has been retained. For academic commentary on the effects of target setting, see references 15–21.

[5] Then known as the Healthcare Commission.

organizations it would affect patient confidence, staff morale and recruitment; and thus have an indirect impact on quality of care.

If a temptation to 'game' could arise out of good intentions (as when managers took the view that other calls on organizational resources were of greater importance to the health of the population that a hospital served) temptation was also the product of bad faith or greed (as when the prospect of earning a performance-related pay award rested on meeting the targets). Some managers and clinicians were tempted into 'gaming', while others succumbed to the temptation of outright fraud [22–26]. 'Gaming' for 'justifiable' reasons may have presented itself at the time as a *bona fides* moral choice – the equivalent of lying to save an innocent life – even if self-interested fraud was always clearly morally insupportable.

Example 2: normative expectations surrounding hospital closure

Dr. George Gulvin is the medical director of Stoneyhill and District NHS Trust; an organization assembled through merger of the several hospitals and health centres that serve a large British city. The city's hospitals had been founded at different times, for different purposes and in different eras of healthcare. The city had grown, modes of transport had changed, medicine had entered a new era, but the old hospitals on their old sites remained, all still attempting to provide a full complement of services in buildings woefully inadequate. The city now had 'beacon' institutions providing secondary and tertiary services and with capacity to serve a wider area, along with outdated general hospitals poorly serving a local, frequently disadvantaged, population.

> Stoneyhill went through a difficult period of restructuring. Each hospital had been providing more or less the full range of services to their local population. But it wasn't sensible to go on doing it that way. The quality of care the weaker hospitals provided was not high enough, they couldn't attract good trainees, and there was too much duplication of provision. Looking at restructuring, it was clear the Trust could not sustain emergency services in all the hospitals. But closing down an emergency service is very hard to justify to local people. The Trust could not argue that emergency care wasn't needed on a particular site, only that there were good organizational or financial grounds for putting it on a different one.

> Although it was a public body the Trust Board decided to implement a plan that went against what local people wanted, what people working in the hospital wanted, and what local politicians wanted, because the Board thought that the plan was right in the long term for the community as a whole. It made them think very hard about whether they were right.

> The public meetings were dreadful. People shrieked and yelled and threw things and shouted that people would die in ambulances on the way to the hospital. All Dr. Gulvin could say was 'Well, no I don't think so, that's just not true'. Some of the doctors were personally vilified. There were accusations that the managers were hiding behind the doctors, which they were. The doctors were the only ones who could talk about safety and staffing and why those were important, and have credibility with the public. It had to be the doctors leading the argument.

> The Trust Board was conscious that they were closing services that people valued in the interests of some greater good. They felt they were making a moral compact with people, asking them to give up services that were of benefit to them in order to achieve better services for the benefit of the city as a whole. It brought out the Trust's responsibility to be clear about what the advantages and disadvantages would be, what the Trust's real intentions were, and what principles they were operating under.
> (Derived from interview with Dr. Gulvin, Stoneyhill and District Hospital NHS Trust)

The normative, empirical and predictive difficulties that Dr. Gulvin and his colleagues had faced when they set about restructuring their hospitals had been reasonably readily resolved, because the options were limited and certain conclusions seemed inescapable. Faced with limited realistic options, the Trust Board drew upon broadly utilitarian principles and calculations to justify the closure of local emergency departments, satisfying itself that its plan would secure the ethical outcome of better care for most of the community.

The Board members were conscious, nevertheless, that they were setting aside the interests of a smaller group in pursuit of advantage to a larger one. This brought to the fore the Trust's accountability – literally, the obligation to render an account – to its community. As well as having responsibility for justly allocating whatever resources were available, the Trust had a responsibility to present itself honestly and openly, to welcome scrutiny, to accept negative reaction, and to hold itself to the principles it promoted.

Analysed from the perspective of normative expectations and reactive attitudes, Dr. Gulvin's is a narrative of patient communities expressing their 'presumption that is also an insistence' that managers and medical leaders live up to certain standards. In the context of the NHS at least, patients' core normative expectation is that resources will be distributed fairly so as to give every individual a reasonable chance of accessing care when they need it. Those for whom existing local services had represented a fair share understandably felt that their normative expectation of fair treatment had been rebuffed. Their reactive attitude was expressed in the angry accusations that Dr. Gulvin attempted to answer.

Expressing this reactive attitude of anger and outrage was a form of 'moral address' [27] through which those attending the public meetings sought to call the organization to account. But Dr. Gulvin's narrative hints at the problem we face when organizational decisions run counter to our normative expectations. To whom should we direct the moral address, and who exactly are we to hold to account? Moral address implies a listener, and a response. Who counts for the purpose of hearing the address? And who has any moral standing to respond to it?

It is telling that in this narrative managers were charged with hiding behind doctors. The normative expectation of health service managers is the normative expectation that we associate with faceless and impersonal bureaucracy: if bureaucracy has a justification it is that bureaucrats manage the organization efficiently, effectively and fairly in the public interest without favouring or disfavouring any particular group. If it is unfair that services are to be closed, it is managers who have failed to meet expectations, and managers to whom morally excoriating address should be directed. Remaining faceless in this example, their absence demonstrated that an impersonal organization was incapable of hearing the moral address.

It is equally telling that the doctors who responded to the address were singled out for vilification. The normative expectation of doctors is that they shall apply their skill and loyalty first and foremost to those patients who most need it. It is precisely that normative expectation, and the trust and hope that accompany it, which gives doctors a mantle of special authority to speak on behalf of healthcare organizations. Surely, the logic goes, these trusted professionals would not agree to something that was not in the interests of patients. But in this example, if doctors were 'conniving' in closing services of value to a few patients in the interests of other patients, had they not betrayed the very expectations that gave them a legitimate position from which to speak? The organizations' demands upon these doctors as managers compromised the moral standing they had as clinicians, and undermined the authority of the response they offered to moral address. There is clearly an awkward paradox at work here. Patients and the public do repose greater trust in doctors than in managers; and greater patient and public trust might be thought likely to bolster medical managers' moral authority to justify hard decisions. But any perception of a 'betrayal' by those most trusted to make decisions on behalf of patients meets with concomitantly deeper sense of outrage.

That Gulvin and his colleagues should have encountered such strength of feeling is a consequence both of the impersonal nature of organizations and of the contradictory aspects of clinical and managerial responsibilities that we noted in Chapter 1. Impersonal bureaucracy may promote fairness, because where goods are allocated impersonally no one will be favoured; but impersonality also thwarts the psychological and social satisfactions afforded by effective moral address. Similarly, good care for individuals rests on good clinical leadership of organizations, which in turn entails forfeiting the interests of some to the interests of the greater number; but patients' first expectation of doctors is that doctors will give priority to treating their own urgent needs. These themes will re-emerge in Chapter 4 when we explore the nature of bureaucratic and medical moralities, and in Chapter 5 when we consider responses to medical harm.

Example 3: normative expectations surrounding clinical innovation

Dr. Nathan Nugen was a member of the first generation of medical directors appointed to lead NHS hospitals. He subsequently experienced the medical director role in more than one organization, and at the time he was interviewed he held advisory roles with several national bodies. One of the issues that had troubled him early in his career, and that he decided to address when he was first appointed as a medical director, was managing clinical innovation.

The object of Nugen's interest was innovation, more particularly surgical innovation that did not amount to clinical research; but which by virtue of being novel carried with it unclear risks and benefits. Nugen's concerns about innovation were both to do with 'innovation through invention' where new procedures might be developed (face transplant, not an issue that concerned Nugen at the time, supplies a clear example of this type of innovation); and also with 'innovation through adoption' where procedures developed elsewhere are introduced locally (as would be the case if face transplants techniques were to be adopted by more surgical teams) [28,29].[6]

Dr. Nugen started by recounting his experience of the impact of surgical innovation on patients and the organization, and went on to describe the policy changes he implemented later in his career.

> In one leading hospital where Dr. Nugen spent time during training, there had been two
> programmes developing new surgical procedures that used a lot of clinical resources. The needs of
> one programme had displaced 'routine' patients from the ITU. Another programme used a lot
> of donated blood. On one occasion when there was no blood left in the blood bank because the
> innovative surgery had used it all, a dozen patients had their operation cancelled; this was for
> the sake of one person who would die anyway, because the early success rate on the programme

---

[6] The ethics of face transplantation are reviewed in references 28 and 29.

was so poor. Some of the doctors who observed the effects of those programmes at the time thought the trade-offs were unacceptable, and that the programmes were unethical. In fact, the second procedure now saves countless lives, and it doesn't cost much in terms of blood and other resources. It could be argued that early failures benefited future populations but, at the time, the procedure was very expensive and very high-risk for the patient.

Later in his career, Dr. Nugen was one of the first medical directors to introduce a Trust policy on innovative procedures. He did so partly in response to the Bristol Inquiry, which identified the harm to patients that could result from poorly managed innovation.[7] The ethical issues that the policy addressed were whether the costs of innovation could be justified, whether innovation would adversely affect other clinical activity, and how harm to patients would be avoided. Some consultants objected to the policy being introduced, but Dr. Nugen justified it on grounds that it was not about stopping innovation but about helping doctors to innovate in a way that reduced risk to patients. The policy engaged all staff groups, because it expected everyone to blow the whistle if they saw new procedures being introduced without permission. The major benefit of the policy was that it made people stop and think about what they want to do, so they would introduce new procedures in a controlled and properly managed way.

(Derived from interview with Dr. Nugen, Former Medical Director of two major NHS Trusts)

Dr. Nugen's narrative is of interest, for itself, as an example of moral entrepreneurship. It is also of interest for the way that, situated in context, it helps us to unpick the association between norms and normative expectations.

Nugen initiated this project because he believed that the norms, and the associated normative expectations, governing surgical innovation in NHS hospitals were misguided. All innovation in medicine – surgical, medical, pharmaceutical or indeed organizational – invites a basic moral question: given that we cannot yet be reasonably sure that doing X will work, or what its side effects may be, do we have adequate justification for proceeding into the unknown? The spectrum of innovation in medicine is vast. If we set aside non-therapeutic research, the spectrum extends from Phase 2 clinical trials, when a new drug compound is used in patients for the very first time; through Phase 3 and 4 clinical trials where the true benefits and risks of new compounds are realized; through the introduction of revolutionary new tools, techniques and devices, such as those underpinning laparo-scopic surgery; to the introduction of new procedures such as laparoscopic cholecystect-omy, and smaller scale innovation such as 'off-label' use of approved medical devices or drugs; through to day-to-day modifications to standard procedures prompted by clinical emergencies such as those encountered on the battlefield; and finally to the adoption of procedures new to a particular team or practitioner but already fully tested elsewhere. The question is how to ensure that innovation at any point on this spectrum results in maximum benefit and minimum harm to patients.

At one end of the spectrum, innovation that falls into the category of clinical research into new drugs and devices has been the object of increasingly robust research regulation and research ethical oversight since the introduction the Nuremberg Code in 1947 and the Declaration of Helsinki in 1964. (Egregious violations continue to be discovered notwithstanding [30].)[8] Around the middle of the spectrum, new procedures that do not

---

[7] The heart surgeons concerned adopted a new approach to repairing heart defects in newborns. The procedure enjoyed reasonable success elsewhere, but the mortality rate at Bristol was high and the surgeons refused to review their practice.

[8] For a brief history of research scandals and a review of research governance in the UK see reference 30.

rely upon new drugs or devices fall outwith the requirements for research ethical review. Here, some combination of professional and organizational responsibility must govern the decision to proceed [31].[9] At the other end of the spectrum small-scale innovation in the guise of improvization is inseparable from surgical practice, and is therefore a candidate for individual professional responsibility.

But where exactly in the spectrum does professional judgement alone suffice to protect patient interests; where should additional oversight be required; and whose responsibility should additional oversight be [31–40]?[10] To put it simply, Nugen believed that oversight should apply to more activity than it did, and that oversight was an organizational responsibility that devolved to all of his staff.

The norm that prevailed at the time that Nugen introduced his policy was that unless it amounted to research, and was thus subject to regulation, surgical innovation was purely a matter of clinical professional responsibility. It was this norm, and the reasoning that underpinned it, that Nugen challenged. He perceived two major issues. One was whether individual professionals were able to make a dispassionate judgement of the balance of risk and benefit to individual patients to whom they offered innovative therapies. The other was the impact of surgical innovation on the organization and on other patients. The ethical justification for trying out hitherto untried procedures frequently turns on potential benefit to the patient offered 'one last throw of the dice' [29]. But when other patients' needs and interests are brought into the picture a 'last throw of the dice' is insufficient justification for organizations to commit resources to innovation. A resource-intensive, high-risk intervention with low probability of individual success comes to be a good use of resources only if there can be a well-founded faith in its future efficacy.

When Nugen introduced his policy, he set out to create a new normative order for surgical innovation. This required the development of new ethical norms, a fresh moral understanding of the risks and benefits of innovation. His policy also entailed new management expectations, most notably that staff would report violations of the new policy. But were these normative expectations in the sense discussed earlier in the chapter? Not, I think, without more. Normative expectations are far more deeply embedded in our moral habits and moral relationships than either norms or expectations alone.

---

[9] Barkun et al. note that 'the introduction of innovative operative procedures is not integrated in any regulatory framework, unless the innovators choose to introduce the procedure in the form of a research study. If they choose not to do so, they are still able to publish the results of their experiment as non-comparative trials (usually series of cases) without special institutional review board requirement, such as that for a randomised clinical trial. For example, surgeons can do highly innovative and untested procedures if these are aimed to improve the health of individual patients. This is the way in which laparoscopic cholecystectomy was introduced.' See reference 31 and also other articles in the same issue, see footnote below.

[10] A landmark series of articles discussing ethics and regulation in surgical innovation appeared in *The Lancet* as recently as 2009 (vol. 374, issue 9695). See references 31–38. The surgical community has lacked a definitive framework for understanding and thus regulating innovation; one proposal has been for a three-level taxonomy of innovation in surgical care, ranging from simple tool modification (e.g. Kocher clamp), to revolutionizing equipment (e.g. Fogarty catheter or video-laparoscopy), to revolutionizing science (e.g. aseptic principles or gene-chip microarrays) (see references 39 and 40).

Walker notes that a 'normative expectation anticipates compliance more or less (and sometimes scarcely at all), but always embodies a demand for that form of behavior [sic] we think we've a right to' [1(p24)]. At the outset the moral behaviour that Nugen anticipated and could demand was not acceptance of the norm, but, rather, acceptance of the managerial and moral authority by which he promulgated the norm. Moreover, staff who complied with his new policy or reported violations would not necessarily be doing so out of a sense of moral obligation or moral affront (some might have); all that he asked was that they do it.

Nugen's conviction that surgical innovation should be scrutinized at organizational level is now widely shared. It has become an organizational norm, although it may not yet be a universal normative expectation among professional groups. Following the Bristol Inquiry in 2001, a complex mesh of protocols and standards has grown up around innovation in the NHS. National guidelines govern Trust-level approval of interventional procedures, a national framework provides for audit of clinical risk management by individual organizations, and innovation has been brought under local managerial control in the form of policies akin to Dr. Nugen's. Activity in the UK has been paralleled by growing concern and further developments in the US and elsewhere [41,42].[11]

The story of the Tuskegee study of untreated syphilis, a study that was once believed to be scientifically worthwhile and morally supportable, now provokes moral outrage.[12] Some commentators have claimed that the Tuskegee research has been misunderstood and misrepresented [43–51].[13] Whether or not that is true, reactions to what is commonly thought to have been done in Tuskegee suggest that moral norms for human research dating back to the Nuremberg trials have now become widely held normative expectations. As moral understandings of the nature of clinical innovation shift, we should expect the specific normative expectations that accompany these moral understandings to be changing too.

---

[11] In the UK relevant standards are contained in the Clinical Negligence Scheme for Trusts; the NICE Interventional Procedures Programme and the associated Health Services Circular 2003/011; NICE technology appraisals; NICE clinical guidelines; National Service Frameworks; and Royal College standards.

[12] The story of the Tuskegee study is a complex one. One way of telling it is as follows. In 1932 the US Public Health Service and the Tuskegee Institute recruited 600 black men, 399 with syphilis, 201 without, for a prospective study of untreated syphilis. At the time of study there was no safe treatment for syphilis, and African Americans had almost no access to medical care. For many men in the trial, examination by the Public Health Service was the first health examination they had ever received. Along with free health examinations, participants received food and transport to a health centre. When subjects died, their families received burial stipends in exchange for permission to perform autopsies. The subjects were not told they had syphilis and received either no treatment or deliberately inefficacious treatment. During WWII, about fifty men in the study were found to have syphilis following screening by army draft boards, and would ordinarily have been expected to undergo treatment. The Public Health Service requested that draft boards exempt the study's subjects from the military's requirement that soldiers be treated. When penicillin became available in 1943, the Public Health Service withheld it from study subjects.

[13] Cave and Holm (see reference 43) argue that the nuances of the research design in these two landmark studies have become lost in bioethical debate so that 'what is discussed is thus often constructions of these studies that are closer to hypothetical examples than to the real studies'. See generally references 44–51.

Example 4: normative expectations surrounding requests for 'exceptional' medical treatment

Dr. William Woodhouse trained as a GP, became intrigued by medical management, and chose to follow his passion by developing a career giving him a strategic role in primary care. When we met, he was the medical director of Meadborough Primary Care Trust. The PCT serves an area where entrenched urban deprivation rubs right up against obvious urban affluence. Meadborough hosts prominent teaching hospitals developing cutting-edge interventions, it has centres of excellence in primary care, and its population includes a fair proportion of well-educated and savvy health consumers. In its less favoured areas, however, Meadborough grapples with faltering general practices and the health problems that accompany inequality, poor education and poverty. The needs of the NHS in Meadborough are enormously varied, and expectations of what the NHS should deliver are high. So there is no simple answer to the question of local healthcare priorities.

As commissioning bodies, PCTs were responsible for planning the supply of medical services in response to local need [52].[14] While the vast majority of services were part of a standard menu of NHS provision, a few services were discretionary and decided on a case-by-case basis. These were for the most part new and costly drugs yet to be approved for use in the NHS by the National Institute for Health and Clinical Excellence;[15] costly drugs that were approved but had marginal benefits; cosmetic procedures that could in some cases be clinically indicated; and procedures that were both costly and controversial, such as in-vitro fertilization (IVF) paired with pre-natal genetic diagnosis (PGD) for avoiding pregnancies where there was a high risk of genetic disease. Dr. Woodhouse was a member of the PCT committee that considered requests for these discretionary treatments [53–57].[16] Each month this committee scrutinized some forty applications for special treatment, and it was these applications that not infrequently elicited a 'reactive attitude' from Dr. Woodhouse.

> Sometimes Dr. Woodhouse just feels cross about applications to the committee. About a third of their special requests each month are for breast enlargement or reduction. He thinks it is absurd that these things are left to be settled at local level, rather than central government being straightforward that the NHS is not there to provide cosmetic breast surgery for anyone who wants it. He is cross that the NHS and the government are not prepared to be candid that fixed resources have to be apportioned, and he is cross that local doctors refer their patients' requests to the committee even though the guidelines are clear that the PCT will not accede to these requests.

---

[14] Commissioning is hard to define. Broadly speaking it is the process by which the supply of publicly funded healthcare (by hospitals and general practices) is shaped by public bodies (PCTs) charged with identifying and funding reasonable patient demands. In the absence of a consumer-driven marketplace for healthcare services, it represents an attempt to rationally plan the type and quantity of medical services available to the population. One fairly authoritative definition is 'the process of specifying, securing and monitoring services to meet individuals' needs at a strategic level'. See reference 52.

[15] NICE's role was not to license drugs or medical devices but to approve and advise on the use of drugs and devices in the NHS, once these had been licensed for use in the UK. Their assessment framework therefore included not just clinical effectiveness but also cost.

[16] As they were making decisions on behalf of a public body such committees were required to comply with proper procedures and their decisions were subject to legal review. See references 53, 55 and 56 for example cases and 60 and 63 for analysis.

In other cases he feels disturbed: sometimes anxious about whether the best care is being offered, sometimes uneasy about the way medicine is going, sometimes troubled by patient expectations that confront his own beliefs.

One set of disturbing decisions relates to 'last chance' therapies, for example for cancer, when the drugs are in the early stages of development or have not yet been assessed by NICE. Often it is apparent that any benefit will be of limited duration and the patient's quality of life will be very poor. He feels that the committee is not in the best position to assess the pros and cons of such therapy; and that an issue not being addressed by doctors who submit the request for special treatment is whether good palliative care could offer more to the patient than a toxic new drug.

Other decisions are deeply uncomfortable because they seem to challenge some fundamental moral norms. It is not unusual for the committee to be asked to approve in-vitro fertilization and pre-implantation genetic diagnosis. Most often, these are cases where the disease would condemn the child to a very short life span or being deeply damaged. But they have had other requests, which are discomfiting because they pose the question where the line should be drawn around 'unacceptable' suffering. Should the NHS routinely offer IVF with PGD to screen for sickle cell disease, an illness that many people lived with?

And one of the cases the committee considered concerned a single mother who had two children severely disabled by a genetic condition. The children were not expected to survive into their teens, and were looked after at home through provision of extensive health and social care. The woman requested IVF using donated sperm followed by PGD so that she could now bear a child of her own, free from genetic disorder, before she was too old to reproduce. It raised a lot of questions for the committee, which took advice from the director of children's services about the wellbeing of the current children and the impact on them. The committee agreed the request in the end but not without misgivings.

(Derived from interview with Dr. Woodhouse, Meadborough Primary Care Trust)

Dr. Woodhouse's account of his committee work helps us to differentiate between the reactive attitude that arises when normative expectations are disrupted, the discomfort that arises from normative equivocality, and the disquiet that arises from normative dissonance.

Woodhouse's resentment of frivolous requests for cosmetic surgery was a reactive attitude. Its source lay for the most part in his normative expectations of healthcare leaders and local GPs, people who are aware of the pressures in a cash-limited, publicly funded healthcare system and should have taken steps to communicate this to patients. Resentment is one of the reactive attitudes that Strawson identified in his first discussion of the phenomenon, associating it with a degree of malice.[17] But Walker has argued that resentment is not only a response to malice: it is also a reaction to those times when when '[s]omeone has made free with what we thought were the rules' [1(p125)]. Woodhouse's resentment was directed towards the leaders, managers and politicians who had, in his view, abdicated responsibility for explaining the constraints of rationing to NHS consumers, and refused to be accountable themselves for the reasonable limits placed on the scope of NHS treatment.

Woodhouse's response to requests for 'last chance' therapies is more complex, reflecting his ambiguous position as the leading doctor within a commissioning body and the normative ambiguity in the decision itself. As a doctor, Woodhouse's first responsibility is to protect and promote the well-being of individual patients. We shall see in forthcoming chapters how medical directors frequently feel most at ease in the leadership role when they

---

[17] See the extract quoted above.

are fulfilling that responsibility, acting as advocates for and protectors of patients. But as a commissioner, Woodhouse's primary responsibility is to help commission the care that will best protect and promote the health of populations within the available budget. How are these two responsibilities to be reconciled? There is no conflict in cases where a last chance therapy offers a reasonable prospect of additional time and acceptable quality of life, because here the patient genuinely benefits; or in cases where therapy would clearly be futile, because here other expenditures ought obviously to take priority. But very few of the requests to Woodhouse's committee were of that nature. They were much more ambiguous.

Assessing more complex and indefinite treatment claims required the tipping point between benefits and burdens to be found, one of many difficulties that observers of medicine have subsumed under the rubric of uncertainty [58–69].[18] When therapies buy time at end of life at the cost of toxic side effects, it is difficult to identify the hour at which the gain in quantity of life outweighs the burdens of the therapy. This task becomes all the more difficult when dying patients' subjective assessments of treatment benefits and burdens are included in the calculation, because patients facing the end of life are inclined to place a different value on days, weeks or months of life, from those who are not [70–80]. If a patient overall believes that extra time would be of value to them, even if only a day, there is no compelling moral equation for settling how much that extra life time is worth to them or their families [81–89].[19]

Where does this leave a local doctor leader, who can see a patient's case for wanting more life time but has a fixed budget to spend? It leaves them with the job of judging a patient's request on grounds that are neither purely clinical, nor truly pragmatic (funds may be limited, but rarely will funds be entirely depleted) nor entirely morally compelling. In commenting on the palliative care dimension missing from such requests, Woodhouse was perhaps turning his attention to the domain in which he felt more comfortable and willing to make a judgement; a 'reactivation' of his clinical assessment of the situation.

Normative equivocality also hangs over the requests for IVF and PGD. Both of the IVF/ PGD requests that Woodhouse described raise the question of what reproductive desires a publicly funded health service should fulfil. The answer depends on both how assisted reproduction and how any right to healthcare are each conceptualized. For example if, as Daniels argues, citizens should have access to health services that restore species-typical normal functioning, does assisted reproduction qualify [90–95]? Some would insist that fertility services are a *sine qua non*; others would respond that a degree of infertility is a part of the human condition. Additionally, commissioners face the same difficulty with assisted reproduction as they do with every other form of treatment, that of allocating a limited healthcare budget between people with incommensurable modes of suffering [96–106].[20] Depending upon how these questions are settled, a second set of ambiguities then arise. As the law stands, clinics providing infertility treatment have a duty to take into account the interests of the child born of a result of treatment, as well as the interests of other existing

---

[18] Following Fox and Atkinson (references 58 and 59). See references 60–69 for further analysis of uncertainty.
[19] QALYS, the most widely known, is heavily contested. See references 81–89.
[20] See, for example, references 96–106.

children [107–112].[21] There are thus empirical uncertainties, such as the mother's existing capacity to care for her current children; and predictive uncertainties, such as her ability to care for her existing two children along with a third.

Finally, Woodhouse, who is a practising Christian as well as a committed medical leader, was obliged to manage a degree of normative dissonance in his work. As a committee member he felt he must defer to the legitimate but different norms and expectations of those making an application. Assisting a single parent to conceive a child through IVF, and then to discard unwanted embryos, did not sit easily with his own moral beliefs. Whatever his personal doubts about how, as a Christian, he should think, Dr. Woodhouse had to set these aside in his role as an impartial arbiter of the request.

When he deferred his own moral beliefs to those of the patients requesting treatment, Woodhouse did so not because other moral beliefs took priority, but because patients' and colleagues' normative expectations did. The normative expectation that counted was the expectation that public functionaries set aside their own beliefs in the interests of fair public administration. In doing this, Woodhouse exhibited the self-discipline and moral neutrality of the good bureaucrat. This is a mode of conduct we consider again in our next example, and that we explore further in Chapter 4.

Example 5: normative expectations surrounding doctors' moral neutrality

The purpose of this chapter has been to understand the nature of normative expectations, and to observe how they differ from and interact with other elements in our moral life. We have seen that Dr. Woodhouse became aware of a conflict between his personal moral beliefs and the moral orientation of others; to deal with that conflict, he complied with the normative expectation that bureaucrats be morally neutral in their public work. Dr Iliffe, whom we will meet below, did broadly the same. In this final section, I consider the place of personal moral beliefs alongside role requirements and ask whether what we are asking of medical leaders is to be moral hypocrites.

Dr. Iliffe works at Graveldene NHS Trust, a well-run, well-supported district general hospital serving a large town and its surrounding area. The town of Graveldene, and the villages it has gradually absorbed, is a surprisingly settled community. It is the sort of place where it is not unusual for people to stay their entire life, or to return and bring up their children in proximity to their extended families. Dr. Iliffe is open about her faith and actively involved in her local church. Though she does not evangelize at work, Graveldene being the sort of town it is Dr. Iliffe assumes that a fair proportion of her consultant colleagues are aware of her Christian beliefs.

Dr. Iliffe has conscientiously objected to any involvement in abortion in the past. She did participate, however, in appointing a consultant to continue running the abortion service in

---

[21] *Human Fertilisation & Embryology Act* 2008 s.14(2)(b), which updated the 1990 Act s. 13(5): an applicant 'shall not be provided with treatment services unless account has been taken of the welfare of any child who may be born as a result of the treatment (including the need of that child for supportive parenting) and of any other child who may be affected by the birth'. The interpretation of the welfare clause and access to assisted conception services have been subject to legal challenge in the cases identified in references 107[3]–112.

her hospital. She could have asked someone to deputize for her on the appointment committee. But the real issue, given that there was a potential break in the provision of the service, was whether it would have been appropriate for her to argue that the hospital should stop providing abortion altogether. Her stance has always been that she will not support abortion, and she would prefer that it was not necessary. But she reasoned that the area relies on having an abortion service, and that people will seek it out elsewhere if they don't provide it. So it seems to her more equitable and just to offer abortion services locally, with local follow-up.

However distasteful it is to medical professionals, the law permits abortion. Part of what you sign up to when you take on the responsibility of being a doctor is accepting that patients' interests come first. If you cannot accept that, then you are free to choose not to become a doctor. She does feel that she is subjugating her personal values for the sake of the hospital and the 'bigger picture'. But she thinks that on balance that is right, and she will continue to argue about issues like euthanasia where there is still disagreement and the law remains unchanged.

(Derived from interview with Dr. Ingrid Iliffe, Graveldene NHS Trust)

Dr. Woodhouse and Dr. Iliffe both experienced a conflict between their faith commitments and the normative expectations of them as medical leaders. Each attempted to reconcile the conflict by developing a narrative that made clear their commitment to patient claims, but neither leader was entirely satisfied with this solution. They found themselves facing the paradox described by political philosopher Michael Harmon, a 'spiritual predicament [that pits] the impulse toward self-creation against the demands for answerability emanating from a world not entirely of our own making' [113]. Public servants experience this paradox particularly acutely, caught as they are between their own individual beliefs and values, the objective impersonality demanded of those who work in a public institution, and the incompatible beliefs and values of those they serve in a pluralist democracy [114–116].[22]

All healthcare staff are bound by ethical and legal rules that prohibit unfair discrimination against patients. Where the issue is not one of discrimination, however, doctors are permitted to act in accordance with their own beliefs if they ensure that patients receive appropriate medical services from others [117–127]. This is not quite as rigorous as the normative expectation that public servants set aside their own moral beliefs when making decisions on behalf of patients and the public. This more rigorous standard is, however, the normative expectation we hold of those in medical leadership roles. Notably, the normative expectation that medical leaders evacuate their own moral beliefs from key decisions is matched by

---

[22] Out of many possible examples of the clash of legally protected equality interests, the case of Mr T Apelogun-Gabriels v London Borough of Lambeth (2301976/05 (5016/62) Feb 2006 is instructive. Mr Apelogun-Gabriels is an evangelical Christian who repeatedly distributed biblical extracts denouncing homosexuality to his colleagues. A number of formal complaints were made. He was dismissed on grounds of gross misconduct and harassment for breaching his employer's equal opportunities policies. He claimed he was subject to direct discrimination on grounds of religion or belief. An employment tribunal rejected that claim, finding that although the source of the material was religious the texts were hostile and offensive to homosexuals. His claim of indirect discrimination was rejected because the employer provided prayer facilities. His claim of unfair dismissal was rejected on the basis employers have a positive duty to take steps to prevent harassment. See references 114–116.

an equally strong normative expectation that medical leaders act in ways that are morally supportable.

What are we to make of Dr. Iliffe's choice to act in a way inconsistent with her Christianity? Dr. Iliffe's decision as a public servant was to defer to the normative expectations of others, an action that she undertook at some personal cost. What is of interest at this stage in my argument is how we characterize the nature of the moral position that she assumed. Was Iliffe morally compromised in doing as she did; or was her action a praiseworthy expression of bureaucratic responsibility? Would others who shared her Christian beliefs be entitled to feel let down – vexed that their normative expectations were disappointed – by her actions?

The charge that might be levelled at Dr. Iliffe, and other 'good bureaucrats', is that of hypocrisy: 'a contrast between a person's activities (in a suitably broad sense of the term) and other aspects of the same person's behavior [sic] and attitudes' [128]. Political philosopher Judith Shklar was among the first to point out that hypocrisy is a vital component in human social affairs, enabling each of us to pursue our own idiosyncratic vision of personal good in complex, radically plural societies [129][136]. So although a charge of hypocrisy is a familiar moral criticism, it is fair to ask whether there is actually anything wrong with medical leaders being hypocritical, holding private beliefs at odds with their public actions or pronouncements. The question I consider below is whether there is anything morally wrong with hypocrisy; it could well be a grave practical mistake if follower disapproval of hypocrisy were to undermine the moral standing of their leader.

Dr. Iliffe found her situation troubling because she perceived a stark contradiction between what she privately believed and the activity that she publicly supported. If we shared her moral disapproval of abortion, we could criticize her for helping to provide it. But as she had reasons for doing as she did, the secondary question is what we make of a medical leader who thinks one thing and does another. Her moral failing, if indeed it was one, would seem to lie in being either inconsistent or inauthentic.

Do inconsistency or inauthenticity matter, morally? According to the moral philosopher R Jay Wallace, consistency in the sense of coherence between one's beliefs and behaviours is 'a trivial virtue, a matter of intellectual bookkeeping or mental hygiene rather than something with independent moral weight' [11(p308)]. Seeking a more robust reason to condemn hypocrisy, he moves on to consider whether inauthenticity provides one.

Hypocrisy evidences a gap between private attitudes and public action. So, assuming 'that one's private attitudes constitute one's "real self"', this dissimulation of private attitudes can be understood as a form of social alienation, a failure to realize or express one's real self in the public social world' [11(p308)]. But Wallace again questions whether it matters morally that our 'true self' fails to find expression in decisions and behaviours. He emphasizes that the moral world is relational and that what really matters morally is what happens in interpersonal relations. Personal authenticity, a sense of being at home with the self, is, arguably, irrelevant to this dimension.

It might be suggested that inauthenticity entails a degree of deception: we withhold our 'real selves' and 'real motivations' from those with whom we interact. While this might be a reasonable moral objection to hypocrisy in some cases, it is clearly not in the case of Dr. Iliffe. She made no effort to conceal her own faith commitment.

Wallace's own view is that some forms of hypocrisy are morally significant, but not because they involve inconsistency, inauthenticity or deception alone.[23] As Wallace's analysis of hypocrisy suggests Iliffe and Woodhouse did little that was morally wrong, how are we to explain the abiding sense of moral trouble that had remained with both medical directors for some time? We can usefully turn here to those accounts of moral life that give prominence to personal narrative as a means of moral orientation or sense-making.

Many moral philosophers, including Margaret Walker, have incorporated a notion of narrative personal identity into their framework of moral understanding. The first and most influential, however, was Alasdair MacIntyre, who treated personal narrative as central to his contemporary theory of virtue. MacIntyre defined virtue as 'an acquired human quality the possession and exercise of which tends to enable us to achieve those goods which are internal to practices' [9(p191)]. The goods that are 'internal' to the practice of medicine are outcomes such as improved health, alleviation of pain or the subjective experience of compassionate care. So the medical virtues are 'acquired human qualities' that allow such goods to be realized: in bioethicist Pellegrino's terms, virtues such as fidelity to trust and promise, benevolence, effacement of self-interest, compassion and caring and intellectual honesty [130].

MacIntyre observed that we are all involved in many 'practices', often simultaneously – the practices of religious faith and medicine for example – so that the problem of multiple practices, and therefore potentially conflicting goods, is omnipresent. The need to choose between conflicting goods is central to MacIntyre's account of the virtues in daily life. He suggests that a certain 'subversive arbitrariness' [9(p203)] threatens to undermine the project of living virtuously, when we find ourselves pulled this way and that by the demands of different practices and goods. Where they appear incompatible, as they do in Dr. Woodhouse and Dr. Iliffe's examples, how should a virtuous agent decide which practice and what good to prioritize? MacIntyre's answer is that the agent should decide by reference to the narrative unity of his own life.

This narrative unity of an individual life is constructed over time, and is built upon foundations of community membership and local 'traditions'.[24]

> [T]he individual's search for his or her good is generally and characteristically conducted within a context defined by those traditions of which the individual's life is a part, and this is true both of those goods which are internal to practices and of the goods of a single life .... What is better or worse for [the agent] depends upon the character of that intelligible narrative which provides [the agent's] life with its unity. [9(p222,225)]

---

[23] His reasoning takes us too far from the current discussion, but his conclusion is that hypocrisy is morally objectionable when it issues forth in the form of censuring others for doing what one does oneself. His view echoes the adage that 'people in glass houses shouldn't throw stones'. Hypocrisy disgusts us when people suffer public moral condemnation for doing something that the speaker does in private. Iliffe may have been justified in deferring her own values to patients' normative expectations; she is only a morally blameworthy hypocrite if she condemns others for doing the same thing. As Iliffe's choice was to place patient and organizational interests ahead of her own personal beliefs, it is hard to imagine her censuring others for doing the same thing.

[24] His concept of a tradition describes a cultural location: e.g. a hospital may have its own tradition.

For MacIntyre, this narrative unity is what supplies the end, or *telos*, that allows us to decide between one good and another. When that is the choice we face,

> by choosing one I do nothing to diminish or derogate from the claim upon me of the other; and therefore, whatever I do, I shall have left undone what I ought to have done. [9(p224)]

Following MacIntyre's account we might, then, understand our doctors' decisions as choices based in the deeply felt, long-held narrative of their lives. These narratives demanded and contained a proper – that is, a virtuous – trace of sorrow for the decisions of the past, choices that left a residue of regret for the path not followed.

Conclusion

In this chapter I have discussed the way that normative expectations, along with the reactive attitudes and insistent presumptions that accompany them, have contributed to instances of moral leadership. Alongside normative expectations and reactive attitudes, we have observed the presence of moral norms, beliefs, values and perspectives that do not amount to normative expectations as such. All of those different ingredients of moral thought nevertheless coloured moral reasoning and moral action.

We noted the possibility that norms, normative expectations, reactive attitudes, beliefs, values and perspectives could be experienced in a narrative form; in the case we considered, it was a narrative of a single life. In forthcoming chapters, we will explore other ways of understanding moral narrative, seeing how moral narratives extend beyond the individual and her concerns to become the guiding force of organizational action.

Normative expectations play a significant role in shaping mutual understanding and mutual negotiation of our responsibilities. Normative expectations and reactive attitudes help to elicit the moral awareness, the will, the determination and the resilience necessary to live up to what we all – healthcare professionals, patients, managers and carers – demand of each other. We now move on to explore exactly what moral leaders do when 'living up to demands' is what has to be done.

Further reading

Walker MU. *Moral Repair: Reconstructing Moral Relations after Wrongdoing.* Cambridge: Cambridge University Press; 2006.

Strawson PF. Freedom and resentment. In: Strawson PF, ed. *Studies in the Philosophy of Thought and Action.* New York: Oxford University Press; 1968.

Lynn J, Baily MA, Bottrell M, Jennings B, Levine RJ, Davidoff F, *et al.* The ethics of using quality improvement methods in health care. *Annals of Internal Medicine.* 2007;**146** (9):666–73.

Jones JH. *Bad Blood: The Tuskegee Syphilis Experiment.* New York: Free Press; 1993.

Daniels N. *Just Health: Meeting Health Needs Fairly.* New York: Cambridge University Press; 2008.

References

1. Walker MU. *Moral Repair: Reconstructing Moral Relations after Wrongdoing.* Cambridge: Cambridge University Press; 2006.

2. O'Neill O. *Autonomy and Trust in Bioethics.* Cambridge: Cambridge University Press; 2002, p. 34ff.

3. Anspach RR. *Deciding Who Lives: Fateful Choices in the Intensive Care Nursery.* Berkeley: University of California Press; 1993.

4. Weitz R. Watching Brian die: the rhetoric and reality of informed consent. *Health.* 1999;3(2):209–27.

5. Bosk C. Irony, ethnography, and informed consent. In: Hoffmaster B, ed. *Bioethics in a Social Context.*

Philadelphia: Temple University Press; 2000, pp. 199–220.

6. Corrigan O. Empty ethics: the problem with informed consent. *Sociology of Health & Illness.* 2003;**25**(7):768–92.

7. Hoeyer K. Informed consent: the making of a ubiquitous rule in medical practice. *Organization.* 2009;**16**(2):267–88.

8. Strawson PF. *Freedom and Resentment. Freedom and Resentment and Other Essays.* London: Methuen; 1974, pp. 1–25.

9. MacIntyre A. *After Virtue.* 3rd edn. London: Duckworth; 2007.

10. Hollis M. *Trust Within Reason.* Cambridge: Cambridge University Press; 1998.

11. Wallace RJ. *Responsibility and the Moral Sentiments.* Harvard: Harvard University Press; 1994.

12. Francis R. The Mid Staffordshire NHS Foundation Trust Inquiry: Department of Health; 2010.

13. PriceWaterhouseCoopers L. Assuring the quality of senior NHS managers: report of the Advisory Group on assuring the quality of senior NHS managers. 2010.

14. A&E Clinical Quality Indicators: Data Definitions. Department of Health; 2010.

15. Elkan R, Robinson J. The use of targets to improve the performance of health care providers: a discussion of government policy. *British Journal of General Practice.* 1998 Aug;**48**(433):1515–8.

16. van Herten LM, Gunning-Schepers LJ. Targets as a tool in health policy: Part I: lessons learned. *Health Policy.* 2000;**53**(1):1–11.

17. Van Herten LM, Gunning-Shepers LJ. Targets as a tool in health policy. Part II: guidelines for application. *Health Policy.* 2000;**53**(1):13–23.

18. Arah OA, Klazinga NS, Delnoij DMJ, Asbroek AHAT, Custers T. Conceptual frameworks for health systems performance: a quest for effectiveness, quality, and improvement. *International Journal For Quality in Health Care.* 2003;**15**(5):377–98.

19. Smith P, Busse R. Learning from the European experience of using targets to improve population health. *Preventing Chronic Disease.* 2010;**7**(5).

20. Smith PC, Mossialos E, Papanicolas I. *Performance measurement for health system improvement: experiences, challenges and prospects.* Tallin: WHO European Conference on Health Systems: Health Systems. Health and Wealth. June 2008.

21. Bevan G, Hood C. Health policy: have targets improved performance in the English NHS? *BMJ.* 2006;**332**:419–22.

22. Gulland A. NHS staff cheat to hit government targets, MPs say. *BMJ.* 2003;**327**:179.

23. Pitches D, Burls A, Fry-Smith A. How to make a silk purse from a sow's ear – a comprehensive review of strategies to optimise data for corrupt managers and incompetent clinicians. *BMJ.* 2003;**327** (7429):1436–9.

24. Yoong KKY, Heymann T. Targets can seriously damage your health…. *BMJ.* 2003;**327**(7416):680.

25. Mason A, Street A. Publishing outcome data: is it an effective approach? *Journal of Evaluation in Clinical Practice.* 2006;**12** (1):37–48.

26. Price L. Treating the clock and not the patient: ambulance response times and risk. *Quality and Safety in Health Care.* 2006;**15** (2):127–30.

27. Watson G. Responsibility and the limits of evil. In: Schoeman F, ed. *Responsibility, Character, and the Emotions: New Essays in Moral Psychology.* Cambridge: Cambridge University Press; 1987.

28. Huxtable RWJ. Gaining face or losing face? Framing the debate on face transplants. *Bioethics.* 2005;**19**:505–22.

29. Freeman M, Jaoudé P. Justifying surgery's last taboo: the ethics of face transplants. *Journal of medical ethics.* 2007;**33**:76–81.

30. Biggs H. *Healthcare Research Ethics and Law: Regulation, Review and Responsibility.* Abingdon: Routledge-Cavendish; 2010, Ch. 2.

31. Barkun JS, Aronson JK, Feldman LS, Maddern GJ, Strasberg SM. Evaluation and stages of surgical innovations. *The Lancet.* 2009;**374**(9695):1089–96.

32. Surgical research: the reality and the IDEAL. *The Lancet.* 2009;**374**(9695):1037.

33. Meakins JL. Surgical research: act 3, answers. *The Lancet.* 2009;**374**(9695):1039–40.

34. Ashrafian H, Rao C, Darzi A, Athanasiou T. Benchmarking in surgical research. *The Lancet.* 2009;**374**(9695):1045–7.

35. Lawrence C. The making of modern surgery. *The Lancet.* 2009;**374**(9695):1055–6.

36. McCullough LB, Jones JW. Unravelling ethical challenges in surgery. *The Lancet.* 2009;**374**(9695):1058–9.

37. Ergina PL, Cook JA, Blazeby JM, Boutron I, Clavien P-A, Reeves BC, *et al.* Challenges in evaluating surgical innovation. *The Lancet.* 2009;**374**(9695):1097–104.

38. McCulloch P, Altman DG, Campbell WB, Flum DR, Glasziou P, Marshall JC, *et al.* No surgical innovation without evaluation: the IDEAL recommendations. *The Lancet.* 2009;**374**(9695):1105–12.

39. Krummel T. What is surgery? *Seminars in Pediatric Surgery.* 2006;**15**:237–41.

40. Riskin DJ, Longaker M, Gertner M, Krummel TM. Innovation in surgery: a historical perspective. *Annals of Surgery.* 2006;**244**:686–93.

41. Reitsma A, Moreno J. Ethical regulations for innovative surgery: the last frontier? *Journal of the American College of Surgeons.* 2002;**194**:792–801.

42. Plumb J, Campbell B, Lyratzopoulos G. How guidance on the use of interventional procedures is produced in different countries: an international survey. *Intenational Journal of Technolog Assessment in Health Care.* 2009;**25**:124–33.

43. Cave E, Holm S. Milgram and Tuskegee – paradigm research projects in bioethics. *Health Care Analysis.* 2003;**11**(1):27–40.

44. Bates BR, Harris TM. The Tuskegee Study of Untreated Syphilis and public perceptions of biomedical research: a focus group study. *Journal of the National Medical Association.* 2004;**96**(8):1051–64.

45. Brandon DT, Isaac LA, LaVeist TA. The legacy of Tuskegee and trust in medical care: is Tuskegee responsible for race differences in mistrust of medical care? *Journal of the National Medical Association.* 2005;**97**(7):951–6.

46. Rockwell DH, Yobs AR, Moore MB, Jr. The Tuskegee Study of Untreated Syphilis; the 30th year of observation. *Archives of Internal Medicine.* 1964;**114**:792–8.

47. White RM. Misinformation and misbeliefs in the Tuskegee Study of Untreated Syphilis fuel mistrust in the healthcare system. *Journal of the National Medical Association.* 2005;**97**(11):1566–73.

48. White RM. Misrepresentations of the Tuskegee Study of Untreated Syphilis. *Journal of the National Medical Association.* 2005**97**(4):564–81.

49. White R. Unraveling the Tuskegee Study of Untreated Syphilis. *Archives of Internal Medicine.* 2000;**160**(5):585–98.

50. White RM, Reverby SM. The Tuskegee Syphilis Study. *The Hastings Center Report.* 2002;**32**(6):4–5.

51. Reverby S. *Examining Tuskegee: the infamous syphilis study and its legacy.* University of North Carolina Press; 2009.

52. Making Ends Meet: *a website for managing money in social services.* Social Services Inspectorate: Audit Commission. [09/02/2011]; Available from: http://www.joint-reviews.gov.uk/money/commissioning/files/CommissioningHardCopy.pdf.

53. R (Ann Marie Rogers) v Swindon Primary Care Trust and the Secretary of State. *EWCA Civ* **392**; 2006.

54. Syrett K. Opening Eyes to the Reality of Scarce Health Care Resources? R (on the application of Rogers) v Swindon NHS Primary Care Trust and Secretary of State for Health. *Public Law.* 2006:664–73.

55. *R on the application of Otley v Barking and Dagenham NHS Primary Care Trust.* EWHC 1927 (Admin); 2007.

56. R (Murphy) v Salford Primary Care Trust. *EWHC* 1908 (Admin); 2008.

57. Jackson E. *Medical Law: Text, Cases and Materials.* 2nd edn. Oxford: Oxford University Press; 2010, pp. 84–86.

58. Fox R. Training for uncertainty. In: Merton RK, Reader G, Kendall PL, eds. *The Student Physician.* Cambridge, MA: Harvard University Press; 1957.

59. Atkinson P. *Medical Talk and Medical Work: The Liturgy of the Clinic.* Thousand Oaks, CA: Sage; 1995, p. 110.

60. Geoffrey HG, Sandra KJ, Jennifer B. Physician expressions of uncertainty during patient encounters. *Patient Education and Counseling.* 2000;**40** (1):59–65.

61. Timmermans S, Angell A. Evidence-based medicine, clinical uncertainty, and learning to doctor. *Journal of Health and Social Behavior.* 2001;**42**(4):342–59.

62. Parascandola M, Hawkins JS, Danis M. Patient autonomy and the challenge of clinical uncertainty. *Kennedy Institute of Ethics Journal.* 2002;**12**(3):245–64.

63. Ogden J, Fuks K, Gardner M, Johnson S, McLean M, Martin P, *et al.* Doctors expressions of uncertainty and patient confidence. *Patient Education and Counseling.* 2002;**48**(2):171–6.

64. Lingard L, Garwood K, Schryer CF, Spafford MM. A certain art of uncertainty: case presentation and the development of professional identity. *Social Science & Medicine.* 2003;**56**(3):603–16.

65. Williams SJ. Parsons revisited: from the sick role to. . .? *Health (London).* 2005;**9** (2):123–44.

66. Pilnick A, Hindmarsh J, Gill VT. Beyond 'doctor and patient': developments in the study of healthcare interactions. *Sociology of Health & Illness.* 2009;**31**(6):787–802.

67. Spafford MM, Schryer CF, Campbell SL, Lingard L. Towards embracing clinical uncertainty. *Journal of Social Work.* 2007;**7** (2):155–78.

68. Fox R. Medical uncertainty revisited. In: Gary L. Albrecht RF, Susan Scrimshaw, eds.

Handbook of Social Studies in Health and Medicine. London: Sage; 2000, pp. 409–25.

69. Ashcroft R. 'Power, corruption and lies': ethics and power. In: Ashcroft R, Lucassen A, Parker M, Verkerk M, Widdershoven G, eds. *Case Analysis in Clinical Ethics.* Cambridge: Cambridge University Press; 2005, pp. 77–94.

70. Richards M. Improving access to medicines for N.H.S patients: a report for the Secretary of State for Health: *Department of Health*; 2008.

71. Chaplin S. How the DoH intends to improve access to medicines. *Prescriber.* 2009;**20**(4):12–6.

72. Raftery J. NICE and the challenge of cancer drugs. *BMJ.* 2009;**338**;b62.

73. Bevan G, Helderman J-K, Wilsford D. Changing choices in health care: implications for equity, efficiency and cost. *Health Economics Policy and Law.* 2010;**5**:251–67.

74. Appleby J, Maybin J. Topping up NHS care. *BMJ.* 2008;**337**:6.

75. Kmietowicz Z. Patients in England are given green light to buy drugs privately alongside NHS care. *BMJ.* 2008;**337**:a2418.

76. O'Dowd A. Top-up fees will lead to two tier NHS, doctors tell MPs. *BMJ.* 2009;**338**: b417.

77. Kmietowicz Z. Think tank calls for withdrawal of guidance allowing top-up payments. *BMJ.* 2009;**338**:b413.

78. Faden RR, Chalkidou K, Appleby J, Waters HR, Leider JP. Expensive cancer drugs: a comparison between the United States and the United Kingdom. *Milbank Quarterly.* 2009;**87**(4):789–819.

79. Weale A, Clark S. Co-payments in the NHS: an analysis of the normative arguments. *Health Economics, Policy and Law.* 2010;**5**:225–46.

80. Jackson E. Top-up payments for expensive cancer drugs: rationing, fairness and the NHS. *The Modern Law Review.* 2010;**73** (3):399–427.

81. Williams A. The value of QALYs. *Health and Social Service.* 1985;**94**.

82. Harris J. QALYfying the value of life. *Journal of Medical Ethics.* 1987;13(3):117–23.

83. Lockwood M. Quality of Life and Resource Allocation. *Royal Institute of Philosophy Supplement.* 1988;23:33–55.

84. Wagstaff A. QALYs and the equity-efficiency trade-off. *Journal of Health Economics.* 1991;10(1):21–41.

85. Broome J. QALYs. *Journal of Public Economics.* 1993;50(2):149–67.

86. Kirkdale R, Krell J, O'Hanlon Brown C, Tuthill M, Waxman J. The cost of a QALY. *QJM.* 2010;103(9);715–20.

87. Tsuchiya A. QALYs and ageism: philosophical theories and age weighting. *Health Economics.* 2000;9(1):57–68.

88. Drummond M, Brixner D, Gold M, Kind P, McGuire A, Nord E, *et al.* Toward a consensus on the QALY. *Value in Health.* 2009;12:S31–S5.

89. Weinstein MC, Torrance G, McGuire A. QALYs: the basics. *Value in Health.* 2009;12:S5–S9.

90. Daniels N. *Just Health Care.* Cambridge: Cambridge University Press; 1985, p. 42ff.

91. Francis LP. Discrimination in Medical Practice: Justice and the Obligations of Health Care Providers to Disadvantaged Patients. *The Blackwell Guide to Medical Ethics.* Oxford: Blackwell; 2008, pp. 162–79.

92. McMillan JR. NICE, the draft fertility guideline and dodging the big question. *Journal of Medical Ethics.*2003;29(6):313–4.

93. Neumann PJ. Should health insurance cover IVF? Issues and options. *Journal of Health Politics Policy and Law.* 1997;22(5):1215–39.

94. Mladovsky P, Sorenson C. Public financing of IVF: a review of policy rationales. *Health Care Analysis.* 2010;18(2):113–28.

95. Bennett R, Harris J. Restoring natural function: access to infertility treatment using donated gametes. *Human Fertility.* 1999;2(1):18–21.

96. Ashcroft R. Fair rationing is essentially local: an argument for postcode prescribing. *Health Care Analysis.* 2006;14(3):135–44.

97. Ashcroft R. Fair process and the redundancy of bioethics: a polemic. *Public Health Ethics.* 2008;1(1):3–9

98. Dawson A. Setting priorities in health care. *Health Care Analysis.* 2006;14(3):133–4.

99. Stanton-Ife J. Resource allocation and the duty to give reasons. *Health Care Analysis.* 2006;14(3):145–56.

100. Devlin N, Parkin D. Funding fertility: issues in the allocation and distribution of resources to assisted reproduction technologies. *Human Fertility.* 2003;6 Suppl 1:S2–6.

101. Peterson MM. Assisted reproductive technologies and equity of access issues. *Journal of Medical Ethics.* 2005;31(5):280–5.

102. Klemetti R, Gissler M, Sevon T, Hemminki E. Resource allocation of in vitro fertilization: a nationwide register-based cohort study. *BMC Health Services Research.* 2007;7(1):210.

103. Pearn J. Gatekeeping and assisted reproductive technology. The ethical rights and responsibilities of doctors. *The Medical Journal of Australia.* 1997;167(6):318–20.

104. Ryan M, Donaldson C. Assessing the costs of assisted reproductive techniques. *BJOG: An International Journal of Obstetrics & Gynaecology.* 1996;103(3):198–201.

105. Pennings G, de Wert G. Evolving ethics in medically assisted reproduction. *Human Reproduction Update.* 2003;9(4):397–404.

106. Ryan MA. *Ethics and Economics of Assisted Reproduction: The Cost of Longing.* Washington DC: Georgetown University Press; 2001.

107. R v Ethical Committee of St. Mary's Hospital, ex parte Harriot. 1 FLR 512 1988.

108. R v Sheffield Health Authority, ex parte Seale. [1996] 3 Med LR 326 1996.

109. R (on the application of Mellor) v Secretary of State for the Home Department. [2000] 2 FLR 951 2000.

110. R (app. Assisted Reproduction and Gynecology Centre and Another v HFEA. [2002] *EWCA Civ* 20 2002.

111. R (app. Rose) v Secretary of State for Health. [2002] *EWHC* **1593** 2002.

112. Dickson v United Kingdom. [2008] 1 FLR 1315 2008.

113. Harmon M. *Responsibility as Paradox: A Critique of Rational Discourse on Government.* London: Sage; 1995, p. 68.

114. Mr T Apelogun-Gabriels v London Borough of Lambeth. *Unreported:* (2301976/05 (5016/62) (ET) 2006.

115. McKevitt T. Employee dismissed for distributing homophobic biblical extracts. *Equal Opportunities Review.* 2007;**163**:28–9.

116. Hambler A. A private matter? Evolving approaches to the freedom to manifest religious convictions in the workplace. *Religion and Human Rights.* 2008;**3**:111–33.

117. GMC. Personal beliefs and medical practice – guidance for doctors 2008: Available from: http://www.gmc-uk.org/guidance/ethical_guidance/personal_beliefs.asp; http://www.gmc-uk.org/static/documents/content/Personal_Beliefs.pdf.

118. Shaw D. Cutting through red tape: non-therapeutic circumcision and unethical guidelines. *Clinical Ethics.* 2009;**4**(4):181–6.

119. Doel M, Allmark PJ, Conway P, Cowburn M, Flynn M, Nelson P, *et al.* Professional boundaries: research report. Project Report General Social Care Council 2009.

120. Rabow MW, Wrubel J, Remen RN. Promise of professionalism: personal mission statements among a national cohort of medical students. *Annals of Family Medicine.* 2009;**7**(4):336–42.

121. Leinum CJ, Trapskin PJ. Writing a personal philosophy of practice. *American Journal of Health-System Pharmacy.* 2011;**68**(2):116–7.

122. Catlin EA, Cadge W, Ecklund EH, Gage EA, Zollfrank AA. The spiritual and religious identities, beliefs, and practices of academic pediatricians in the United States. *Academic Medicine.* 2008;**83**(12):1146–52. 10.097/ACM.0b013e31818c64a5.

123. Frader J, Bosk CL. The personal is political, the professional is not: conscientious objection to obtaining/providing/acting on genetic information. *American Journal of Medical Genetics Part C: Seminars in Medical Genetics.* 2009;**151C**(1):62–7.

124. Dyer C. Doctors must put patients' needs ahead of their personal beliefs. *BMJ.* 2008;**336**(7646):685.

125. MacDonald J, Sohn S, Ellis P. Privacy, professionalism and Facebook: a dilemma for young doctors. *Medical Education.* 2010;**44**(8):805–13.

126. Gold A. Physicians' 'right of conscience' – beyond politics. *The Journal of Law, Medicine & Ethics.* 2010;**38**(1):134–42.

127. Whiting D. Should doctors ever be professionally required to change their attitudes? *Clinical Ethics.* 2009;**4**(2):67–73.

128. Wallace RJ. Hypocrisy, moral address, and the equal standing of persons. *Philosophy & Public Affairs.* 2010;**38**(4):307–41.

129. Shklar J. *Ordinary Vices.* Harvard: Belknap Press; 1984.

130. Pellegrino ED. Toward a virtue-based normative ethics for the health professions. *Kennedy Institute of Ethics Journal.* 1995;**5**(3):253–77

Prologue to Chapters 4 and 5

In the next two chapters I shall be arguing that an important element in the practice of moral medical leadership is distinctive patterns of behaviour giving effect to important values. I call these patterns of behaviour 'propriety', and I shall be examining five such ways of acting: fiduciary propriety, bureaucratic propriety, collegial propriety, inquisitorial propriety and restorative propriety.

Propriety makes an important contribution towards the work of orchestrating organizational moral narrative, demonstrating approved ways of acting and signalling significant moral commitments. But medical leaders owe many overlapping moral responsibilities, and have to take into account the multiple needs of different individuals and different groups at different times. The complexity of their moral responsibilities occasionally results in the emergence of apparently irreconcilable aims and contradictory moral goods. There are insoluble moral tensions to be found at the heart of medical management and these come to the surface, I believe, in conflicting proprieties.

The argument so far

I have argued that the best way to conceptualize moral leadership in medicine is as a process of orchestrating organizational moral narratives. Organizational moral narratives are the form in which groups express their moral values, and realize their moral decisions. Moral leaders in organizations play a significant role in the emergence of such narratives: instigating, investigating, sense-making, influencing, supporting, promoting and enforcing groups' story-making activities. Moral leadership actively promotes collaborative efforts to formulate, test, modify and express a fitting moral narrative.

In Chapter 2 I described three phases in the making of an organizational moral narrative. In the first phase, the leaders became aware of the need for moral action, by starting to make moral sense out of the data of their experience. During a second phase, they involved others in their group in understanding what was going on, and in making deeper moral sense of the situation. In the third and final phase, the leaders worked with colleagues to continue to develop and act out their agreed moral narrative. Then in Chapter 3 I examined how normative expectations and reactive attitudes contribute to the process of moral sense-making. Normative expectations give rise to a keen sense that we 'have a right' to demand certain actions of others. Normative expectations are accompanied by strongly felt 'reactive attitudes' of anger, outrage, resentment, disgust, dismay when we perceive that we have been let down.

The presence of normative expectations, and the reactive attitudes that accompany them, prompts us to notice a 'gap' in the moral order of things. It is propriety that helps us to do something about it. The next two chapters are, then, about what moral leaders can (and ought) concretely to do so as to make healthcare organizations work better for everyone.

Introducing propriety

As I use the term in this book, 'propriety' refers to distinctive social practices that give expression to a set of related moral understandings. When propriety is being practised, moral understandings inform and shape skilful behaviours, while skilful behaviours protect and serve moral goals.

Propriety means something other than simply acting according to moral principle. Relevant actions and behaviours serve to communicate particular moral values, just as employing a compassionate tone of voice serves to communicate a compassionate purpose in the speaker. Propriety is clearly situation specific. Situations in which medical leaders must act as patients' representatives call for fiduciary propriety; situations in which they must act as custodians of collective interests call for bureaucratic propriety; situations in which they serve the community of practitioners call for collegial propriety; situations in which they must investigate harm or wrongdoing call for inquisitorial propriety; and situations in which moral repair must be done call for reparative propriety. Many situations will call for a combination of two or more proprieties. Acting with propriety is more or less expected in many situations, so that failing to act with propriety can bring forth a reactive attitude in much the same way that failing to live up to a normative expectation would do. Finally, propriety is a performance of moral understanding. As a performance it is sometimes consistent with, and at other times quite at odds with, the dispositions or self-identities of the performer. For example, medical leaders may feel very much at home with the behaviours of fiduciary propriety, where they act as patients' representatives; but ill at ease with the behaviours of bureaucratic propriety, which tend to be less preferred ways of thinking and acting.

Although I have given the word propriety a specific meaning, this has its roots in common understanding. The Oxford English Dictionary tells us that the word was in use by the seventeenth century to refer to 'fitness, suitability, conformity with requirement, rule, or principle' and that it came later to include 'conformity with good manners or polite usage; correctness of behaviour or morals' [1]. There is evidence that medical morality was thought of in these terms. Interestingly, this usage faded as the nineteenth century progressed, as Fissell noted.

> By the later part of the eighteenth century, medical manners and morals became unglued; no longer were codes of conduct based on courtesy functional. [2]

Most of these meanings accord with the way I have used propriety, particularly those senses of conformity with requirement and principle, and correctness of behaviour. The themes of conformity and correctness capture, first, how propriety aligns an individual's behaviour with the normative expectations that others hold; and second, how propriety signals a positive moral intent through correct forms of behaviour [3,4].[1]

Conventional use of the word makes apparent that propriety matches behaviour with situation, and that actions deemed morally praiseworthy in one set of circumstances are iniquitous in others. For example, in most democratic societies we expect special solicitude to be shown towards family, dependants and friends, but have no difficulty condemning nepotism by public officials as corruption. Interestingly, practices of propriety may develop ahead of a theoretical understanding of the normative principles that underpin them. So

---

[1] Notably, Margaret Walker refers to propriety in passing but does not supply any definition, (see reference 3). Nikku and Eriksson discuss behaviours similar to propriety, but do not argue that patterns of behaviour correspond to normative expectations (see reference 4).

while bureaucratic propriety had long forbidden public officials from favouring family members however urgent their needs, philosophers were continuing to debate the moral principles that justified partiality towards those close to us or impartiality towards all moral agents [5,6(p66ff),7–15].[2,3]

All in all, practices of propriety tend to cultivate trust and confidence, support relationships of reliance and responsibility, and build community. The converse is also true. Practices that have about them the whiff of impropriety raise suspicion and distrust, threaten to undermine reciprocal reliance, and jeopardize community. Individuals may find one of the proprieties to be more congenial than others; but versatility in all of them is what is required of medical leaders, who become virtuoso performers of propriety.

In the next section I briefly introduce each of the five modes of propriety. This introduction substantially reproduces the overview that I provided in Chapter 1 so some readers may prefer to go directly to Chapters 4 and 5, where I have organized discussion of the proprieties around the moral concerns most prevalent in the study data. Chapter 4 considers how fiduciary, bureaucratic and collegial propriety come to the fore when problems arise around allocating resources and designing services so as to fairly and efficiently meet healthcare needs. Chapter 5 looks at the emergence of inquisitorial and restorative propriety as a response to actual or possible medical injury. However, propriety is more in the way of a range of practices than it is a particular response to a particular problem. We will see that fiduciary, bureaucratic and collegial propriety are used to orchestrate organizational moral narratives around medical harm, just as reparative proprieties may be mobilized in response to issues of rationing or organizational improvement.

In each of the two chapters a conceptual discussion precedes a detailed examination of practices of propriety as medical directors described them. It might therefore appear as though the data from the study are illustrating an a priori conceptual framework. This is not the case. The notion of propriety was developed by examining the ways that medical leaders talked about their moral experience. Its existence became apparent because I adopted an iterative, interpretative process which placed the data about practice into context alongside normative theory. Formal conceptions of fiduciary responsibility, bureaucracy, collegiality, inquiry and moral repair are discussed here because medical directors narrated informal accounts of fiduciary, bureaucratic, collegial, inquisitorial and restorative propriety.

An overview of propriety

Margaret Urban Walker comments that the concrete behaviours through which we practise our responsibilities towards one another are 'as marvelously intricate as philosophical accounts of responsibility have tended to be austere' [6(p100)]. They run the gamut from A to W, if not quite to Z: they include such behaviour as apologizing, blaming, conciliating and excusing; through praising, quizzing or reprimanding; to voicing one's values and

---

[2] See, for example, reference 5. Goodin is also discussed in reference 6.

[3] The philosophical debate has considered the implications of the moral grounding of partiality for several areas, such as justice in global ethics (between citizens of different countries), within one society, and also in relation to moral proximity; i.e. the significance of the closeness of our relationship with another moral agent to our moral obligations. For instance, this has implications for our duties to future generations as well as those currently living. See the work of Williams, Singer, Glover and Rawls (identified in references 7–10), and also references 11–15 for further discussion.

whistleblowing [16].[4] We would expect to find in medicine a special subset of practices of responsibility, practices geared towards protecting particularly vulnerable people from harm. The propriety that I discuss in the following chapters is that particular subset of practices of responsibility apparent in medical leadership.

'Fiduciary propriety' will perhaps need least introduction. Doctors stand in a fiduciary relationship to their patient beneficiaries, and the essence of the fiduciary role is to promote the beneficiary's interests. Fiduciary propriety thus exhibits in action the principle that attending to their patients' needs must be doctors' first priority. Learning the skills of fiduciary propriety begins in medical school, and developing them is a life's work.

Fiduciary propriety fuels noble dreams and selfless endeavour. It has motivated courageous action on behalf of patients around the world: patients stigmatized by HIV/AIDS, mutilated during war, incarcerated by state authorities, abandoned by their families. In the normal run of things however, fiduciary propriety is most evident in how it grants a licence to speak very assertively on behalf of patients; indeed, to speak in ways that would be thought unacceptable if interests other than those of patients were at stake. It is fiduciary propriety that frequently underpins rhetorical sorties into 'shroud-waving' or other regions of the moral high ground.

'Bureaucratic propriety' has as its first concern the needs of the organization, in so far as the organization is the repository of collective interests. Bureaucracy might seem an unlikely place to go looking for moral goodness. But bureaucracy has a legitimate purpose and a positive ethical intent, in the form of supporting equitable, efficient and effective distribution of community goods such as healthcare. A virtuous bureaucracy serves us very much better than nepotism, for example. Equally, vicious bureaucracy can do great evil. The difference between the two is, to some degree, dependent upon whether bureaucrats act with bureaucratic propriety or bureaucratic impropriety.

The hallmarks of bureaucratic propriety are the behaviours of the good bureaucrat: impartiality in deed and in demeanour, transparency and a willingness to be held to account, abnegation of personal interests and moral predilections, support for rules and protocols as a way of distributing public goods, conscientiousness in office. These practices do not come naturally. They have to be learned, and it takes self-discipline to exercise them, especially in the face of provocation.

'Collegial propriety' is a way of behaving suited to an enterprise in which participants rely not upon hierarchy, but upon goodwill and cooperation, to meet their professional and moral responsibilities. No healthcare professional can meet the needs of their patients singlehandedly, nor can they do so without the moral support of others. Collegial propriety is a bond that sustains the medical professional community, and in doing so it also serves patients.

The bonds of collegiality have been the subject of sustained criticism from commentators critical of self-serving professional alliances and their tendency to operate, in George Bernard Shaw's memorable phrase, as a 'conspiracy against the laity' [17]. In the positive form of collegial propriety, we see behaviours that help doctors to understand what they can reasonably ask of others, to express what they owe to each other, and see where they stand in relation to their professional community of practice. Collegial propriety is visible in values and practices such as fellowship, reciprocity, support for and mentoring of juniors,

---

[4] The practice of voicing values refers to Gentile. (See reference 16.)

service to a professional body such as a Royal College, arbitration of clinical standards and empathy with fellow professionals.

'Inquisitorial propriety' is a set of moral practices called upon when allegations of harmful treatment, poor performance or misconduct arise. Misconduct, misbehaviour and medical mistakes presented many of the medical leaders in the study with their most intractable moral troubles. The informal and formal inquiries that follow in the wake of actual or alleged misconduct, and actual or alleged mistakes, call for active moral leadership. Inquisitorial propriety facilitates the expression of 'proper behaviour' by everyone involved in an investigation. Medical leaders will typically have experience of several inquiries, while individual doctors or witnesses will be unlikely to experience more than one or two. Leaders therefore become the repository of understandings of how things ought morally to be done, and their own practice of inquisitorial propriety encourages others to comply.

Inquisitorial propriety reflects considerations of natural justice and due process, but goes somewhat beyond them. For the person leading an investigation, 'inquisitorial propriety' demands demeanours that demonstrate objectivity, neutrality, fairness, openness to 'hearing the other side', prudence and sound judgement. For the person under investigation, 'inquisitorial propriety' calls for candour, regret and, where appropriate, frank confession. In a complainant, 'inquisitorial propriety' demands truthfulness and, if not forgiveness, then mercy towards the transgressor. Inquiries are capable of either rebuilding or destroying patient trust, collegial relationships, clinician self-confidence, team dynamics and respect for medical management. The answers to apparently pragmatic questions such as who should be told about an allegation, and when, carry a significant moral load: telling the wrong people at the wrong time in the wrong way can cause real pain and injustice.

'Restorative propriety' is the fifth and final propriety. It is conduct that seeks to restore moral relations after harm and it turns on acknowledgement: acknowledging that a harm has occurred, acknowledging that certain persons or bodies are responsible, acknowledging that a complaint is legitimate, acknowledging that the person who was harmed has a 'moral right' to define the situation in their terms, acknowledging that steps must be taken to respond.

'Restorative propriety' is a familiar element in our everyday lives, apparent in such behaviours as contrition, the performance of apologies, or making financial restitution. Restorative propriety becomes much more problematic in institutional settings. In organizations, it raises questions such as who has standing to 'perform' gestures such as apology, whether there is sincere regret, whether and what changes to practice may be made, and how such changes can be monitored.

One of the most potent sources of moral anxiety in medical leadership roles is that these five proprieties not infrequently conflict with one another. Each propriety promotes a particular moral good, permitting – to recall the philosopher Margaret Urban Walker – 'people and valued things to be kept out of unnecessary harm's way' [6(p101)]. But precisely because each propriety gives priority to a singular good, medical leaders find the proprieties pulling in different directions. They may find they have to choose between enacting the good of partiality towards their own patients in fiduciary propriety or enacting the good of impartiality towards patients in general in bureaucratic propriety; between enacting the good of fellowship in collegial propriety and enacting the good of neutrality in inquisitorial propriety; or between enacting the good of 'hearing the other side' in inquisitorial propriety and enacting the good of acknowledging a patient's perception of harm in 'restorative propriety'.

Medical leaders have many moral responsibilities: to individual patients, to the general population, to their political masters, to their colleagues, and to those who may be or become the victims of medical harm. Choosing between proprieties when they conflict may be even more demanding than choosing between moral principles. This is because the proprieties are not necessarily consciously recognized forms of behaviour; whatever knowledge medical leaders have of the proprieties tends to be tacitly held. This means that the basis for a strongly-felt decisional bias may not always be apparent; and that a customary behaviour may take hold of the situation before there is any conscious deliberation about how best to proceed.

I noted in Chapter 1 that Immanuel Kant placed the capacity to reason, and compliance with moral duty, at the centre of his account of morality. For Kant, being 'moral' meant to align one's actions with universal and absolute moral laws. If this meant unwillingly surrendering to the demands of moral duty, against one's inclinations, all the better [18,19].[5] This rather austere view encouraged Kant to argue that 'accessibility, affability, politeness, refinement, propriety, courtesy, and ingratiating and captivating behaviour ... call for no large measure of moral determination and cannot, therefore, be reckoned as virtues' [20]. In the next two chapters I set out further evidence for my argument that Kant's emphasis on reason and duty tends to narrow the scope of morality and virtue too far. I have proposed a broader view of morality, one that includes social behaviours that could appear, superficially, to be no more than accessibility, politeness, refinement and so on. In the form of propriety, such behaviours constitute highly disciplined moral accomplishments that help to build ethical healthcare organizations.

---

[5] For a helpful exposition see reference 19.

References

1. Baker R. Medical propriety and impropriety in the english speaking world prior to the formalization of medical ethics. In: Baker R, Porter D, Porter R, eds. *The Codification of Medical Morality: Historical and Philosophical Studies of the Formalization of Western Medical Morality in the Eighteenth and Nineteenth Centuries, Volume One: Medical Ethics and Etiquette in the Eighteenth Century.* Dordrecht: Kluwer Academic; 1993, pp. 15–17.

2. Fissell ME. Innocent and honourable bribes: medical manners in eighteenth-century Britain. In: Baker R, Porter D, Porter R, eds. *The Codification of Medical Morality: Historical and Philosophical Studies of the Formalization of Western Medical Morality in the Eighteenth and Nineteenth Centuries, Volume One: Medical Ethics and Etiquette in the Eighteenth Century.* Dordrecht: Kluwer Academic; 1993, pp. 32–7.

3. Walker MU. *Moral Repair: Reconstructing Moral Relations after Wrongdoing.* Cambridge: Cambridge University Press; 2006, p. 25.

4. Nikku N, Eriksson BE. Microethics in action. *Bioethics.* 2006;20(4):169–79.

5. Goodin R. *Protecting the Vulnerable.* Chicago: University of Chicago Press; 1985.

6. Walker MU. *Moral Understandings: A Feminist Study in Ethics.* 2nd edn. New York: Oxford University Press; 2007.

7. Williams B. *Persons, Character and Morality. Moral Luck: Philosophical Papers 1973–1980.* Cambridge: Cambridge University Press; 1981, pp. 1–19.

8. Singer P. *One World: The Ethics of Globalisation.* New Haven: Yale University Press; 2002.

9. Glover J. *Moral Distance. Causing Death and Saving Lives.* London: Penguin; 1977, pp. 286–97.

10. Rawls J. *A Theory of Justice.* Revised edn. Cambridge, MA: Harvard University Press; 1999.

11. Goodin RE. Vulnerabilities and responsibilities: an ethical defense of the welfare state. *The American Political Science Review.* 1985;79(3):775–87.

12. Donaldson T. Morally privileged relationships. *The Journal of Value Inquiry.* 1990;**24**(1):1–15.

13. Friedman M. The practice of partiality. *Ethics.* 1991;**101**(4):818–35.

14. Coleman D. Partiality in Hume's moral theory. *The Journal of Value Inquiry.* 1992;**26**(1):95–104.

15. Vernon R. *Friends, Citizens, Strangers: Essays on Where We Belong.* University of Toronto Press; 2005.

16. Gentile MC. *Giving Voice to Values: How to Speak Your Mind When You Know What's Right.* New Haven: Yale University Press; 2010.

17. Shaw GB. *The Doctor's Dilemma.* London: Constable; 1911, p. xxii, Act 1: p. 28.

18. Kant I. *Fundamental Principles of the Metaphysic of Morals.* New York: Prentice Hall, Library of Liberal Arts Press; 1949.

19. Norman R. *The Moral Philosophers.* 2nd edn. Oxford: Oxford University Press; 1998.

20. Kant I. *Lectures on Ethics 1875–1880.* New York: Harper; 1963.

Expressing fiduciary, bureaucratic and collegial propriety

In this chapter we will be examining practices of responsibility through which medical leaders seek to ensure that their organizational systems allow patients the best care possible, within the constraints of the resources available to them.

Following the account set out in my prologue to Chapters 4 and 5, I shall be discussing practices of responsibility that are recognizable in distinctive clusters of activity called 'propriety'. Propriety expresses values and beliefs about the right way to do things, values and beliefs that surface in response to the particular issue or problem in hand. In this chapter I shall be focussing on issues that for the most part have to do with effective use of resources. But I should make very clear at the outset that the three proprieties I discuss here – fiduciary, bureaucratic and collegial – are relevant across the entire span of medical management activity. They do not apply only to resource-related concerns. This will be particularly clear in the discussion of fiduciary propriety, but it is a point that might be overlooked when we concern ourselves with bureaucratic propriety.

In healthcare ethics, when the word 'resources' appears it typically signals ethical problems concerning allocative justice [1,2].[1] Allocative justice is about ensuring that finite resources such as drug treatment budgets are fairly shared, which is frequently taken to mean that one way or another they are dispensed so as to secure the greatest possible net benefit. Ethical debate over problems to do with allocative justice has exposed the indeterminacy of medical criteria in allocative decisions. A typical example, expenditure on reproductive technologies, was considered in Chapter 3. We noted that the medical status of infertility does not supply a ready answer to questions of entitlement to treatment, and nor does it indicate who might be most deserving of treatment should limited resources be available. Moreover, reproductive technologies beg a host of questions about social management of reproduction; whether all adults have a right to become parents, for example, and whether, if collective resources help to create children, the collectivity has a legitimate say in who may reproduce [3–9]. A second example concerns the allocation of healthcare resources to those towards the end of the expected human lifespan. Is it intergenerational justice, or is it ageist, to argue that those who have enjoyed a fair innings have a lesser claim on collective resources [10–16]?[2]

These debates surrounding allocative justice already present seemingly intractable questions about the proper scope of medicine, about how we measure quality of life, about

---

[1] I use Rawls's terminology; see references 1 and 2.

[2] In the UK people over 60% of hospital bed days are accounted for by patients 65 and older. It has been predicted that the number of people over 65 will increase by nearly 50% in the twenty years from 2006 to 2026, with concomitant rises in disability and dependency.

what social criteria to include in allocative calculations, about how we formulate inter-generational justice, and so on. Ethical conundrums regarding the right use of resources are difficult enough to resolve in principle, but they become almost absurdly complex in leadership practice.

Ethical use of healthcare resources in and by organizations means not just allocating financial resources fairly. It means squeezing the greatest possible benefit out of every kind of organizational asset: time, expertise, culture, organizational memory, research, learning environment, buildings, land, stakeholder relationships, reputation and so on. There are economies of scale to be secured through closures and mergers that promote important clinical aims, while relegating social concerns (such as proximity to home and family) that others judge equally valuable; departments whose output is low may have to be reorganized in the face of opposition from patients and professionals who value the personal quality of service they receive and provide; patients and professionals conspire to secure treatments that yield slender evidence of effectiveness in many cases (e.g. tympanostomy tubes or 'grommets' for children with middle-ear infections [17]); national initiatives or new drug marketing campaigns promise undoubted healthcare benefits but threaten to divert budgets and professional energies away from meeting pressing but low-profile local needs. These are the sorts of issues that supply the everyday moral anxieties and matching moral action that I discuss in this chapter.

Providing the best care possible with the available resources

I will be using excerpts from more than a dozen different narratives of resource manage-ment to ground the discussion in this chapter, but these excerpts give little sense of the larger issues that medical directors were dealing with. To provide a clearer idea of the background concerns, in the following paragraphs I describe some of the circumstances that medical leaders recounted to me. I have chosen to retell the stories, rather than present a version of the transcripts, in an attempt to recapture some of the vitality of the original interviews. The text of an interview narrative rarely reveals the character of the narrator, and the emotions apparent in the original telling. But character and emotions are a part of the moral quality of real life. When character and emotion are absent it is tempting to treat these stories as just tales of the everyday business of medical management, and overlook their moral dimension; but it is important to remember that these were medical leaders talking about moral trouble. This was what they thought about when they wondered whether they were good people and virtuous leaders. Later in this chapter I discuss medical leaders' awareness of the moral dimension in how patient experiences are retold in organizational narratives; so it is important to emphasize that I have myself retold medical leaders' stories in order to convey their emotional tone as well as their factual content. The stories are theirs, but the retelling is my responsibility.

Dr. Gulvin (Stoneyhill and District NHS Trust) and Dr. Quinn (Bankside Hospitals NHS Trust) had both led their organizations through bruising periods of structural change. There had been months first, extending into years, when plans for reconfigur-ation were formulated, discussed, opposed, rejected, modified, opposed again, rejected again, modified again, and finally partially implemented in less than optimal circum-stances. Both doctors had grappled long and hard with their own consciences, their colleagues and their public representatives over the question of how to secure the best care for patients in the long term.

Their organizations had had little choice but to confront the issues of industrialization, institutionalization and 'diffusion of the health agenda' that we noted in Chapter 1. They had aimed to secure economies of scale, maximize clinical efficiency, enhance patient safety and configure more responsive services. The most stark, fear-inducing and contentious changes they tried to introduce concerned proposed closures of outlying clinical services, particularly services that provided a response to emergencies. Dr. Gulvin and Dr. Quinn had endured trial by media, trial by politician, trial by colleagues and trial by public consultation. Their accusers said that by downgrading local hospitals and centralizing emergency services they would be putting patient lives at risk. According to their opponents, the blood of every patient who died before they reached a hospital would now irrevocably stain their hands. But what was the point, Dr. Quinn reflected, in 'scooping someone off the road and rushing them to a hospital which hasn't got the infrastructure or the staff or the equipment to cope with their needs'?

Dr. Vaisey (Riverdale Primary Care Trust) had also decided to support the reorganization of emergency care, this time across a number of community hospitals. She found not only her clinical judgement but also her good intent called into question. In Vaisey's case, money and the need to modernize were contributory factors but they were not the only issue. A succession of Serious Untoward Incidents[3] [18] had cast doubt on the strategy of trying to maintain several local emergency centres each on a limited budget. In cases that brought home the clinical risks involved, parents had rushed their children to the Minor Injuries Unit of a nearby community hospital, where staff had treated them to the best of their ability. But these small hospitals did not have the facilities or expertise found in full-scale emergency departments. More than one child had come close to dying as a consequence of well-intentioned but inexpert care. The PCT faced an unenviable choice. It could keep the Minor Injuries Units in their present form knowing that the community valued them for what they could offer, but also believing that little could realistically be done to make them safer in similarly difficult cases. Alternatively, it could further restrict or close the service and direct patients to more distant hospitals with full emergency departments. Keeping the local units going in their current form looked to Dr. Vaisey an implausible option. Her moral and managerial duty, as she saw it, was to minimize harm to patients by making the clinical argument for closures and reorganizations. But this argument provoked a furious response from patients and their supporters, and it was a source of deep disagreement between Dr. Vaisey, staff in the community hospitals and senior PCT colleagues.

Rather differently, Dr. Alex Adrien (Greenborough Hospital Trust) described intervening in conflicts around 'bedside rationing'. He faced the challenge of settling arguments over patient admission to intensive care, disputes that erupted sometimes between clinicians from different specialties, sometimes between clinicians and patient families, and sometimes between all at once. Although Dr. Adrien's hospital, along with others, had

---

[3] Management of Serious Untoward Incidents (SUIs) is part of clinical governance in every NHS Trust. NHS London defines SUIs as 'something out of the ordinary or unexpected, with the potential to cause serious harm, and/or likely to attract public and media interest that occurs on NHS premises or in the provision of an NHS or a commissioned service. This may be because it involves a large number of patients, there is a question of poor clinical or management judgement, a service has failed, a patient has died under unusual circumstances, or there is the perception that any of these has occurred'. See reference 18.

adopted protocols to help determine who should be admitted to their fixed number of intensive care beds, borderline cases and clinician and family advocacy continued to challenge doctors' technical and moral judgements. Was the clinician who argued for cessation of treatment, on grounds that the patient had only a minimal chance of recovery to enjoy tolerable quality of life, correct in his judgement; or were those arguing for continuing treatment on grounds of a more optimistic prognosis the better judges? Was it right to turn away a 'marginal' patient who needed care now, in favour of preserving resources for future patients with more realistic chances of survival? To a clinician managing resources on behalf of all those who might benefit, a slender chance of survival – say 5% – could seem too small to place a patient ahead of other contestants in the competition for limited care; to the individual or their family, a 5% chance of survival contained the hope that all 100% of a life may yet be saved, creating a moral claim on treatment. How could these gaps in technical and moral perception be navigated?

Clinical effectiveness is about achieving the best patient care possible within the available budget. It means improving, standardizing, reconfiguring, renewing and reinventing healthcare organizations. Much of medical leaders' time is spent contending with the prosaic and obdurate task of husbanding the resources they have at their command. And so it is that endlessly inventing, reiterating, renewing and reordering organizational narratives of resourcing and improvement are part of the mundane 'moral housekeeping' [19] that has be done in ethical healthcare organizations. The basic moral responsibility to use shared healthcare resources wisely comes to be expressed in enacted organizational narratives. The somewhat dreary, turgid, bureaucratic necessities that such narratives entail, and their tendency to lack dramatic, sublime or cathartic conclusions, frequently make this moral activity, as Dr. McGregor (Remembrance Hospitals Trust) commented, 'a difficult sell to the doctors'. It is easier to get doctors (and, it has to be said, ethicists) morally exercised by rare cases concerning face transplants, assisted death and the right to refuse life-saving interventions, than it is to focus their attention on the moral dimensions of budgets, treatment protocols, reorganizations and methods for monitoring chronic disease. But routine and un-dilemmatic though they may be, these are the sorts of moral trouble that tax medical leaders' ethical skill and moral determination.

We now move to look in turn at each of the three proprieties that concern us in this chapter: fiduciary, bureaucratic and collegial. I examine each one by first setting out a conceptual background indicating how we might understand the (often tacit) values that inform actions performed with propriety. I then describe practices of propriety that were present in the study data, illustrating them with examples from the interviews.

Fiduciary propriety: voicing moral responsibility for patients

Each of the 'proprieties' gives first priority to one dimension of medical leadership responsibilities. Fiduciary propriety gives first priority to patients.

In one of the earliest English-language texts on medical ethics, Thomas Percival wrote that doctors

> should minister to the sick with due impressions of the importance of their office, reflecting that the ease, the health and the lives of those committed to their charge depend on their skill, attention, and fidelity. (from ref. 20, cited in ref. 21)

Percival's preoccupation in the passage quoted appears to have been with the *manner* in which doctors attended to the sick. Patients sought technical expertise (such as it was at the time), undivided attention and loyal service. The doctor's obligation to his patient was to care for that patient to the best of his ability, and to do so to the exclusion of other concerns. Percival called upon doctors to comport themselves in such a way that their patients could be assured they were indeed skilful, and that they were committed to their patients' interests above all else. In doing so he encapsulated an understanding of professional propriety that has prevailed for centuries. Percival's exhortations to his fellows illustrate that a sense of fiduciary propriety has long been a component of medical professional culture.

Latterly, however, in the bioethical literature, the notion of the doctor as a fiduciary, with associated fiduciary duties, has tended to be attributed to the law of trusts [22,23].[4] Legal trusts arose as a way of ensuring that valuable property could be well managed by someone who knew what they were doing, but be available for the use of others who could benefit from it (typically, women and feckless offspring). The trustee is duty bound to use his skill and judgement to manage the property in the interests of the beneficiaries. Viewing doctors as 'trustees' of patient interests follows from doctors having a specialized expertise; having control of medical resources to which patients may have a claim; and, in consequence of the first two, having anxious and relatively powerless patients in a position of dependency upon them.

My aim in this chapter is to examine how doctors' sense of fiduciary responsibility is expressed in a pattern of behaviour that I recognize as fiduciary propriety. I start by outlining a theoretical understanding of fiduciary obligation. This outline reveals the potential of the fiduciary concept to shape personal, professional and organizational narratives. Examination of the concept also suggests, though, that it is only a partially accurate description of the exigencies of medical practice. I then go on to trace in the data how the sense of being a fiduciary permeates medical management. We will see that fiduciary propriety shapes the conduct of doctors as leaders, but is also subject to the constraints imposed by other modes of propriety.

The conceptual background to fiduciary propriety

Moral responsibilities of a fiduciary nature arise when one person is dependent upon another to take action on their behalf. The general nature of a fiduciary obligation is clear, at least to lawyers who use the term. The beneficiary – in this case, the patient – trusts the fiduciary – in this case, the doctor – to use their skill and judgement to further the beneficiary's interests. They must rank the interests of the beneficiary ahead of the fiduciary's own, and – strictly speaking – should spurn opportunity for personal or professional gain while acting on the beneficiary's behalf [24].[5] Interestingly, the fiduciary must act as it is assumed the beneficiary would – that is, selfishly – by placing the beneficiary's interests before all other claims or considerations.

---

[4] 'The patient-physician relationship presupposes patients entrusting physicians to act on their behalf and physicians remaining loyal to their patients.' See reference 22 and 23.

[5] The Charter on Medical Professionalism: 'This principle is based on a dedication to serving the interest of the patient. Altruism contributes to the trust that is central to the physician–patient relationship. Market forces, societal pressures, and administrative exigencies must not compromise this principle.' See reference 24.

The fiduciary discharges their moral responsibility for the patient's welfare by having recourse to two types of fiduciary practice [25].[6]

The first type of practice is taking action to aid patients as beneficiaries. This practice is associated with the duty to give care. This duty to give care is open-ended and uncertain. The extent of it is ascertained largely by reference to professional and organizational convention. It alters according to circumstance, most notably the resources available for care (which are quite different for a Nigerian doctor in Nigeria and the same doctor in the UK or USA). The duty to give care means that a doctor must undertake activities that are in the best interests of her patient, but how she does so is a matter of judgement and discretion. It is clear that she is to dedicate herself to her patient; but is that for 24 hours a day, or four? Four may be all that is affordable. It is clear that her patients' interests must come first; but is she to attend to her patients' interests to the exclusion of all else? This is simply not possible: all doctors use one of their most precious resources – time – to fulfil other priorities than treating patients. They rightly take time for medical education and training, for medical research and for medical management, for example.

The second type of fiduciary practice is avoiding taking action that might run counter to the interests of patient beneficiaries, a practice more in the way of a negative duty of loyalty. These negative duties are tolerably certain, more closed and less negotiable in nature than the open-ended duty of care. They include negative injunctions such as those against disclosing confidential information, using the beneficiary's rights or entitlements to advantage oneself or others, and entertaining financial conflicts of interest.

Although I have suggested that the two kinds of practice express positive and negative duties, these labels are apt to mislead. The positive duty may entail what doctors sometimes describe as 'masterly inaction', a conscious decision not to intervene when a person's body or mind might better heal itself or die. Equally, the negative duty of loyalty may only be satisfied by an outlay of positive and expensive effort. The organizational resources involved in maintaining patient confidentiality – developing secure information systems, appointing 'Caldicott guardians', disseminating information policies, investigating breaches of confidentiality and punishing lapses – are all evidence of the definite steps that must be taken in order to avoid compromising patient interests.

It is widely accepted that fiduciary obligations are not absolute. There is a broad consensus that the fiduciary obligation to individual patients is a prima facie duty: that is, one where significant obligations to others may occasionally trump doctors' obligations to individual patients. Framing the fiduciary relationship as a prima facie duty inevitably prompts the difficult question of what other interests might be capable of 'trumping' the obligation. This is where consensus breaks down.

The first set of difficulties arises when doctors face the competing moral interests of another individual. So, for example, most accept that the moral good of confidentiality may be trumped by the moral requirement to prevent serious harm befalling another. But whether confidentiality ought to be breached in order to warn a third party of a risk of contracting HIV/AIDS is a debatable point [26].[7]

---

[6] The duty of loyalty is akin to Kant's 'perfect duty' while the duty of care is Kant's 'imperfect duty'. See reference 25.

[7] One of the most stimulating discussions of the problems around HIV transmission is cited in reference 26.

A second set of difficulties arises where doctors feel the tug of competing moral claims asserted on behalf of the general good. If fidelity to patients' interests means putting one's own patient first, how can it be consistent with the fiduciary role to settle what one patient will get by taking into account what other patients need? Some commentators have insisted that fidelity to patients' interests forbids the doctor from acting as a 'double agent', taking into consideration the best interests of an organization or an abstract public as well as the best interests of the patient [27–38].[8] Against this it has been argued that organizations represent a collective interest in resource allocation that cannot be ignored, and that Hippocratic individualism [39,40][9] is ultimately self-defeating:

> An appeal to the perspective of 'My patient comes first' is a formula for uncontrolled costs and for the undermining of the very fiduciary obligations that the perspective was originally proposed to protect. Uncontrolled costs will exhaust organizational resources, leaving some physicians – including some who put their patients first – without access to the resources that their patients need. Adopting a 'My patient comes first' perspective is thus a self-defeating strategy for any physician attempting to deal with the scarcity of resources in a manner consistent with the fulfilment of fiduciary obligations to his or her patients .... [21]

A convincing claim can almost always be made that a patient or group of patients will be disadvantaged by a service change or by budgetary restraint. So the notion of a fiduciary duty to patients is always on hand to fuel morally loaded arguments: against cutting a service budget, altering current treatment regimes, reorganizing services, rationing new or costly treatment, restraining innovation, and so on. The notion of a fiduciary duty might also be used, of course, to argue for salary restraint in the NHS or against doctors being paid substantial fees by patients, but infrequently is.

Are those medical leaders who argue the case for budgetary restraint, service redesign and so on really failing in their moral obligation to patients? If being a fiduciary really does mean putting ones' patients' interests first at all times, doctors are perpetually in contravention of their fiduciary role. They are bound to be, if they are to manage their responsibility to care for one individual patient alongside caring for other patients, alongside their responsibility for clinical audit, alongside their responsibility to educate the next generation of doctors, alongside their responsibility to advance clinical science through research, and so on.

So either the concept of fiduciary responsibility is untenable, or it means something other than 'putting a patient's interests first at all times'. The key lies in differentiating between the open-ended, positive duty of care and the prima facie, negative duty of loyalty. Doctors cannot always, all the time, care single-mindedly for a single patient, and the duty to care does not require them to do so. They can, most of the time, avoid actively injuring their patient's interests, and this is what the duty of loyalty demands. There is a point, of course, at which the negotiable duty to provide care meets the non-negotiable duty of loyalty: that is, when the care that is or can be offered falls so far short of expectations that it

---

[8] See references 27–36 on double agency. Clinician and researcher perceptions of the fiduciary role are readily apparent in Hedgecoe's discussion of the politics of prescribing Herceptin. See references 37 and 38.

[9] See references 39 and 40.

begins to seem that patients are suffering an avoidable harm. In this situation the meaning of fiduciary responsibility is clear: it means taking action to avoid harm befalling the beneficiary. This is the situation that medical leaders confront when shortage of resources puts the minimum reasonable standard of care in jeopardy.

Given the open-ended negotiability of the duty to care, every argument concerning allocation of limited resources is vulnerable to assertions that certain patients' interests are in jeopardy; and that fiduciary responsibility mandates they be defended. Identifying the point at which there is a 'genuine' breach of fiduciary responsibility is thus a matter of clinical, political and situational judgement. Moreover, the 'tipping point' is relative. Medical leaders in the study recognized that they would react and argue differently were they running hospitals in developing countries or dealing with a health crisis such as pandemic influenza. But wherever they reckoned the 'tipping point' to be, that was the point at which fiduciary propriety should be – and was indeed – mobilized.

The continual interplay of negative and positive duties partly explains why committed clinicians robustly defend a fiduciary account of clinician-patient relations, even though meeting any one individual patient's needs comes second for a great part of their working lives. Another part of the explanation is, straightforwardly, the ideological importance and narrative potential of the fiduciary model. Underlying the notion of a fiduciary obligation is an appealingly selfless narrative that sees professional skill and personal virtue knit together in pursuit of some higher purpose. It is this narrative that prompts the behaviours we will recognize below as fiduciary propriety. Purity of motive, disinterestedness and loftiness of aims all supply an idiom in which to frame narrative action, as well as granting licence to claim the moral high ground.

It is a persuasive argument that while the notion of doctors' unqualified fidelity to patients' interests is, on close inspection, a naive myth, the concept has also served as an important regulative ideal [29]. This 'regulative ideal' is expressed in practice as fiduciary propriety. Arguments emanating from fidelity are certainly mythological and idealistic. However, they function as a powerful rhetorical trope through which to express significant normative expectations and elicit the practice of responsibility.[10] When patients' interests are threatened, fiduciary propriety demands advocacy on behalf of patients and their needs. When doctors' own interests are threatened it is tempting, naturally, to have recourse to the same rhetorical practices.

---

[10] Normative expectations were discussed in detail in Chapter 3. For readers who have turned directly to this chapter, normative expectations fuse what we think ought to happen with what we think will actually happen. They are concerned with 'norms' in the sense that moral theorists use the word, referring to morally significant standards for behaviour. 'Respect patient autonomy' is a norm familiar to doctors. The existence of norms elicits expectations from those with an interest in them. So 'respect patient autonomy' elicits expectations from healthcare professionals, as well as from patients, carers, regulators and others. Such expectations are 'expectations' in two senses. First we 'expect' others to adhere to certain standards, taking the view that they ought to respect these standards because the standards embody values important to us. Second we 'expect' that much of the time others will observe these standards, because they have demonstrated a willingness to abide by them or because they have expressed sentiments suggesting they support them. So we expect (in a moral sense) doctors to respect patient autonomy, and we expect that (in a predictive sense) doctors will for the most part try to do so.

Practices of fiduciary propriety

In medical leadership, advocacy on behalf of patients is the paradigmatic mode of fiduciary propriety. (In medical practice, as we have seen, it is giving care.) The essence of the fiduciary role is to do for another what he cannot do for himself; when the beneficiary cannot speak for himself, the fiduciary becomes his advocate. Thus, in the corridors of power, where patients cannot freely walk, medical leaders must faithfully represent patients' interests and concerns.

A fiduciary is not, however, a mere agent for the patient, acting according to the patient's will. The fiduciary is a trustee for the patient's interest, acting to promote their welfare. Fiduciaries are not charged simply to act upon or speak the beneficiary's view: rather, fiduciaries are to use their expertise and judgement to decide what to speak and how to speak on their beneficiaries' behalf. Trustees do not always judge their beneficiaries' welfare as their beneficiaries would. One tension in the fiduciary relationship is that patient-beneficiaries may disagree with their doctor-fiduciaries about how their interests are best served, and how they should be represented. Moreover, medical leaders act as fiduciaries not just for individual patient interests, but also for collective patient interests. The two are not always in concordance.

So sometimes it falls to the fiduciary to be faithful to a patient's voice, to carry it to places the patient cannot be. Other times the fiduciary must speak from authority, in a voice of their own. Sometimes she must speak on behalf of the individual interest. Other times he must speak on behalf of the group interest. Using the best voice, in the best way, at the best time, figured prominently in medical leaders' accounts of ethical action, whether or not they consciously conceived of their role in fiduciary terms.

Re-presenting patient narratives

Clinician leaders compose their moral narratives around the echoes and reverberations of many patients' described experience. Patients entrust their stories to clinicians because they believe clinicians have the power to act on those stories. Clinicians thus become a repository of patient narratives of experience: in significant ways, they become trustees for their patients' narratives of experience as well as trustees of their patients' interests.

We should not underestimate the moral and psychological intensity of the stories that clinicians hear, and the power they have to influence clinical thinking and activity. Patients narrate with a purpose. They aim to exhibit their identity, to earn approval, to secure sympathy, to absolve themselves of responsibility for being unwell, to portray their case as deserving, to convince that they are worthy of consideration, to persuade that they are entitled. They narrate to express fear, hurt, anger, blame, disappointment, relief, and all the other emotions of their sick role or illness trajectory. The emotional notes in these narratives carry to clinicians in subtle and unpredictable ways: clinicians may be captured by patients' stories, sometimes moved, sometimes repelled, rarely untouched.

If moral leadership is, in the end, about formulating and implementing organizational moral narrative, then how individuals' interests come to be included within those narratives is of considerable importance.

In narrative terms, fidelity to patients' interests commands a degree of fidelity in the representation of patients' interests. A sense of what is proper and improper attaches to the terms in which patients' interests are discussed. Dr. Vaisey recognized too late that she and PCT colleagues had chosen the wrong way to represent patient experience when they set out to justify the stringent financial savings that circumstances required of them. Using the wrong language, they provoked moral condemnation, dissent, and distrust.

> What we did was say things like, 'This is our financial envelope. These are the pressures. These are the targets' . . .. That word 'pressures', to me, is one of the key issues . . . I've heard it used in clinical settings, and local authority ones. To a manager, it's a way of expressing 'a very difficult problem'. To a clinician it might mean 'an old lady who doesn't get meals on wheels on Sunday and hasn't got anybody else to cook for her'. It might mean 'a patient who's dying who's not going to get night nursing'. And that word 'pressures' used to represent *those* problems almost sounds abusive, really. (Dr. Vaisey, Riverdale Primary Care Trust)

All doctors – even those who have become jaded or inured to patient distress – carry with them traces of the complex sorrows that they have heard. They know intimately the pain, sadness, self-destruction, hopelessness, anxiety or frank terror that life, illness and death invoke. To reduce this to 'pressures' is to fail to respect the moral gravity of this experience. Proper use of language is, then, about more than 'the pleasure and charm of social intercourse' as Kant might have it. Language is the chief means leaders have at their disposal to identify, represent and negotiate the moral responsibilities of institutions. It matters whether the language that is used – 'collateral damage' instead of 'indiscriminate killing', 'pressures' instead of 'hunger and pain' – conceals or reveals them. The words leaders use contribute to collective moral perception.

There are ethical choices to be made in how medical leaders go about representing patient experience. Sometimes it will be right to encode experience in precise technicalities, selecting from its richness only those details that serve the immediate purpose, and stripping out emotional superfluity. Lawyers reformulate their clients' narrative of experience, stripping them of superfluous detail to reveal their legal resonance. Doctors reformulate patient narratives of experience to reveal a clinically relevant history, retelling them in a methodical and precise formula that organizes clinical thinking [41].[11] And healthcare leaders reformulate patient narratives to promote patient interests in the organization. Individual patients themselves, and their complex life stories, may be virtually absent from organizational narratives; their interests portrayed as 'clinical risk'. In the following example, Dr. Dillon recalled his response to a non-executive member of the hospital Board – a person of considerable business experience and acumen – who had argued that the solution was simple: close down areas of activity until such time as they had money to reopen them.

> Perhaps it was easier for me to say it than it was for a manager to say it: 'You can't do it. It is a demand led service! We don't have electives; you can't just say, "well, we don't do your hip operation for six months". Most of what comes onto this ward is very emergency driven. So unless you can stem the tide of the emergencies, you can't close the ward, because we're still left with a clinical risk . . .. We can change the system to try and stem the flow of emergencies, which might *then* enable you to close the ward. But you don't start by closing the ward.'
> (Dr. Dillon, Five Bridges Mental Health Trust)

What made it easier for Dr. Dillon to argue the case for keeping wards open was that, as a doctor, he was normatively expected to argue from a fiduciary perspective. Although

---

[11] A recent observational study reveals how morally salient concerns are subsumed into a clinical profile; see reference 41.

Dr. Dillon depersonalized the argument on this occasion by adopting the terminology of 'clinical risk' and 'emergency driven', there are times when moral leadership of organizational narrative calls for the opposite approach. When lawyers relate their clients' stories to a jury they may choose to reinsert telling personal detail; and when doctors narrate patient experience in order to mobilize organizational action, 'repersonalizing' the story may be the most effective way of doing so. There are times when it is right to return to the emotional timbre, the richness of individual and situation, that were present in the patient's own narrative. Retelling patient stories with the vivid detail that lends authenticity, and in the powerful language of fiduciary responsibility – using the power of narrative persuasion [42–44][12] – may be a powerful way to secure general assent to the leaders' preferred action.

Intuitively aware of the persuasive quality of patient stories, medical leaders give voice to the urgency of patient need. Dr. Quinn, for instance, recalled how sometimes the need to confront a sceptical Board had called forth impassioned advocacy:

> I probably don't recognize the strength with which I put over some of the arguments. I'm not by nature a particularly forceful character. But I suppose at times I do invest quite a lot of emotional involvement in the way that I will put across difficult issues at [Board] level, particularly to the non-execs where they're not necessarily aware of . . . . Well it goes back to that patient thing. You know what the effect on individuals could be.
>
> (Dr. Quinn, Bankside Hospitals NHS Trust)

Patient stories are a cornerstone in clinicians' understanding of patients' interests. They are, of course, only a small part of clinicians' professional knowledge; but they supply the raw material on which clinicians' expertise is brought to bear. They are thus intimately bound into clinicians' reasoning and into their explanations of the courses of action that they urge.

The rich informational and emotional possibilities of stories of patient experience can create significant difficulties when, for reasons of patient confidentiality, parts of the story cannot be told. The moral leader then finds herself in the role of advocate, speaking up for patients' interests and speaking out of patients' experience, but prevented from faithfully representing it. The moral narrative based in patient experience then loses both its fidelity and its force. Dr. Vaisey's support for the reconfiguration of Minor Injury Units was based on her 'insider' knowledge of the patients' stories, and her fear of potentially catastrophic clinical risk was based on them. But she was defending an unpopular proposal. To objectors, the plan appeared to be designed to cut costs and to pave the way for the closure of community hospitals. If she was to earn their trust, Dr. Vaisey needed to narrate the experiences that underpinned her reasoning. But:

> I found it difficult to anchor my argument because of the bits I had to generalize. For instance, to say that 'We had a child that had an injury which was inappropriately treated, and if we were unlucky, that child would have suffered an amputation of their limb' is quite frightening. But it's not the same as saying: 'The child broke their leg. Their blood supply was cut off. And if they hadn't got to [a proper emergency department at another] hospital in time, they would have had to have their leg amputated' . . . . If you say: 'There's a 3-year-old child who attended Minor Injury one evening with a mild injury. And then another evening with some other mild injury. And we didn't identify that those injuries weren't [accidental]. The next time they came in they had a skull

---

[12] A useful recent overview is reference 42. See also references 43 and 44.

fracture'. [That is more compelling than] saying 'We found we weren't picking up repeat incidents and we had a child who suffered a life-threatening injury because of that'. So we tried to explain the reality but nothing is quite as gripping as the real story is it? You can't really make up a story in those circumstances ... (Dr. Vaisey, Riverdale Primary Care Trust)

As it appears in the extract above, the comparison Dr. Vaisey was making is not quite as stark as she intended to convey. For understandable reasons, she was reluctant to tell the 'real' stories in interview too. Rather than name the child's injuries, Dr. Vaisey carefully withheld detail and used the abstraction 'mild injury' instead. (I have also removed some elements of the story to further preserve anonymity.)

Re-prioritizing patient narratives

It is not only *patients'* experiences that feature in the highly charged moral narratives that circulate in clinical settings. Narratives about the patient experience often also refer to professionals' normative expectations and how they reacted. In this emotionally febrile arena, patient stories become part of other equally urgent professional and personal narratives. Particular patient stories may contribute to clinicians' own narratives of rescue, or of fidelity, or of professional pre-eminence [45].[13] When things go wrong, patient stories can become the reference point in professional narratives of blame, recrimination, resolution, reparation or redemption. But precisely because patient narratives do call forth responses from professionals, the patient narrative itself can be all too easily lost in the surrounding confusion. The initial narrative, and patients' normative expectations, may disappear in the swirl of reactive attitudes. It is the role of moral leaders, acting as fiduciaries, to press the patient-beneficiary's claim upon the attention of others and ensure it receives due precedence. When the moral and personal narratives of patients, carers, clinicians and others come into conflict, fiduciary propriety insists that a patient narrative be brought to the fore.

Dr. Alex Adrien gave an example of just such a conflict, and just such a response, when he described intervening in disputes between his colleagues around patients' admission to intensive care. Typically, he will be called to arbitrate when his 'crash team' has resuscitated a patient, endeavours to admit the patient to intensive care, but find the intensivists of the view that the patient does not satisfy their criteria for intensive treatment.

This frequently gets us into areas of conflict .... You can come at it from the intensive care unit/ trust management end and say 'Well we absolutely must be using these resources appropriately, if we don't they're not available for other people'.... You have the family perspective which is 'Yes I accept that my mum's got Alzheimer's, she's also got kidney failure, we know she's going to die some time soon, but she's got pneumonia and we want you to put her on a ventilator if she needs it, okay'. You've got the doctors looking after the patient, and the nurses looking after the patient, who may have their own views in one direction or another .... The intensive care doctors are saying 'They don't fulfil the criteria, we're not going to take them'.... And the doctors in charge of the patient are saying 'Well we've saved them. Now we want them to go to intensive care'. (Dr. Adrien, Greenborough Hospital Trust)

The challenge to moral leadership is to locate a single moral narrative capable of reconciling the normative expectations embedded in these three perspectives. There is a complex family

---

[13] See, for example, reference 45.

narrative of care. It is one that may more or less clearly articulate the value of this person, or of life itself; carry more or less rational reactions to doctors, medical authority or hospital technology; encode a sense of entitlement, disempowerment, grief, guilt, relief or responsibility. Next there is a clinical narrative of rescue. It is one that may be founded purely in seeking to act on behalf of an individual patient; it may arise from clinical inexperience; or be bound up with a desire for redemption, or fear of death; it probably reflects a sense of professional identity, purpose or ambition. Finally there is a clinical-managerial narrative of triage. It conveys, perhaps, the onus of being the designated gate-keeper and the weariness of negotiation; expresses maybe a sense of rectitude in working to protocol, a degree of professional seniority or a view on best use of valuable resources. Each of these narratives recognizes a particular moral responsibility, and expresses a view on how that moral responsibility should be discharged. From the point of view of fiduciary propriety, circumstances such as these call for the moral leader to assert a narrative of fiduciary responsibility: that is, a clinical decision made on the basis of the patients' best interests in light of the available resources.

> You discuss it through, make sure the right people are talking to each other, make sure that you've got the patient's views as much as you can into that conversation, and then usually everyone comes to agree a direction of travel. I do the 'Let's get everyone to take a step back' approach here, because very often you come in and it's quite heated ... I say 'Look I'm not interested in any of that. I don't care who said what to whom. What I want at this moment in time is to say we've got a patient here, let's start again and let's make a clinical decision'. ...
> Very often I find ... the most appropriate senior people haven't been involved. For example it will have been the emergency on-call medical team that would have resuscitated the patient, but they haven't called the consultant who actually is in charge of that patient. The intensive care team would have spoken to their intensive care unit consultant on the phone, who ... may not have come to see the patient .... What I find is interesting, in most areas of ethical conflict in the health service if you just get the right people rationally discussing the problem around the table for a short period of time, you come up with a solution that everyone's comfortable with. (Dr. Adrien, Greenborough Hospital Trust)

We can see here how, even where there are treatment protocols to govern a situation, there is a continuing need for practices of fiduciary propriety. Protocols are a bureaucratic means of channelling behaviour so that harm is avoided, and as such are a bureaucratic form of morality (I discuss this further in the next section of this chapter). But protocols, clear at their core, are inevitably surrounded by a penumbra of uncertainty: how to interpret rules that may be unclear in some circumstances; whether this patient fits the rules; how to deal with borderline cases. Such uncertainty calls for the exercise of judgement. At the edges of protocol, where bureaucratic control tapers off, what is called for is a judgement made on grounds of fiduciary propriety (and collegial consensus, which we examine at the end of this chapter). The fiduciary's aim must be to reassert the primacy of the narrative of patient interest. When different moral narratives come into conflict, and the question of 'who said what to whom' threatens to wrest attention away from basic moral responsibilities, fiduciary propriety plays its ace: a 'clinical decision'.

When Dr. Adrien reflected on the implications of fiduciary propriety, he acknowledged the difficulty in maintaining an appropriate stance within his leadership role. Implementing a conscionable balance between individual patients' needs and interests, and the needs and interests of the patient community as a whole, was both taxing and troubling.

A typical thing a clinician will do is to wear blinkers in terms of 'I have my patient in front of me now and I want to do the best for my patient. If that involves a drug that costs £40,000 a year that's what I want, or if that involves putting them in intensive care when everybody else thinks they're not going to survive well actually I want to give them that chance'. Once you become more managerially involved, you've also sat in the Critical Care Network meeting where it's been discussing the real problem of critical care bed capacity in the [region]. So you're just more aware of that bigger picture. Sometimes that's to the good. Sometimes it might take you in a direction where you don't want to be taken, and then you find yourself . . . making decisions where, when you reflect on them afterwards, you think 'Gosh, was that really the right thing for the patient?'

(Dr. Adrien, Greenborough Hospital Trust)

Re-asserting patient narratives

Dr. Adrien described his exercise of fiduciary propriety as mediation. But his aim was clear and explicit: a measured reaffirmation of a fiduciary narrative. There are many occasions, however, when the reaffirmation of a fiduciary narrative is anything but measured. In fact, fiduciary propriety gives licence to practices of advocacy that might, in other situations, be regarded as impolite, excessive or unacceptable. Describing the difficult arguments around closing one of her Minor Injury Units, Dr. Vaisey recounted a discussion with her chief ally, an experienced Director of Nursing:

I'd been sitting there thinking my way through it: how am I going to manage the politics?. . . . So I briefed her . . . . She said to me, 'Have we got to close this unit?' And I thought, 'Maybe we have'. She said to me, 'Look, we're clinicians. And we have to go in there and tell [the Chief Executive]: "Shut up". Because we've got to close the unit'. [We were] allies in terms of 'Hang on a minute. Let's just get back to our roots and think what we've got to do as clinicians'.

(Dr. Vaisey, Riverdale Primary Care Trust)

Of course we cannot know exactly how these two allies put their view to the CEO; when people recount their experiences they may sometimes claim to have been more assertive than they actually were [46,47].[14] The point, however, is that Dr. Vaisey and her colleague conceptualized 'what we've got to do as clinicians' as being implacably persuasive. They understood their duty to be to plant their feet firmly on the perceived fiduciary high ground and stand firm in the face of opposition. 'Getting back to our roots' as clinicians meant it was proper to set aside bureaucratic, consultative, managerial or collegial considerations and make a stark declaration of clinical prerogative on behalf of patients. It meant insisting on the fulfilment of a fiduciary responsibility for minimizing clinical risk, even in the face of considerable hostility from the patients on whose behalf they acted.

It is fiduciary propriety that prompts, literally, fighting talk. As Dr. Seddon (Saxonvale University Hospitals Trust) put it, there were only two things in his job that he 'would die in a ditch' to defend, and they were patient safety and fairness towards his staff. We shall see in the next chapter, especially, that medical leaders may experience difficulty balancing their moral responsibility to protect patients with their moral responsibility for procedural fairness. But when it comes to cost-cutting exercises, the battle lines are starkly drawn and far easier to defend. Even Dr. McGregor, who was throughout his interview a staunch advocate of cost containment and clinical efficiency, described himself as most a medical leader on those occasions when he had found it necessary to dig in his heels:

---

[14] Classics of medical sociology include references 46 and 47.

Protecting our patients against [excessive cost-cutting] is the thing that probably worries me the most . . . . On many occasions, I've had to put my foot down and say, 'No. I can't do this. Because I'm just not confident it's not going to adversely affect patients'. . . . That's the time I've got it right.

(Dr. McGregor, Remembrance Hospitals Trust)

In protracted conflicts, when fiduciary rhetoric proceeds with ever greater energy, urgency and dramatic momentum, medical leaders may find the narrative stakes being raised ever higher. Finally, they have to decide whether to gamble on their 'face', pledging their professional credibility and moral authority in the name of patients' clinical interests. This can mean threats of resignation, taking the argument outside the organization to press or politicians, or even open disobedience. What can be gained by doing so has to be weighed against what might be lost or left behind. Fiduciary propriety suggests the occasions for 'shroud-waving', but also draws attention to the risks associated with it. Dr. Edward Evans, whose hospital had been embroiled in months of punishing financial retrenchment and whose consultant body had been close to mutiny, had given it serious consideration.

When you start any post like this there has to be time when you say 'No, you've taken me [too far]'. . . . Alongside that shroud-waving is what you leave behind. There's no doubt your ability to wave that shroud is only possible if you know it's going to be effective . . . . If all you've done is resigned and left . . . you may have made things worse for . . . the whole, the reason you did it in the first place . . . . There's even an ethical [dimension] when you are in your deepest, darkest moments. (Dr. Evans, Brickvale Hospital NHS Trust)

Fiduciary propriety, as we have begun to see, is very tightly bound in to clinicians' sense of personal and professional identity. Earlier, Dr. Vaisey described how the logic of fiduciary propriety grew out of her 'roots' as a clinician. Learning the basic elements of fiduciary propriety is part of doctors' socialization to their profession so that – once it is prompted – it is perhaps one of the easiest idioms to mobilize.

I have at board level had to hold the line . . . . We were proposing that we would restrict or even close services on the basis of safety and I did have to stand up for that. Funnily enough I didn't find that particularly difficult. I mean the Chief Exec did take me to one side and say, 'Are you telling me this is unsafe? Is there any other way?' and I said, 'Well not any other way you've come up with'. . . . It was very clear to me that a child had nearly died, and that's not hard is it?

(Dr. Vaisey, Riverdale Primary Care Trust)

And Dr. Alex Adrien captured precisely that logic of fiduciary propriety when he described his practice of turning 'rogue doctor':

There's times, and I'd always warn my Chief Executive about this, I'll be in a meeting or something . . . and I say 'Now I'm going to turn rogue doctor'. . . . Because there's a time as a medical director you have to be the conscience or the voice of the medical staff, to tell unpalatable and difficult facts to the executive. And the other way round. (Dr. Adrien, Greenborough Hospital Trust)

Thus, where one of the demands of fiduciary propriety is faithfully to represent the patient voice, another is to represent the clinician voice. We should be very clear that this does not mean simply representing clinicians. Medical leaders were quite emphatic that to represent clinicians was not their role. To them, to represent the clinician voice meant to vocalize the imperatives of clinical fiduciary responsibility. This they did forcibly with the power and authority of their own voice and position. As Dr. McGregor described it:

it's not a veto. But you have a strong voice; which you expect to be listened to.

(Dr. McGregor, Remembrance Hospitals Trust)

Moderating patient narratives

Inevitably, those who live in fiduciary roles eventually cultivate aspects of a fiduciary identity. Central to it is a sense of integrity intimately bound up with their capacity to act on their patients' behalf.

Fiduciary integrity implies a willingness to speak up for beneficiaries, even where it invites opprobrium or punishment or some other form of penalty. This is not the same as being moved by patient stories or patient needs. Fiduciary integrity is integrity as a discipline, and it arises from a recognition that patient beneficiaries assert a claim on the conscience as much as on the heart. Dr. Quinn distinguished the 'rational' discipline of integrity, which meant standing up to his Board, from the 'emotional' connection to patients grounded in narrative.

> I have a view of my own integrity, which I accept others may not share. But I hold it very strongly . . . . It's got me into occasional hot water with the Board, when I've said 'Look, you know I can't accept this; this; etc., etc., etc.'. . . . Rationalization and integrity are fine. But if I didn't allow myself to feel humanly affected by the personal accounts of some of the people's illness . . .
>
> (Dr. Quinn, Bankside Hospitals NHS Trust)

The fiduciary role supplies a moral warrant for a particular kind of communication: clinical, authoritative, emphatic, zealous, even bellicose on occasion. The danger, however, is that of excess: an excess of advocacy, an excess of clinical fervour, an excess of authority, an excess of assertiveness, an excess of rhetoric that mutates into symbolic violence or verbal aggression. Fiduciary propriety may become fiduciary impropriety. Perhaps (my data can only hint at this) a kind of fiduciary excess shapes and excuses the bullying of colleagues that is endemic in healthcare organizations [48–53].[15] I do not mean to imply that the participants in my study bullied their colleagues; rather, I suggest that in some circumstances fiduciary fervour can get out of hand. Fiduciary impropriety might be a partial explanation of some of those occasions when otherwise good and compassionate people behave with brutal disregard for the feelings of colleagues.

If the overuse of inflammatory rhetoric threatens to spark conflagration between colleagues, incautious or over-zealous advocacy can be even more hazardous for patients. Dr. Gulvin cited the controversy surrounding the MMR vaccine as an example of advocacy getting out of control. (The General Medical Council has since concluded that the claim the MMR vaccine was unsafe was founded in dishonest research, but at the start of the affair it appeared to be merely an example of imprudent campaigning.) [54–61] But even though they acknowledged the problems caused by excessive advocacy, medical directors generally tended to approve of fiduciary oratory. It seems to offer, as Dr. Gulvin reasoned, a singularly important benefit that could only be acquired at the cost of a smaller disadvantage.

---

[15] References 48–52 evidence how widespread bullying is in healthcare, and also how the serious harm done to professionals who work in bullying cultures has yet to be adopted as a topic of discussion in healthcare organizational ethics. Those two observations reveal a striking gap between the real harm that bullying represents and recognition by scholars and leaders of its moral significance. Compare, however, reference 53.

It's very important that [doctors] are advocates for [patients] because who else otherwise will be?. . . If we have people dying, as we did, from this unknown virus infection – HIV – it's absolutely right that the doctors looking after those patients, and the virologists, got up and . . . insisted something got done about it . . . . There's a price to be paid for that kind of advocacy model, and you saw it very well in the MMR controversy . . . . A very good example of somebody who passionately believed in something, that happened to be completely wrong. There was a disastrous effect on the health of people. So it can go badly wrong. But I would much rather have that . . . than to have people keep silent. (Dr. Gulvin, Stoneyhill and District NHS Trust)

Bureaucratic propriety: enacting impartial moral responsibility

Fiduciary propriety gives first priority to patients. Bureaucratic propriety, by contrast, gives first priority to the needs of the organization.

In this section I discuss how a bureaucratic mode of propriety functions alongside the fiduciary behaviours we have already examined, and consider how these two modes may occasionally conflict. I start by briefly outlining a concept of bureaucracy, and argue against the familiar charge that bureaucracy is a morally bankrupt domain. I describe the ethical comportment of the good bureaucrat, and then go on to discuss how behaviours described by the participants in the study are consistent with this portrait of a bureaucratic ethic.

In one of the great classics of sociology, Max Weber set out a typification of the bureau, of bureaucracy, and of the identity of the bureaucrat that has supplied the foundation for almost all subsequent analyses of bureaucracy. It is to Weber that we owe this understanding of an archetypical bureaucracy:

(i) an official jurisdictional area where the order of formal rules prevails;

(ii) governance through a strict hierarchy of office with precisely regulated avenues of appeal against decisions of lower officials;

(iii) meticulous record-keeping;

(iv) reliance on the specialized technical expertise of officials;

(v) the appointment of career bureaucrats who view their office as a vocation; and

(vi) the use by officials of extensive procedural expertise [62].

Weber's early analysis has supplied the impetus for a huge corpus of scholarship. The later contributions consider the maturation of bureaucracy, and its manifestation in contemporary public and corporate administration. So as to understand the demands of bureaucratic propriety in medical leadership, in the next section I sketch the discernible and largely agreed features of bureaucracy in the current age.

Contemporary conceptions of bureaucracy

Although some bureaux of state have quite closely fitted Weber's ideal type – the interwar British Civil Service perhaps – more commonly, bureaucratic organizations blend elements of bureaucracy and professional collegiality, bureaucracy and managerialist freedoms, or bureaucracy and entrepreneurship [63(p191)]. Importantly, bureaucracy is not the exclusive preserve of the great machineries of state administration. In contemporary societies, significant social and welfare functions are discharged by a plethora of private bodies providing services vital to a stable community. The extent to which these bodies are normatively expected to comply with requirements of administrative fairness depends in part on what goods they allocate. The more vital the good, the greater is the expectation of administrative fairness. Healthcare is just such a good, and healthcare insurers as well as providers are subject to just such normative expectations. Thus bureaucracy is perhaps best viewed as a set of principles and practices that may be found alongside others in a range of organizational settings. These principles and practices ensure that formal rationality is the dominant means of making and implementing decisions.

Where formal rationality prevails, responsibilities are discharged according to laws, codes, rules, guidelines, protocols and administrative procedures. The tools of formal rationality aim to settle in advance contentious principles of entitlement, stipulating what is relevant and what irrelevant to future claims. It follows that the central principle of administrative 'reasonableness' is that decision-makers take into account only those matters that are relevant, and all of those matters that are relevant [64].[16] Formal rationality is characterized above all else by adherence to impersonal administration: kith and kin, lords and paupers, friends and enemies are all equals under its rules. Formal rationality thus promises a degree of certainty in decision-making, a domain of apparent value neutrality, and administrative decisions based on formal equality for all.

The frank evils of formal rationality have been amply rehearsed, most famously by Hannah Arendt [65,66]. The value neutrality of formal rationality has supplied, in the twentieth century, the means by which horrible ends have been achieved. There are those who argue, therefore, that formal rationality implies the wholesale evacuation of morality from the bureaucratic domain. If the only value in bureaucracy is the pursuit of efficient means of administration, so the argument goes, then it has abandoned all claims on the judgement of ends. It is available to be a tool of whatever regime it serves, and both bureaucracy and the bureaucrat are morally destitute. But this is not, I shall argue shortly, the whole story.

A second criticism of formal rationality renders bureaucracy liable to the same objection as the law: which, as Anatole France famously observed, 'in its majestic equality forbids the rich as well as the poor to sleep under bridges, to beg in the streets, and to steal bread' [67]. Formal rationality promises the advantages of universalism; that is, it dispenses justice by treating all in the same class of claimants as alike. Furthermore, it resists particularism, refusing to treat claimants in the same class as in any way different or worthy of special consideration. In the final analysis, whether this is a good or a bad thing is a matter of perspective. An administrative system that resists the special pleading of privileged individuals or sub-groups will appear at times to be fair and equitable, a vehicle indeed of radical reform. In other circumstances, spurning the claims of the underprivileged who are unfairly lumped into the same class as the privileged, it will appear to be harsh and inflexible.

Although an efficient bureaucracy would seem to be an effective mechanism through which a ruling elite (either political or organizational) might exert its will, we should be wary of seeing it as a simple mechanism. First, as I observed in my earlier discussion of fiduciary propriety, all rules contain both a certain core and an uncertain penumbra. Bureaucratic rules are no different, so that bureaucratic governance is intrinsically reliant upon the exercise of bureaucratic discretion. How that discretion is exercised, and how it is controlled, are therefore matters of great importance to ruler and subjects alike. A great deal

---

[16] Legal principles first enunciated in the case identified in reference 64.

of the distrust of bureaucracy derives from a well-founded fear of bureaucratic discretions that it seems practically impossible to fetter.

Moreover, although formal rationality embodies value neutrality in the processes of administration, bureaucracies may be compelled to manage value conflicts that rulers are unwilling to resolve. Studies of welfare bureaucracies in action have noted that legislators are inclined to leave to bureaucratic discretion just those contentious issues most likely to provoke dissent. Far from settling value conflicts in advance, rulers deliberately leave them to be resolved by 'street-level' bureaucrats, either case-by-case or by locally developed rules [68,69]. The implications of this analysis for rationing healthcare are obvious. Organizations such as the UK's National Institute for Health and Clinical Excellence (NICE) exist to settle the value conflicts politicians would rather avoid; and doctors function as street-level bureaucrats resolving similar issues through bedside rationing [37,38].[17] It is the fate of the front-line bureaucrat to wrestle with the intractable conflicts that political and organizational elites avoid.

Weber's analysis of bureaucracy preceded a notable development of late twentieth-century public administration: extensive surveillance of bureaucratic action. Bureaucracy is now subject to broadly democratic apparatuses of accountability. Weber's analysis anticipated some of this, in his reference to avenues of appeal against bureaucratic decision, meticulous record-keeping and the separation of public monies from the private property of the official. But the constant and repetitive scrutiny by internal and external audit, evaluation, oversight, quality assurance, public consultation and other legal and bureaucratic mechanisms, all significant features of contemporary welfare bureaucracy, are recent developments.

In the field of ethics, the critics of bureaucracy are legion. The leading lights, including MacIntyre and Bauman, allege that bureaucracy is morally bankrupt [70,71]. Sympathetic analysts of bureaucracy are far fewer. Cooke, Du Gay, Hoggett and Minson [12,63,72–74] are among them, and these scholars see a positive ethical content in its values. Hoggett celebrated four positive clusters of administrative value underlying contemporary bureaucracy:

> [K]eep it visible and accountable, keep it lean and purposeful, keep it honest and fair, keep it robust and resilient . . . . Each set of core values has its own standard of failure – imperviousness (avoidance of responsibility, opacity of authority), waste, malversation (unfairness, bias, corruption) and catastrophe (risk, breakdown, collapse).[73(p165)]

The pro-bureaucracy analysts argue for the advantages of a formalist and impersonal ethic, and make the point that any substantive ethic set against it will contain its own moral risks and disadvantages. The extensive debate surrounding the ethics of bureaucracy cannot be further rehearsed here, but the ethical value of formal rationality and proceduralism will be observable in this chapter and the next.

Accepting the validity of a positive account of bureaucratic ethics enables us to move to the next part of this introduction to bureaucratic propriety: the ethical comportment of the bureaucrat.

---

[17] The function of NICE is to evaluate therapeutic options for their clinical and cost effectiveness and produce guidelines for their use in the NHS. On the politics of NICE see references 37 and 38.

In Weber's account the impersonal, expert, procedural and hierarchical character of bureaucratic reason and action is not treated as a symptom of moral deficiency; instead the bureau is represented as having its own distinct ethic of existence. The ethical attributes of the good bureaucrat – strict adherence to procedure, acceptance of hierarchical sub- and superordination, abnegation of personal moral enthusiasms, commitment to the purposes of the office – are the product of definite ethical practices and techniques. [72(p29)]

Practices of bureaucratic propriety

The figure of the good bureaucrat emerged out of this research, too, as a person of moral accomplishment. Bureaucratic propriety brings into leadership a commitment to definite moral values. One of those values is value-neutrality. It brings to leadership a commitment to definite principles of personal conduct. One of those principles is impersonality. And it expresses a commitment to definite administrative techniques. Such techniques discipline the leader to serve public moral values at odds with his own moral preferences. The characteristics associated with bureaucratic propriety are not an abandonment of authentic personhood, but an expression of a (frequently highly valued) identity:

> a positive moral achievement requiring the mastery of a difficult ethical milieu and practice. They are the product of definite ethical techniques and routines – 'declaring' one's personal interest, developing professional relations with one's colleagues, subordinating one's ego to procedural decision-making – through which individuals develop the disposition and ability to conduct themselves according to the ethos of bureaucratic office. [75]

My argument concerning bureaucratic propriety is not that moral leaders in the UK NHS should embrace a public sector ethos. It is a much larger argument. I propose that bureaucratic propriety is a coherent set of ethical techniques that help moral leaders to establish a compelling organizational moral narrative.

What is described below is the enactment of bureaucratic virtuosity. There is, first of all, corporate comportment, an acceptance of the disciplines of collective decision-making. We see next a 'non-sectarian comportment': that is, independence of ties to families, friends, factions and all other self-interested groups; and commitment to the purposes of office, independent of personal passions or political preferences [72(p44)]. We also see expert comportment, the use of technical knowledge and procedural expertise in service of ethical decision-making. And finally we observe a comportment of accountability, perhaps one of the most fundamental moral responsibilities that it falls on leaders to discharge.

Corporate comportment

In this study, bureaucratic propriety became most visible when it acted as a constraint on the rampant Hippocratic advocacy sometimes associated with fiduciary propriety. The core values of bureaucratic propriety were consistently likened to responsible stewardship of collective resources.

> I think [doctors] need to understand – particularly in a publicly funded organization – that there is a stewardship that we all share. We all share the stewardship of the public purse, very important. People say that money isn't health. It is . . .. And there's clearly the stewardship of quality. And the stewardship of access; and so on.
>
> (Dr. Richard Rosenberg, St. Frideswide Hospitals NHS Trust)

The first aspect of bureaucratic propriety that I consider here is the discipline in acknow-ledging, and binding oneself to, the corporate interest. Corporate entities matter, morally, because they are a tangible representation of collective need. Corporate comportment matters because it enables individuals to transcend personal or sectional interests, and put the corporate entity first. It means contributing one's expertise (in ways we examine below) to a collective decision and then supporting the decision. And it means adhering to the normative expectations that govern organizational relationships, having due regard for the responsibilities of office even if one lacks personal regard for the office-holder.

Dr. Gulvin accepted that the Trust Board had a responsibility to express this kind of moral leadership in its own behaviour, and had been impressed by the two principles adumbrated by a senior colleague:

> [I]f we're going to succeed, then what we walk out of the room having agreed, we have to go out and deliver. And so this is about being corporate. Agreement is agreement, and we can't leave rooms and meetings and not do what we've said we would do . . . . The second one is that we should always speak well of each other. In other words, in a large public service like this which has its own difficulties, you can't allow internal dissension to distract from doing the job in hand.
> (Dr. Gulvin, Stoneyhill and District NHS Trust)

Bureaucratic discipline, Dr. Vivian Vaisey pointed out, required commitment and assur-ance. Corporate loyalty did not mean spinelessly following orders. It meant having the courage of one's convictions, and being prepared to participate in a continuing process of 'challenging and stretching and discursive debates' about corporate values and plans.

> I understand now what it means to be corporate and retain your integrity; which, as a clinician, I would probably have thought was a very long stretch! I think clinically if you work for an organization, you have to be prepared to identify yourself as a member of that organization; and that means espousing certain values and plans. GPs particularly are notorious for being kind of bags of ferrets . . . . When I started I thought [corporate loyalty] was something that you paid lip service to . . . I don't think I appreciated how those values and plans are hammered out . . . and people decide that 'A is what is to be done. . .'. Through that debate and discussion you reach a point where you can say, 'A is to be done – I have these reservations'. Either it's recognized that you have those reservations and they need to be integrated into [the solution], or you need to be having a discussion with somebody to say, 'I cannot go out and [implement this]'. It's that thing that says you are open about your problems, and you have to resolve them. But you cannot keep them until you're on the [public] stage [representing the organization]. It's that commitment to the organization that says you'll be honest. But equally that trust, that you will work together on it. (Dr. Vaisey, Riverdale Primary Care Trust)

Corporate loyalty is owed to organizations because they are the repository of collective expectations and shared goods. It is this overarching collective interest – not loyalty to the institution as such – that justifies asking clinicians to compromise their specialty loyalties, advocacy of behalf of special groups of patients, and professional differences.

In so far as 'the corporation' represents the sum of common interests, serving 'the corporation' can be a meaningful and productive way of serving the common good. Problems arise, however, where the organizational good becomes an end in itself, and leaders defer to the needs of the organization ahead of the needs of patients. This is clearly a concern for clinician leaders working in private healthcare businesses, where the interests of financial stakeholders in making a profit may conflict with the interests of patients in consuming healthcare resources. It is equally a risk for clinical leaders in publicly or charitably owned organizations such as those in the NHS. Here, the interests of employees and other stakeholders in organizational continuity may come into conflict with changing patient needs or with the interests of a wider health economy; and the system has witnessed more than once how clinical failure has been concealed in misguided attempts to protect organizational reputation [11,76].

An excess of loyalty to the organization as a certain sort of entity, or an excessive focus on competitive success, can do grave harm to the moral interests the organization exists to serve. So it is that corporate loyalty, a component of bureaucratic propriety, has to be balanced by fiduciary advocacy, a component of fiduciary propriety.

'Non-sectarian' comportment

Dr. Quinn had discerned early in his career that a 'non-sectarian' technical rationality was a right and proper way to proceed, but it was not his preferred way of being. Bureaucratic propriety was plainly, for him, a self-disciplined performance of responsibility. When we spoke, he described one of the episodes in his journey to becoming a medical leader:

> I was asked to undertake a project looking at the background to a new piece of equipment, whether it was appropriate, whether there were alternatives . . . I presented a paper to my colleagues. And they all – there was dead silence! And then one said 'Have you ever thought of becoming a manager?'

> *What was it that they saw in you?*

> I've thought seriously about it . . . I think undoubtedly it was the logical approach, the completeness. And the failure to be swayed by 'decision-making-by-decibel-level', which is something my consultants and colleagues employed. I just thought about it and said 'This is the issue. Here are the problems. That breaks down into this, bmm, bmm, bmm, bmm, bmm. Therefore, what I suggest is the following. . . . It's strange because I've always hated detailed process and I still hate it with a vehemence. (Dr. Quinn, Bankside Hospitals NHS Trust)

'Decision-making-by-decibel-level' was supplanted by 'decision-making-by-technical-rationality'. In Quinn's example, technical rationality had the effect of subordinating the sectional preferences of influential consultant colleagues to the clinical needs of the organization. Quinn's ends were those of clinical effectiveness, and using technical rationality those ends prevailed. In other circumstances, a similar technical rationality will serve other priorities. It is a condition of participating in a bureaucratic order that leaders are expected to further the ends of those in a position to determine what they should be. Dr. Gulvin remarked of his Trust Board members:

> [T]heir concern primarily has to be driven by what the Minister wants. And currently the Minister wants waiting times reduced, he wants financial balance, and he wants inequalities tackled. Those are the big three. So the conversation starts with 'Well, what's the contribution of this to reducing waiting times?' 'What's the contribution of this to reducing inequalities?' 'What's the contribution of this to achieving (or not) financial balance?' – Decisions are shaped by those as much as by any purist argument around the relative [clinical] merits of a particular programme. (Dr. Quinn, Bankside Hospitals NHS Trust)

It is a feature of non-sectarian technical rationality that, whilst it is a definite ethical value in and of itself, it locates 'political' values as external to it. The value that bureaucracy places on value-neutrality has spawned a familiar narrative, the cautionary tale of the evil done by those who are blindly following orders. But there is also virtue in deferring to the purposes of beneficent organizations, in accepting that justifiable rules serve to procure the greatest good for the greatest number so long as they are consistently applied. Moreover, compliance with bureaucratic decision procedures serves to limit idiosyncratic moral judgement. Bureaucratic decision procedures quite literally 'rule out' expressions of individual conviction, moral desert or patient worth.

The value of value-neutrality serves to *support* purely clinical decision-making, at least as much as it threatens to subvert it through implementing ministerial or managerial edict. In the last chapter, we considered Dr. Woodhouse's example of deciding the allocation of discretionary funds for non-standard treatment. Dr. Woodhouse has his own views, as a Christian and public servant, on what he would like the NHS to fund. But this was not the basis on which he was expected to exercise his discretion. He and his colleagues had adopted the ethical framework commonly used by such committees, one that aims to exclude from deliberation potentially discriminatory non-medical criteria [77–81].[18] Whilst being apparently value free, this framework nevertheless reinforces adherence to the medical values of the organization. It exists to ensure that all applicants receive equal consideration according to medically relevant criteria. Accepted and internalized, it guides the 'street-level bureaucrats' in the proper exercise of their discretion.

> We try to have a very simple ethical framework around our decision-making. The treatment requested; is there evidence that it will do any good? A remarkable number of them don't. Is there any evidence that it will actually do harm? Just recently someone asked for hypnotherapy for weight reduction. Not very good evidence around that, but the patient also had bi-polar affective disorder and manic depression and it's actually contraindicated in that. So there you would have absolutely clear harm. Look at patient choice. And then the other big one that we look at is ... equity or equality but it's really about, if we make a decision to say 'Yes' what's the impact on the rest of that population? So if you said that any ... couple who've got sickle cell trait could have pre-implantation [genetic diagnosis] you would be [obliged to provide that to everyone]. [82][19]
>
> (Dr. Woodhouse, Meadborough Primary Care Trust)

A comportment of expertise

Fiduciary propriety demands partiality and vigorous argumentation in favour of sectional interests. Bureaucratic propriety, conversely, demands impartiality and the contribution of expertise to collective decision-making. Dr. Gulvin made apparent the difference between the two modes when he described how he contributed as a clinical scientist to Board discussions.

> Although I work in a particular clinical area I'm not there to represent the patients with heart disease or the patients with depression or the patients with learning disabilities, I'm there to assist the Board in making defensible decisions . . .. From time to time Boards are asked to

---

[18] Local NHS committees with essentially the same function have gone under different names: e.g. 'Interventions Not Normally Funded' (INNF); 'Exceptional Treatment Arrangements' (ETA). They tended to converge, however, on similar ethical frameworks, in part in order to comply with legal requirements. See references 77–81.

[19] The NHS Sickle Cell & Thalassaemia Screening Programme offers antenatal and newborn screening. See reference 82. The only choice following antenatal genetic diagnosis is whether to abort. The example exposes the limitations of localism in the NHS: if the costs of PGD and IVF for thalassaemia carriers were shared nationally, they would not be prohibitive.

fund extremely expensive individual treatment and you have to make a judgement about that. I'm able ... to bring to bear on that a scientific approach ... the methodology of an N=1 trial .... If that treatment has demonstrably worked for that individual then it doesn't matter what the rest of the literature says, it's probably important for that individual to continue treatment. There is demonstrable benefit that will cost the Board X-amount so the Board has to then decide whether it's willing to do that. Equally if ... that individual is not benefiting from treatment, and there'd be no worthwhile improvement, then despite there being a wealth of evidence from larger trials that it was in general worthwhile ... there's no point in the Board spending it's scarce resources on that. (Dr. Gulvin, Stoneyhill and District NHS Trust)

What kind of expertise is to be found in the 'comportment of expertise' associated with bureaucratic propriety? It is not scientific expertise alone that medical directors contribute. It is the ability to make a procedural judgement informed by technical considerations. This expertise, and the need for it, is closely associated with the phenomenon of standardization in healthcare.

Timmermans and Berg have observed that standardization in healthcare is replacing 'disciplinary objectivity' with 'mechanical objectivity'. Disciplinary objectivity 'typifies powerful, specialist disciplinary communities', whose members are trusted to make expert decisions on a case by case basis. Mechanical objectivity displaces trust in experts 'by trust in mechanical rules, procedures and numbers' developed and enforced by the disciplinary community [83].

Standardization requires clinical and scientific acumen, to assess the evidence base and identify the optimum approach; and it requires procedural acumen, to codify and implement standards of care in practice. Weber saw resort to technical and procedural expertise as characteristic of bureaucracy. From a bureaucratic perspective, the fact that case-by-case professional judgement produces inconsistent outcomes presents an obvious problem. The bureaucratic solution is to encode approved technical expertise in guidelines and protocols, and hold professionals accountable for implementing these standards. In such a system, proper and improper professional behaviour is defined by acceptance of and compliance with the rules.

Standardization and bureaucratic propriety are thus close cousins. Standardization calls for a bureaucratic mode of propriety; bureaucratic propriety expresses the ethical values embedded in standardization.

Many creative (and frustrated) clinicians will contend that making a fetish of protocols is not the best means of achieving high standards. But the moral aims of evidence-based, protocol-guided medicine are clear: greater medical benefit, reduced medical harm, cost-effective care and better translation of research findings into practice [84]. It is unsurprising therefore that Dr. Patrick Phelps considered his work on introducing treatment protocols to have been a significant ethical achievement during what had been a difficult period for his organization:

If you look back over the last few years, would you say that you've had some important ethical wins?

Ethical wins: yes ... I've set up a [life-threatening condition X] Working Party. We've set up protocols for the management of [life-threatening condition X] across the Trust. We now have a uniform practice ... I've written a number of [other] protocols which are working .... You don't want to spend a lot of time on things that aren't important. But if it's high profile, with large volumes, that's the stuff you've got to try and get into.

(Dr. Phelps, Valleyshire University Hospitals Trust)

A comportment of accountability

Protocols hold out the promise of control over future action, and control over others' exercise of their discretion. They also serve to manage the demands of accountability.

A comportment of accountability is not unique to bureaucratic propriety. All normative expectations, we noted in Chapter 3, contain assumptions about, and an insistence on, accountability in a loose sense. This insistence may be expressed in many different ways, through different mechanisms and in different social relationships. Organizational hierarchies, however, contain expectations of accountability that are as often as not expressed and vindicated through bureaucratic propriety.

The first discipline of bureaucratic propriety is taking responsibility for ensuring that difficult decisions are made in accordance with expectations of fair and reasonable process.

> You have to make decisions that people are uncomfortable with. It's inevitable. If you've got 4,000 staff not every decision's going to be one that people like. And hey-ho, that's part of the job. But I think if it's open on what basis you've made it, and what considerations you've taken into account, and what consultation you've had, what kind of awareness you have of the downside of what you're proposing, then I think most people can live with it.
>
> (Dr. Dillon, Five Bridges Mental Health Trust)

The second discipline is holding oneself personally answerable for decisions in which one has participated. This is aptly described as a discipline. It is not hard to be accountable for a decision that will benefit vulnerable people. It is extremely uncomfortable to be held accountable for a decision that will deprive them of something they value, even if it has been made on the basis that it is the lesser of two evils.

> Well at one level I feel it's, it is my job to do that. Having come to that decision, it is my job to try and make sure that people understand why I've come to that decision; and try and encourage them to accept that I've come to that decision for good reasons; and to question me. Not 'This is the best solution, you've got to lump it guys'. I tend to talk through the thought processes, and the balancing act that we've had to try and achieve. And I do see it as my role because [these decisions have unpleasant consequences for clinicians and patients].
>
> (Dr. Ingrid Iliffe, Graveldene NHS Trust)

We started this discussion of bureaucratic propriety with consideration of corporate comportment; and we noted Dr. Vaisey's conviction that clinical leadership calls for commitment to the organization, alongside genuine honesty and trust between colleagues. The theme of honesty and trust between colleagues brings us to the third propriety: that of collegiality.

Collegial propriety: enacting norms of community

Fiduciary propriety gives first priority to patients; bureaucratic propriety gives first priority to the needs of the medical corporation; and we shall shortly see how collegial propriety gives first priority to the needs of the medical 'collegium'. In this section I start by considering the meaning of collegiality and what this implies for the practices of collegial propriety. I then examine the significance of collegial propriety in moral medical leadership.

The notion of collegiality can be traced back to antiquity, where references to the 'collegium' of the priesthood can be found in the works of the Roman philosopher and statesman Cicero. Following its adoption by the scholar-priests of Oxford, the values of the 'collegium' gradually came to be associated with the values of academic community [85].

The meaning of collegiality has broadened in contemporary use, to signify the informal reciprocal relationships and formal internal regulations governing communities of professional practitioners. Contemporary references to collegiality in medicine emanate from diverse sources, but have much in common with Weber's sociological analysis of collegiality.

In Weber's scheme, his analysis of collegiality was offered as a contrast to his analysis of bureaucracy. Collegiality was the organizational structure that best served the emergent professions, while bureaucracy was the organizational structure that best served corporations and the state. Since Weber's time the professions have become central to welfare bureaucracies; so what now differentiates collegiate from bureaucratic modes of organization? Waters has characterized the relationship between bureaucracy, collegiality and professionalization, as follows:

> some characteristics are common to the ideal-typical bureaucracy and the ideal-typical collegiate organization: each emphasizes technical competence and rationality in pursuit of ends, each has a highly specialized task structure, and each has a professional career structure that embodies security of tenure.[20] The crucial area of difference is the *structure of authority relations*. Collegiality emphasizes processes of equality, consensus and autonomy in which decisions emerge as a collective process and are morally binding only on members; bureaucracy emphasizes processes of hierarchy, delegation, and accountability in which decisions are matters of individual responsibility and are imperatives for subordinates. [86] (emphasis added)

Bureaucracy and collegiality thus differ, crucially, in the area of moral authority; that is, how they uphold normative expectations and render individuals accountable to a joint enterprise. In that sense, they are different moral schemes. To lead colleagues towards a goal in a collegial culture entails marshalling the activity of presumptively equal and autonomous professionals through collaborative decisions they feel morally obliged to accept. In a bureaucratic culture, contrastingly, leadership entails mobilizing the resources of hierarchical command to implement decisions that emanate from the top of the organizational hierarchy, and which may or may not be consistent with a collegiate consensus. The difficulty is of course that while we can differentiate these two moral schemes in principle, in medical practice they are coterminous. The collegial culture of medicine intersects with the bureaucratic culture of healthcare corporations. While collegiality and bureaucracy can serve to reinforce each other, their demands also on occasion collide.

Collegiality in medicine

Collegial authority has been extensively explored in sociologies of the professions. For many sociological observers, the single most significant feature of a profession is the prerogative of self-regulation [24,87–92]. This prerogative is claimed by the 'collegium' on the grounds that those with specialist knowledge and expertise are best held to account by their peers. The single greatest failing of collegial bodies, observers note, is the failure to properly hold their members to account.

Self-regulation is a social good, proponents of professional collegiality argue, because it is grounded in aspirations to excellence; and it is necessitated, they claim, by the esoteric knowledge base of professional collegial communities. Sceptical observers, Freidson among

---

[20] Not so in modern bureaucracies.

them, counter that the more enticing benefits of self-regulation are maintaining profes-sional monopoly, avoiding external determination of the standards of practice and minim-izing external scrutiny of actual performance.

Freidson argued that aspects of collegial organization (the work setting) and collegial culture (a 'clinical mentality') were major impediments to effective medical self-regulation. The 'collegium' signally failed, in his observation, to protect patients from incompetent professionals. Freidson's findings have been echoed ever since in socio-logical, professional and governmental inquiries into failures of professional perform-ance, and failures in professionals' management of professional performance. The grim catalogue of ineptitude, indifference, imperviousness, protective practice, inappropriate blame, rebuffed whistleblowers, victimization and failure of moral repair compiled in the forty years since Freidson published his work makes for depress-ing reading [93–120].[21] In light of it, it is all the more disconcerting to realize that a similar story has been told since at least the 1930s when Carr-Saunders and Wilson reported the collegial rationale by which British doctors avoided confronting problem colleagues and adopted informal sanctions to deal with them (ref. 121, cited in ref. 87, p. 161).

It is tempting to conclude from all of these studies and reports that collegiality is a vice to be extirpated from medical practice. But it is hard to know whether it is collegiality itself or a regrettable permutation of collegiality that is the problem. Equally, it is difficult to assess whether a non-collegial bureaucracy would have served patients any better. Perhaps the collective and collaborative loyalties of medical collegiality have allowed more or different problems to be identified and managed, where the hierarchical controls of a clinical bureaucracy would have suppressed some or all of them? Perhaps collegiality affords compensatory benefits to doctors and patients that bureaucracy would deny them? In the terminology of this chapter, is it collegial propriety or collegial impropriety that is to blame?

The problem is that we have no controls with which to compare the findings from studies of medical professionalism. There is therefore little way of knowing whether collegiality's failures are intrinsic to it, whether they are an avoidable by-product, or whether collegiality is, overall, better or worse for patients than the alternatives.

Since collegiality remains, for good or ill, central to the organization of medical practice we need to consider what normative expectations it embodies, and how these appear to be enforced.

The reciprocal vices and virtues of collegiality

In her review of research into the management of incompetent doctors, sociologist Marilynn Rosenthal described the dualistic role of collegial culture, how it sustains doctors for good and ill through the arduous demands of medical practice:

> A circle of esteem and mutual respect. A circle of support in the face of great responsibility for patient care. A circle of comfort in a stressful work environment. A protective retreat in the face of difficult cases, complications, and inevitable fallibility. And then there is the other side of collegiality. Closing ranks against outsiders, including patients. Reticence to criticize and

---

[21] Inquiry reports are identified in references 93–102. See references 103–102 for further analyses.

protection of the questionable. How to balance the absolutely legitimate need for collegiality with the need to help (and stop) faltering fumbling and failing fellow doctors [*sic*]. [122]

I have quoted Rosenthal because she aptly captures something of the emotional tenor of collegiality, as well as hinting at its many meanings. But there is also a suggestive imbalance in her description. When she writes of its goodness, collegiality seems spontaneous and unforced, an empathetic response to the plight of colleagues. When she writes of the nastiness in collegiality, it seems deliberate, a knowing abdication of responsibility that results in serious health risk and moral harm to patients. There is no doubt that this picture is correct in part, but significant elements are missing. One is the 'moral discipline' involved in conjuring up positive collegiality, a practice that I believe is more than a non-moral habit of 'mere affability'. A second is the way that virtuous collegiality contributes to care for patients.

A less jaundiced view than Rosenthal's would be that the practice of medicine is underpinned by the way in which reciprocal collegial expectations bind medical practitioners into a community committed to the pursuit of a shared ideal. Those reciprocal expectations serve to elicit positive behaviours in pursuit of the shared ideal, and they constrain negative behaviours that might damage it. As such, they promote patient interests, and protect patients from harm. Collegiality imports into mere fellowship a set of normative expectations and reactive attitudes that benefit colleagues, patients and the enterprise as a whole. Collegial propriety is then the behaviour through which the positive moral benefits of collegiality are secured. Mangiardi and Pellegrino expressed a similar thought when they argued, from the perspective of virtue ethics, that the pursuit of (academic) medicine imposed specifically collegial ethical obligations on its participants:

> The source of obligations derives from the ethical constraints of the ideal pursued, responsibility to the society to which the groups belongs, and the individual's obligation to maximize efforts to fulfil the stated goals of the group . . . Collegiality derives from certain obligations that are in fact duties, not from camaraderie, fellowship, or even familial feeling. Only when the duties of collegiality are observed in a gracious, caring spirit of mutual respect, friendship, or family does duty become transformed into virtue. But even without virtue, the moral strictures of collegial duty apply. [123,125][22]

Moral leadership in medicine is thus, in part, concerned with mobilizing the moral ideals associated with a supportive and productive community of practice, working for patient benefit. In this chapter, where the focus is on the proprieties as they become apparent in organizational narratives around best use of resource, we see moral leaders harnessing the collegial ideal in broadly two ways. In some interactions with colleagues they emphasized mutuality of engagement, upholding expectations of professional civility such as reciprocity, consensual decision-making and respect for multi-professional interdependence. In other interactions, they were attentive to the shared meanings that bind practitioners in tacit understandings of the moral dimension of their work.

Practices of collegial propriety

The central criticism of collegiality is a telling one: it is that professional colleagues attend to one another's interests and needs and not those of the people they serve. This is telling

---

[22] Their view echoes MacIntyre's claim that we formulate moral goals by locating 'goods internal to a practice'.

because at the heart of collegial propriety is indeed the practice of truly attending to colleagues, and to others who participate in the joint enterprise. To attend in this way means to hear, recognize and respect the needs of those with whom one works in relationships of mutual interdependence. To attend to colleagues in such a manner is to act with collegial propriety; to attend only to *colleagues* with recognition and respect, to the exclusion of others, is to act with collegial impropriety.

Attentiveness to reciprocity

Leaders in a collegiate culture are first among equals, fellows in a shared enterprise. It is right, then, that they demonstrate an ethic of reciprocity in their own actions. Reciprocity here means doing that which you expect others to do: voicing the concerns of the community, and standing up to be counted when it matters. As Dr. Seddon expressed it in a military metaphor:

> You're not sitting up there and saying 'Go on, there you go over the trenches but I'm not following . . . I'll be standing in safety several miles back while you all get shot, and it's different for me'.
> (Dr. Seddon, Saxonvale University Hospitals Trust)

This symbolic willingness to participate in potential moral hazard signifies the mutuality that collegial propriety is built upon.

Attentiveness to expertise

In theory, the project of improving health services would not seem to present much of an ethical dilemma. Better healthcare would appear to be self-evidently good. But in practice, there are many morally loaded decisions to be made. There are questions of priority: for example, the different weight to be given to 'output' targets, maintaining patient dignity, or reducing rates of hospital-acquired infection when each is easier to achieve at the expense of others. There are questions about standards: for instance, identifying what ought to be achieved with the resources available; what care, in the circumstances, is 'good enough' care. There are questions about dissent: for example, whether objectors are fiduciary advocates begging to be heard, or self-interested opponents positioning themselves on the moral high ground. And there are questions about what a reasonable compromise might be: whether the morally praiseworthy ends are sufficient to justify the costs in achieving them. Collegial propriety demands that such questions be answered, as far as possible, by seeking a consensus.

Dr. Matthew McGregor described how he set about negotiating improvements in services by assiduously attending to colleagues:

> [T]here's no point in having great ideas that you just can't deliver. And the biggest thing that determines whether you can achieve it or not is whether you can win over support of the people in the organization. In my case, particularly the doctors, but wider than that . . . . The way I do that is to have informal discussions, conceptual discussions, with the people I work closely with and say, 'Look, how do you think this will go down? Did that work well with the consultant body? Would they support this? Do you think there'll be a lot of resistance? Who do you think the resistance groups will be? Is there any way we can meet that?'
> (Dr. McGregor, Remembrance Hospitals Trust)

Dr. Ingrid Iliffe spoke of navigating the sensitivities inherent in a collegial culture based on specialist expertise, equality between peers, professional autonomy and consensual decision-making. She had sought to maintain a stable balance between giving support and setting high expectations. In common with several other medical directors, she believed her clinical experience in a 'support' speciality (by which I mean specialties such as haematology, radiology, palliative care and intensive care) had taught her how to elicit collegiality in clinical collaboration.

> We work with virtually every other specialty in the hospital . . . going round helping and advising and working in collaboration with other consultants . . . . We're always having to tread quite carefully, not offending people, or seeming to be muscling in, or telling people how to do their job properly . . . I was seen as somebody who was honest, who didn't tend to be judgemental, was generally supportive, but also not afraid to tackle the difficult situations.
>
> (Dr. Iliffe, Graveldene NHS Trust)

Compare Dr. Iliffe's description with leadership in a bureaucratic mode. There, the emphasis lies on following procedure, following instructions from superiors and maintaining order. Collegial cultures, and collegial propriety, normatively expect individuals to take responsibility for the ideals of the enterprise. Because bureaucracy emphasizes regularity and order, rule-breaking is always a matter of concern, notwithstanding any claim that breaking the rules has beneficial effects. With its emphasis on individual responsibility, collegial propriety is perhaps more tolerant of rule-breaking so long as it is in the service of the good. Bureaucratic propriety is a source of standards and protocols; collegial propriety defends the ideals of the enterprise and permits forgiveness of those who fulfil them in idiosyncratic ways.

> I have a couple of people here . . . who drive me absolutely round the bend. Because they'll do things all the wrong ways, they'll break all the rules; but actually they deliver phenomenally well . . . . You can be enormously forgiving of people who are slightly maverick, slightly eccentric, do things the wrong way, providing they're not doing anything that's dangerous, or anything that's terrible. Because they give rise to enormous innovation and service delivery, and they do everything you want them to do. I think you can be very, very forgiving of that.
>
> (Dr. Adrien, Greenborough Hospital Trust)

So long as mutuality is present in collegial relations, much difficult negotiating can be accomplished. It is when mutuality breaks down that behaviour begins to be judged unacceptable, and the practices of collegial propriety are liable to be displaced by a more authoritarian approach.

> Where I've found it most difficult is with a small number of individuals who appear to be on board, agree with you what the problems are, agree to work with you to take them forward and just never keep their end of the bargain. You realize after a period of time that you've been very skilfully and very carefully manipulated . . . and that it's extremely unlikely that you'll ever effect any lasting change by consensus. The only way that you'll get lasting change and the situation fixed is by a much more aggressive performance management approach, which isn't my style at all and therefore I hate it. (Dr. Adrien, Greenborough Hospital Trust)

Negotiations of mutuality must sometimes give way to an insistence that individuals acknowledge they are participants in, and accountable to, a joint enterprise.

Attentiveness to voice

Medical practitioners have normative expectations around interaction with members of their practice community, and also around interactions with those outside their practice community. These expectations are a component of collegial propriety, and may be a source of collegial impropriety. They define who may say what to whom; how it may be said; and who will be listened to. These are, morally speaking, important matters. Who may say what to whom and be heard indicates what interests are believed to be morally significant, and who is worthy of respect.

Attentiveness to voice means acknowledging the community's view of what matters, what deserves attention and what should be done. Some voices carry special weight; others may be silenced. Who participates in healthcare decisions, and how, is a contentious matter. More voices than ever – patients, carers, nurses, members of the 'multi-professional team' as well as doctors – seek to be heard, and speak in a sometimes discordant chorus.

If collegiality places a higher value on expertise than on status, then collegial propriety implies that a person with the right clinical expertise, irrespective of status, ought to be recognized and respected for their ability to contribute to the clinical enterprise. The demands of true collegial propriety thus become visible in collective deliberations: in clinicians from different specialties respecting differing expertise; in senior clinicians paying attention to junior healthcare professionals; in practitioner experts paying attention to patient experts, recognizing them as partners in, while not full members of, the practice community.

In Dr. Fox's organization, as elsewhere, nurses had felt belittled and excluded from full participation in the caring enterprise. Aside from the harm to them as individuals, this had damaged efforts to bring about organizational improvements on behalf of patients. Dr. Fox and senior colleagues had embarked on an extended organizational development project that attempted to address both the underlying cause in status and professional distinctions and the effects this had on patient care. Fox reflected on how issues of voice and status became apparent to the executive in a series of workshops and seminars:

> [the executive team] had to learn to shut up, which was quite difficult. You would often find that the finance director, the director of nursing and myself, say, would do most of the talking and then [the facilitator would] say 'Shut up' … [One time] one of the ward sisters started to speak and her voice was quavering. She really was extremely nervous about speaking her mind about what the problem was on the ward. I was struck by that. I just thought 'Wow. What is going on in this organisation that the ward sister's nervous?'
>
> (Dr. Fox, The Three Spires Hospital)

Dr. Vivian Vaisey spoke to a different circle of exclusion, this time of GP's from strategic decision-making within the PCT. In a period when many difficult decisions had to be made, the PCT opened the debate to local clinicians.

> It's been a seminal moment in my career really. We held a clinical pathway event to disseminate this strategy to clinicians, and people were saying before, 'I bet you get loads of managers there. [Clinicians] won't come.' … Actually we had between 80 and 100 clinicians and they were just, it was as if they couldn't get the words out fast enough in the workshops. They were brimming over. I think this feeling that they know what is right, and that they haven't been able to communicate on the service level what they know, seems to me to be a very powerful one. Their wish to participate constructively in that discussion seems very powerful as well.
>
> (Dr. Vaisey, Riverdale Primary Care Trust)

Finally, Dr. Quinn reflected on the complexity of attending to patient voices during protracted political and legal battles that had accompanied his Trust's attempts to reconfigure local services. During this process, there had been extensive local consultation. But opinion had been strongly divided around the best way to reorganize several hospitals. By and large, expert opinion was in favour of concentrating services on fewer sites for reasons of efficiency and safety. Popular opinion was in favour of maintaining dispersed services in the interests of local access. Collegial propriety invited the question of who qualified as an 'expert' in the 'enterprise', and where responsibility and accountability lay. According the right weight to lay and expert opinion was where Dr. Quinn located the ethical challenge:

> (Interviewer) *I'm wondering what for you gives this work an ethical flavour?*
>
> Trying to improve patient care, and recognizing that patients have a sensible voice . . . . Ethically, that's where the whole issue comes from . . . . Do you translate that into saying that the patient view of what should happen is the absolute driver? I always say to clinicians: 'That's not to say that you're abdicating your professional responsibilities. You're here as a healthcare professional. We've got to take a view, [but one] which is hugely informed by the patient view.' To say we won't take any notice of it is stupid. (Dr. Quinn, Bankside Hospitals NHS Trust)

To the extent that collegial propriety involves negotiating the boundaries of inclusion in decisions, it also implies that once voices have been heard and views considered, the outcome should be treated as morally binding. Dr. Jonathan Jay and his colleagues had faced several rounds of opposition to their attempts to implement 'The Hospital at Night', a national policy reorganizing how patients were cared for overnight necessitated by the reduction in junior doctors' hours of work. Recognizing the fiduciary quality in the objections that had been raised, but still needing to make progress, Dr. Jay's latest plan was:

> a very detailed, targeted consultation. We're going to pick off the groups that are making the most noise and meet with them and say 'This is what we're doing, what's the problem with it?' Instead of allowing the noise, we actually pin them down to what are the problems with this? And then address them one by one . . . .. And that way at the end of the three months I will be confident that we've one, got a rota that'll work; two, we've consulted fully; and three, we've done everything we can to mitigate the risks. Then I'd be prepared to take them on.
>
> (Dr. Jay, The Charter NHS Trust)

Attentiveness to meaning

Medical leaders, I noted in Chapter 1, are 'boundary crossers', passing and re-passing across the borders of several practice communities: management, doctors, nurses, other health professionals, local politicians and expert patients for example. The moral narratives that bind these different communities – around the basic good of health – have much in common. But they also differ in their emphasis, and in their expression. For senior non-clinician managers, the emphasis resides in efficiency, and the idiom in which their organizational narratives are expressed is words such as targets, conversion rates and follow-up ratios. For clinical leaders, the emphasis is meeting individual clinical need, and their fiduciary aims are expressed in the idiom of clinical case management or patient narrative. Interpretation, translation and attentiveness to meaning are thus central to the task of leading through collegial propriety.

We have seen throughout this chapter that language and propriety are intimate associates. Improper language invites the suspicion that what is afoot is improper action. We noted earlier Dr. Vaisey's concern that the language of service 'pressures' was used to refer to 'an old lady who doesn't get meals on wheels on Sunday and hasn't got anybody else to cook for her' or 'a patient who's dying who's not going to get night nursing'. She reflected on how her organization had endeavoured to protect and promote patient interests in a difficult period of change, but provoked disquiet among clinicians by describing their aims in the wrong language.

> We ended up with things clinicians would want to do, expressed in terms that would make them want to walk away from it . . . . General practitioners understand what the problems are. They know the issues around waiting times, around unnecessary follow ups . . . . They would have subscribed to that. But: 'to give them that target'; 'to change that ratio'. . .! We encapsulated the problem in management terms, and my God, we had a turbulent time.
>
> (Dr. Vaisey, Riverdale Primary Care Trust)

As Dr. McGregor observed:

> If we were asking [doctors] to be more efficient in terms of reducing the quality of service, yes, they would think that [we're asking them to do something a bit unethical] . . . . So you've got to go in there, and you've got to say, 'Actually, first and foremost, this is about providing the best care we can, and as efficiently as we can'. So yes, there is an ethical issue there. I'm on the side of the doctors in terms of clinical quality, and the management in terms of efficiency, and [my aim is] bringing them together. (Dr. McGregor, Remembrance Hospital Trust)

Concluding remarks

Here I have explored three modes of 'proper conduct' governing relationships of moral responsibility in healthcare organizations. I have shown how propriety is found in leadership behaviours that give expression to distinctive clusters of value and belief, and how these behaviours contribute to the construction of organizational moral narratives. In this chapter, we considered values and beliefs that emerge to deal with the everyday activity of leading healthcare organizations in such a way that they use their finite resources to greatest effect.

Propriety is not limited to the three modes of conduct we have considered here: fiduciary, bureaucratic and collegial. We shall see two more modes of propriety, inquisitorial and restorative, in the next chapter. Neither is propriety only relevant to situations where there are challenging questions of resource use. In the forthcoming chapter we see propriety in how leaders conduct investigations into medical harm and rebuild moral relationships in the aftermath of it.

Each mode of propriety serves valuable purposes, offering an appropriate template of values and behaviours from which medical leaders may design a response to characteristic challenges. We have seen, however, that each propriety foregrounds certain values and asserts their pre-eminence. There is therefore ample scope for the proprieties to come into conflict. This is a potent source of moral tension in medical leadership roles. Medical leaders must juggle the demands of fiduciary propriety, in which the patient comes first, with the demands of bureaucratic propriety, in which the organization comes first, and with the demands of collegial propriety, in which the practitioner community comes first. Similar difficulties arise in balancing the imperatives of inquisitorial and restorative propriety.

I have noted that for every propriety there is a matching impropriety. We have seen that fiduciary propriety mandates doctors to act as emphatic advocates of individual patient, or patient sub-group, interests. When it is unrestrained, however, advocacy leads to 'decision-making-by-decibel-level', to moral grandstanding, and possibly even to bullying. We have seen that bureaucratic propriety emphasizes corporate loyalty, and impartial and objective decision-making in the communal interest. The risk in un-tempered bureaucracy is that individual needs will be subordinated to corporate interests, ends will be subordinated to means, and personal morality be lost from sight. And we have seen that within a professional community, collegial propriety mandates consensual decision-making on grounds of expertise and relatively autonomous clinical responsibility. An excess of collegiality carries with it the danger of misplaced loyalty, so that the interests of those in the 'collegium' come to be placed before the interests of patients and carers.

We shortly move on to consider the final two proprieties, inquisitorial and restorative. Where the focus for this chapter has been on best use of resources, the focus in the next will be the moral management of medical harm.

A note on 'accountability for reasonableness' as a means of resource allocation

Dealing as it does with narratives of resource utilization and allocation, this chapter invites comparison with other analyses of allocative processes in healthcare settings. The best known of these is the 'accountability for reasonableness' framework [126]. Daniels and Sabin argue that in the face of intractable normative argument and perhaps incommensurable values, healthcare priorities can best be settled by procedural means. The 'accountability for reasonableness' (A4R) framework supplies just such an approach to democratic deliberation.

A4R requires allocative decisions to be compliant with four procedural conditions. Decisions must be made for reasons that are relevant in the circumstances; be transparent and publicly accessible; be open to review or challenge; and regulated so as to ensure that the first three conditions are met. Although the A4R framework has been described as innovative in applying deliberative theories to the problem of priority-setting [127–133], it draws on principles that would be familiar to Weberian bureaucrats. They would recognize its standard of impersonal, technical assessment; the meticulous record-keeping mandated by open decision-making; the mechanisms of review and appeal. The requirements of transparency, and further regulation, are all too familiar to the public-sector bureaucrats of today.[23]

Here I want to consider the framework in light of my account of fiduciary, bureaucratic and collegial propriety. Daniels and Sabin proposed the A4R model in order to address the problem of inconclusive and interminable moral debate about healthcare priorities. Moral theorizing had not led ineluctably to a single conclusion; rather, further controversies arose as the merits of reasonable alternatives were endlessly disputed. In practice, however, the A4R framework may be vulnerable to exactly the deficiencies and excesses of propriety that I summarized above.

Organizational ethicist Gibson and her colleagues have reported a brave attempt to engage some sixty-five healthcare leaders in a priority-setting exercise based on A4R, using open debate and open voting by clinicians and administrative staff [127]. Several factors

---

[23] Daniels and Sabin concentrate on private Health Maintenance Organizations (HMOs) so their argument may be construed as meaning that private companies distributing welfare goods should be bound by principles of public administration.

significantly undermined the process. Clinical leaders advocated strongly for their patients' (and departments') interests; they were swayed by others' passionate advocacy; they found it difficult to adopt a 'whole organization' perspective; they were discomfited by different levels of knowledge and expertise, and by lay input into clinical priority-setting; and they did not relish disrupting relationships of patronage and dependence by bluntly expressing their disagreement with colleagues through open voting procedures. From the perspective of the proprieties it is hard to avoid the conclusion that the experiment revealed the limited capacity of structural solutions (the A4R framework) to contain conflicts grounded in the principled behaviours and valued identities of fiduciary and collegial propriety.

Gibson and her colleagues concluded that a fifth 'accountability for reasonableness' condition – 'empowerment' – should be added:

> The empowerment condition states that there should be efforts to minimize power differences in the decision-making context, and to optimise effective opportunities for participation in priority setting .... Leaders have an indispensable role in setting the tone, establishing clear expectations for fair deliberation, and aligning the process and their actions accordingly. [127]

As a quasi-bureaucratic procedure, what 'accountability for reasonableness' seems to call for is mutual restraint as much as, if not more than, empowerment. Would this exercise have succeeded with better-informed, more expert, impartial, disinterested, dispassionate, decision-making behaviour? If so, what it needed was a touch more bureaucratic propriety. Perhaps if 'bureaucracy' carried the same positive connotations as 'empowerment' the value of bureaucratic propriety would be more readily acknowledged [134–137].[24]

---

[24] See also references 134–137.

Further reading

Baker R, Fissell ME, Harley D, Porter R. Part One: Medical propriety and impropriety in the English-speaking world prior to the formalization of medical ethics. In: Baker R, Porter D, Porter R, eds. *The Codification of Medical Morality: Historical and Philosophical Studies of the Formalization of Western Medical Morality in the Eighteenth and Nineteenth Centuries, Volume One: Medical Ethics and Etiquette in the Eighteenth Century*. Dordrecht: Kluwer Academic; 1993.

Savulescu J. Rational non-interventional paternalism: why doctors ought to make judgments of what is best for their patients. *Journal of Medical Ethics.* 1995;21:327–331.

Fadiman A. *The Spirit Catches You and You Fall Down: A Hmong Child, Her American Doctors, and the Collision of Two Cultures*. New York: Farrar, Straus and Giroux; 1998.

Jackall R. *Moral Mazes.* New York: Oxford University Press; 1988.

Wenger E. *Communities of Practice; Learning, Meaning, and Identity*. Cambridge: Cambridge University Press; 1998.

References

1. Rawls J. *A Theory of Justice.* Revised edn. Cambridge, MA: Harvard University Press; 1999, p. 50, p. 56ff.

2. Rawls J. *Justice as Fairness: A Restatement.* Cambridge, MA: Harvard University Press; 2001.

3. McMillan JR. NICE, the draft fertility guideline and dodging the big question. *Journal of Medical Ethics.* 2003;29(6):313–4.

4. Mladovsky P, Sorenson C. Public financing of IVF: a review of policy rationales. *Health Care Analysis*. 2010;**18**(2):113–28.

5. Bennett R, Harris J. Restoring natural function: access to infertility treatment using donated gametes. *Human Fertility*. 1999;**2**(1):18–21.

6. Ashcroft R. Fair rationing is essentially local: an argument for postcode prescribing. *Health Care Analysis*. 2006;**14**(3):135–44.

7. Devlin N, Parkin D. Funding fertility: issues in the allocation and distribution of resources to assisted reproduction technologies. *Human Fertility*. 2003;**6** Suppl 1:S2–6.

8. Peterson MM. Assisted reproductive technologies and equity of access issues. *Journal of Medical Ethics*. 2005; **31**(5):280–5.

9. Klemetti R, Gissler M, Sevon T, Hemminki E. Resource allocation of in vitro fertilization: a nationwide register-based cohort study. *BMC Health Services Research*. 2007;**7**(1):210.

10. Wanless D. *Securing Good Care for Older People: Taking a Long-Term View*. London: King's Fund; 2006.

11. Oliver D. Age based discrimination in health and social care services. *BMJ*. 2009;**339**:b3378.

12. Farrant A. The fair innings argument and increasing life spans. *Journal of Medical Ethics*. 2009;**35**(1):53–6.

13. CPA. *Selected Readings: Ageism and Age Discrimination*. 'A literature review of the likely costs and benefits of legislation to prevent age discrimination in health, social care and mental health services and definitions of age discrimination that might be operationalised for measurement' [serial on the Internet]. 2010: Available from: http://www.cpa.org.uk/information/readings/age_discrimination.pdf; http://www.cpa.org.uk/information/reviews/reviews.html.

14. Williams A. Intergenerational equity: an exploration of the 'fair innings' argument. *Health Economics*. 1997;**6**(2):117–32.

15. Harris J. *The Value of Life*. London: Routledge; 1985, pp. 87–102.

16. Shaw AB. In defence of ageism. *Journal of Medical Ethics*. 1994;**20**(3):188–94.

17. Lous J, Burton M, Ovesen T, Rovers M, Williamson I. Grommets for hearing loss associated with otitis media with effusion. *Cochrane Database of Systematic Reviews*. 2005(1).

18. NHS L. Serious Untoward Incident (SUI) reporting guidance. [21/02/11]; Available from: http://www.london.nhs.uk/webfiles/tools%20and%20resources/NHSL_SUI_Guidance.pdf.

19. Warren VL. Feminist directions in medical ethics. *Hypatia*. 1989; **4**:73–87.

20. Percival T. *Medical Ethics*. London: John Churchill; 1849, pp. 13–14.

21. McCullough L. Power, integrity and trust. In: Frankel PE, Miller Jr. F, Paul J, eds. *Bioethics*. Cambridge: Cambridge University Press; 2002, p. 203.

22. Rodwin MA. Strains in the fiduciary metaphor: divided physician loyalties and obligations in a changing health care system. *American Journal of Law and Medicine*. 1995;**21**:241.

23. McCullough LB. A basic concept in the clinical ethics of managed care: physicians and institutions as economically disciplined moral co-fiduciaries of populations of patients. *Journal of Medicine and Philosophy*. 1999;**24**(1):77–97.

24. Brennan T. Medical professionalism in the new millennium: a physician charter (Project of the A.B.I.M Foundation, A.C.P-A.S.I.M Foundation, and European Federation of Internal Medicine). *Annals of Internal Medicine*. 2002;**136**:243–6.

25. Laby AB. Resolving conflicts of duty in fiduciary relationships. *American University Law Review*. 2004;**54**:75–149.

26. Weait M. *Intimacy and Responsibility: The Criminalisation of H.I.V. Transmission*. London: Routledge-Cavendish; 2007.

27. Angell M. The doctor as double agent. *Kennedy Institute of Ethics Journal*. 1993;**3**(3):279–86.

28. Menzel PT. Double agency and the ethics of rationing health care: a response to Marcia Angell. *Kennedy Institute of Ethics Journal*. 1993;3(3):287–92.

29. Murray TH. Divided loyalties for physicians: social context and moral problems. *Social Science & Medicine*. 1986;23(8):827–32.

30. Daniels N. *Just Health: Meeting Health Needs Fairly*. New York: Cambridge University Press; 2008.

31. Beach MC, Meredith LS, Halpern J, Wells KB, Ford DE. Physician conceptions of responsibility to individual patients and distributive justice in health care. *Annals of Family Medicine*. 2005;3(1):53–9.

32. Tauber AI. Medicine, public health and the ethics of rationing. *Perspectives in Biology and Medicine*. 2002;45(1):16–30.

33. Alexander GC, Hall MA, Lantos JD. Rethinking professional ethics in the cost-sharing era. *The American Journal of Bioethics*. 2006;6(4):17–22.

34. Weingarten MA, Guttman N, Abramovitch H, Margalit RS, Roter D, Ziv A, *et al*. An anatomy of conflicts in primary care encounters: a multi-method study. *Family Practice*. 2010;27(1):93–100.

35. Spece R, Shimm D, Buchanan A. *Conflicts of Interest in Clinical Practice and Research*: Oxford University Press; 1996.

36. Morar S. Ethical aspects of the physician-society relationship (Aspecte etice ale relaţiei medic-Societate). *Revista Romana de Bioetica*. 2007;5(2):37–42.

37. Hedgecoe A. *The Politics of Personalised Medicine: Pharmacogenetics in the Clinic*. Cambridge: Cambridge University Press; 2004.

38. Hedgecoe A. It's money that matters: the financial context of ethical decision-making in modern biomedicine. In: de Vries R, Turner L, Orfali K, Bosk C, eds. *The View From Here: Bioethics and the Social Sciences*. Oxford: Blackwell; 2007.

39. Brooks S. Dignity and cost-effectiveness: a rejection of the utilitarian approach to death. *Journal of Medical Ethics*. 1984;10(3):148–51.

40. Harris J. Arresting but misleading phrases. *Journal of Medical Ethics*. 1984;10(3):155–7.

41. Agledahl KM, Førde R, Wifstad A. Clinical essentialising: a qualitative study of doctors' medical and moral practice. *Medicine, Health Care and Philosophy*. 2010;13:107–13.

42. Petraglia J. The importance of being authentic: persuasion, narration, and dialogue in health communication and education. *Health Communication*. 2009; 24(2):176–85.

43. Green MC. Research challenges in narrative persuasion. *Information Design Journal*. 2008;16(1):27–52 (6).

44. Green MC, Brock TC. In the mind's eye: transportation-imagery model of narrative persuasion. In: Green MC, Strange JJ, Brock TC, eds. *Narrative Impact: Social and Cognitive Foundations*. Mahwah, NJ: Lawrence Erlbaum; 2002, pp. 315–41.

45. Robinson WM. The narrative of rescue in pediatric practice. In: Charon R, Montello M, eds. *Stories Matter: The Role of Narrative in Medical Ethics*. New York, London: Routledge; 2002, pp. 97–108.

46. Stimson G, Webb N. *Going to See the Doctor*. London: Routledge & Kegan Paul; 1975.

47. Baruch G. Moral tales: parents stories of encounters with the health profession. *Sociology of Health and Illness*. 1981;3(3):275–96.

48. Quine L. Workplace bullying, psychological distress, and job satisfaction in junior doctors. *Cambridge Quarterly of Healthcare Ethics*. 2003;12:91–101.

49. Quine L. Workplace bullying in nurses. *Journal of Health Psychology*. 2001;6(1):73–84.

50. Hutchinson M, Vickers M, Jackson D, Wilkes L. Workplace bullying in nursing: towards a more critical organisational perspective. *Nursing Inquiry*. 2006;13(2):118–26.

51. Vanderstar ES. Symposium: introduction to the symposium on workplace bullying:

workplace bullying in the healthcare professions. *Employee Rights and Employment Policy Journal.* 2004;455.

52. Randle J. *Workplace Bullying in the NHS.* Radcliffe; 2006.

53. Yamada JDD. Workplace bullying and ethical leadership. *The Journal of Value Based Leadership* [serial on the Internet]. 2008;**1**(2). Available from: http://www. valuesbasedleadershipjournal.com/issues/vol1issue2/yamada.php

54. Wakefield AJ, Murch SH, Anthony A, Linnell J, Casson DM, Malik M, *et al.* Retracted: Ileal-lymphoid-nodular hyperplasia, non-specific colitis, and pervasive developmental disorder in children. *The Lancet.* 1998;**351**(9103): 637–41.

55. Burgess DC, Burgess MA, Leask J. The MMR vaccination and autism controversy in United Kingdom 1998–2005: inevitable community outrage or a failure of risk communication? *Vaccine.* 2006;**24**(18):3921–8.

56. Bedford HE, Elliman DAC. MMR vaccine and autism. *BMJ.* 2010;**340** (c655).

57. Lewis J, Speers T. Misleading media reporting? The MMR story. *Nature Reviews Immunology.* 2003;**3**(11):913–8. 10.1038/nri1228.

58. Offit PA, Coffin SE. Communicating science to the public: MMR vaccine and autism. *Vaccine.* 2003;**22**(1):1–6.

59. Casiday RE. Children's health and the social theory of risk: insights from the British measles, mumps and rubella (MMR) controversy. *Social Science & Medicine.* 2007;**65**(5):1059–70.

60. Dyer C. Lancet retracts Wakefield's MMR paper. *BMJ.* 2010;**340**:c696.

61. Kmietowicz Z. Wakefield is struck off for the 'serious and wide-ranging findings against him'. *BMJ.* 2010;**340**: c2803.

62. Weber M. *Economy and Society: An Outline of Interpretive Sociology.* Based on 4th German ed. Berkeley: University of California Press; 1978, pp. 956–958.

63. du Gay P. *The Values of Bureaucracy.* Oxford: Oxford University Press; 2005.

64. Associated Provincial Picture Houses v Wednesbury Corporation. 1 KB 223 1948.

65. Arendt H. *The Origins of Totalitarianism.* New York: Harcourt, Brace; 1951.

66. Canovan M. *Hannah Arendt: A Reinterpretation of her Political Thought.* Cambridge: Cambridge University Press; 1992.

67. France A. *Le Lys Rouge.* 1894, Ch. 7.

68. Lipsky M. *Street-Level Bureaucracy: Dilemmas of the Individual in Public Services.* New York: Russell Sage Foundation; 1980.

69. Blau PM. *The Dynamics of Bureaucracy.* Chicago: University of Chicago Press; 1955.

70. MacIntyre A. *After Virtue.* 3rd edn. London: Duckworth; 2007.

71. Bauman Z. *Postmodern Ethics.* Oxford: Blackwell; 1993.

72. du Gay P. *In Praise of Bureaucracy.* London: Sage; 2000.

73. Hoggett P. A service to the public: the containment of ethical and moral conflicts by public bureaucracies. In: du Gay P, ed. *The Values of Bureaucracy.* Oxford: Oxford University Press; 2005, pp. 167–90.

74. Minson J. *Questions of Conduct: Sexual Harassment, Citizenship, Government.* London: Macmillan; 1993.

75. Hunter I. *Re-thinking the School.* Sydney: Allen & Unwin; 1994, p. 157.

76. Francis R. The Mid Staffordshire NHS Foundation Trust Inquiry: Department of Health; 2010.

77. R (Ann Marie Rogers) v Swindon Primary Care Trust and the Secretary of State. *EWCA Civ* 392; 2006.

78. Syrett K. Opening eyes to the reality of scarce health care resources? R (on the application of Rogers) v Swindon NHS Primary Care Trust and Secretary of State for Health. *Public Law.* 2006:664–73.

79. R on the application of Otley v Barking and Dagenham NHS Primary Care Trust. *EWHC* 1927 (Admin); 2007.

80. R (Murphy) v Salford Primary Care Trust. *EWHC* 1908 (Admin); 2008.

81. Jackson E. *Medical Law: Text, Cases and Materials.* 2nd edn. Oxford: Oxford University Press; 2010, pp. 84–6.

82. NHS. NHS Sickle Cell & Thalassaemia Screening Programme. [22/02/11]; Available from: http://www.kcl-phs.org.uk/haemscreening/default.htm; http://sct.screening.nhs.uk/.

83. Timmermans S, Berg M. *The Gold Standard: The Challenge of Evidence-Based Medicine and Standardization in Health Care.* Philadelphia: Temple University Press; 2003, p. 138.

84. Rogers W. Are guidelines ethical? Some considerations for general practice. *British Journal of General Practice.* 2002;**52**:663–9.

85. Petro JA. Collegiality in history. *Bulletin of New York Academy of Medicine.* 1992;**68**(2):286–91.

86. Waters M. Collegiality, bureaucratization and professionalization: a Weberian analysis. *American Journal of Sociology.* 1989;**94**(5):945–72.

87. Freidson E. *Profession of Medicine: A Study in the Sociology of Applied Knowledge.* Chicago: University of Chicago Press; 1970.

88. Blank L, Kimball H, McDonald W, Merino J, for the ABIM Foundation AF, EFoIM. Medical professionalism in the new millennium: a physician charter 15 months later. *Annals of Internal Medicine.* 2003;**138**(10):839–41.

89. Wear D, Aultman JM. *Professionalism in Medicine: Critical Perspectives.* New York: Springer; 2006.

90. Davies M. *Medical Self-Regulation: Crisis and Change.* Aldershot: Ashgate; 2007.

91. Cruess RL, Cruess SR, Johnston SE. Professionalism: an ideal to be sustained. *The Lancet.* 2000;**356**(9224):156–9.

92. Emanuel L, Cruess R, Cruess S, Hauser J. Old values, new challenges: what is a professional to do? *International Journal For Quality in Health Care.* 2002;**14**(5):349–51.

93. Learning from Bristol: The Report of the Public Inquiry into Children's Heart Surgery at the Bristol Royal Infirmary: *Cm* 5207; 2001.

94. An inquiry into quality and practice within the National Health Service arising from the actions of Rodney Ledward. Department of Health; 2000.

95. Independent investigation into how the N.H.S handled allegations about the conduct of Richard Neale. *Cm* 6315; 2004.

96. Independent investigation into how the N.H.S handled allegations about the conduct of Clifford Ayling. *Cm* 6298; 2004.

97. Independent investigation into how the N.H.S handled allegations about the conduct of William Kerr and Michael Haslam. *Cm* 6640; 2005.

98. Shipman Inquiry. Safeguarding patients: lessons from the past – proposals for the future. *Cm* 6394; 2004.

99. Davies G. Queensland Public Hospitals Commission of Inquiry: Report 'The Davies Inquiry'. *Queensland* 2005.

100. The Bundaberg Hospital Commission of Inquiry: 'The Morris Inquiry'. 2005.

101. Stewart J. *Blind Eye: How the Medical Establishment Let a Doctor Get Away With Murder.* New York: Simon and Shuster; 1999.

102. Baucus M, Grassley C. Staff report on cardiac stent usage at ST. Joseph Medical Center. 2010.

103. Rosenthal M. *Dealing with Medical Malpractice: The British and Swedish Experience.* Durham, NC: Duke University Press; 1988.

104. Rosenthal M. *The Incompetent Doctor.* Buckingham: Open University Press; 1995.

105. Rosenthal M, Mulcahy L, Lloyd-Bostock S, eds. *Medical Mishaps; Pieces of the Puzzle.* Buckingham: Open University Press; 1999.

106. Hart E, Hazelgrove J. Understanding the organisational context for adverse events in the health services: the role of cultural censorship. *Quality & Safety in Health Care.* 2001;**10**(4):257–62.

107. Øvretveit J. Understanding and improving patient safety: the psychological, social and cultural dimensions. *Journal of Health Organization and Management.* 2009;**23**(6):581–96.

108. Jorm C, Kam P. Does medical culture limit doctors' adoption of quality improvement? Lessons from Camelot. *Journal of Health Services Research & Policy.* 2004;**9**(4):248–51.

109. Ehrich K. Telling cultures: 'cultural' issues for staff reporting concerns about colleagues in the UK National Health Service. *Sociology of Health & Illness.* 2006;**28**(7):903–26.

110. Henriksen K, Dayton E. Organizational silence and hidden threats to patient safety. *Health Services Research.* 2006;**41**(4p2):1539–54.

111. Thompson F. How culture influences the reporting of unethical behaviour in the workplace. In: Tschudin V, Davis AJ, Hancock C, eds. *The Globalisation of Nursing.* Oxford: Radcliffe; 2008, pp. 206–20.

112. Waring JJ. Beyond blame: cultural barriers to medical incident reporting. *Social Science & Medicine.* 2005;**60**:1927–35.

113. Lawton R, Parker D. Barriers to incident reporting in a healthcare system. *Quality and Safety in Health Care.* 2002;**11**(1):15–8.

114. Vincent C, Stanhope N, Crowley-Murphy M. Reasons for not reporting adverse incidents: an empirical study. *Journal of Evaluation in Clinical Practice.* 1999;**5**(1):13–21.

115. Espin S, Lingard L, Baker GR, Regehr G. Persistence of unsafe practice in everyday work: an exploration of organizational and psychological factors constraining safety in the operating room. *Quality and Safety in Health Care.* 2006;**15**(3):165–70.

116. Waring JJ. Doctors' thinking about 'the system' as a threat to patient safety. *Health.* 2007;**11**(1):29–46.

117. Waring JJ. Patient safety: new directions in the management of health service quality. *Policy & Politics.* 2005;**33**:675–92.

118. Pfeiffer Y, Manser T, Wehner T. Conceptualising barriers to incident reporting: a psychological framework. *Quality and Safety in Health Care.* 2010;**19**:1–10.

119. Braithwaite J, Westbrook MT, Travaglia JF, Hughes C. Cultural and associated enablers of, and barriers to, adverse incident reporting. *Quality and Safety in Health Care.* 2010;**19**(3):229–33.

120. Moumtzoglou A. Factors that prevent physicians reporting adverse events. *International Journal of Health Care Quality Assurance.* 2010;**23**(1):51–8.

121. Carr-Saunders EM, Wilson PA. *The Professions.* Cambridge: Clarendon Press; 1936.

122. Rosenthal M. How doctors think about medical mishaps. In: Rosenthal M, Mulcahy L, Lloyd-Bostock S, eds. *Medical Mishaps: Pieces of the Puzzle.* Buckingham: Open University Press; 1999, p. 152.

123. Mangiardi JR, Pellegrino ED. Collegiality: what is it? *Bulletin of the New York Academy of Medicine.* 1992;**68**(2):292–6.

124. Rosenthal M. Medical uncertainty, medical collegiality, and improving quality of care. *Research in the Sociology of Health Care.* 1999;**16**:3–30.

125. Medical Collegiality. Finnish Medical Association; 2002 [19/02/11]; Available from: http://www.laakariliitto.fi/e/ethics/code_of_collegiality.html.

126. Daniels N, Sabin J. *Setting Limits Fairly: Can We Learn to Share Medical Resources?* New York: Oxford University Press; 2002.

127. Gibson JL, Martin DK, Singer PA. Priority setting in hospitals: Fairness, inclusiveness, and the problem of institutional power differences. *Social Science & Medicine.* 2005;**61**:2355–62.

128. Gibson JL, Martin DK, Singer PA. Evidence, economics and ethics: resource allocation in health services organizations. *Healthcare Quarterly.* 2005;**8**(2):50–9, 4.

129. Bruni RA, Laupacis A, Martin DK, for the University of Toronto Priority Setting in

Health Care Research Group. Public engagement in setting priorities in health care. *CMAJ.* 2008;**179**(1):15-8.

130. Chen DT, Werhane PH, Mills AE. Role of organization ethics in critical care medicine. *Critical Care Medicine.* 2007;**35**(2):S11-S7. 0.1097/01. CCM.0000252913.21741.35.

131. Spicker P. What is a priority? *Journal of Health Services Research & Policy.* 2009;**14**(2):112-6.

132. Platonova EA, Studnicki J, Fisher JW, Bridger C. Local health department priority setting: an exploratory study. *Journal of Public Health Management and Practice.* 2010;**16**(2):140-7. 10.1097/ PHH.0b013e3181ca2618.

133. Kapiriri L, Martin D. Successful priority setting in low and middle income countries: a framework for evaluation. *Health Care Analysis.* 2010;**18**(2):129-47.

134. Friedman A. Beyond accountability for reasonableness. *Bioethics.* 2008;**22**(2):101-12.

135. Rid A. Justice and procedure: how does 'accountability for reasonableness' result in fair limit-setting decisions? *Journal of Medical Ethics.* 2009;**35**(1):12-6.

136. Syrett K. Health technology appraisal and the courts: accountability for reasonableness and the judicial model of procedural justice. *Health Economics, Policy and Law.* 2010. Epub ahead of print.

137. Lauridsen S, Lippert-Rasmussen K. Legitimate allocation of public healthcare: beyond accountability for reasonableness. *Public Health Ethics.* 2009;**2**(1):59-69.

Chapter 5

Expressing inquisitorial and restorative propriety

When medical care goes wrong, what are the moral responsibilities that fall to medical leaders? This chapter is an examination of the proprieties involved in managing medical harm. It is concerned with the moral repair necessitated by tragic mischance, damaging errors, catastrophic omissions, unwanted side effects, organizational dysfunction, management failure, and more [1–3].[1] Exploring how medical leaders practice propriety to support the restoration of trust in people and organizations, the discussion offers a fresh perspective on medical failure and its place in organizational ethics [4–8].[2]

It is striking to find that the leading texts on healthcare organizational ethics have canvassed scant discussion of medical harm [9–14].[3] This is surprising for several reasons. Organizational ethics has reasonably been defined as 'the study of personal and organizational moral norms and choices as they contribute to the activities and goals of an organization and to the integral human fulfilment of persons and communities' [9(p15)]. Preventing medical harm from occurring, and morally responding to it when it does, would appear to be pivotal to this goal. The worldwide patient safety movement has made preventing and responding to medical harm a fiduciary concern for all doctors, and for medical leaders in particular [15–29].[4] Along with harm to patients, the financial and human costs for institutions following medical harm are a significant burden, so the topic might be expected to be prominent in institutional ethics. Finally, if a good first principle for medical professional ethics is 'first do no harm', a corollary principle might be expected to play a central role in healthcare organizational ethics.

---

[1] I have avoided using the term accident as it has been argued for some three decades that there is no such thing as a true accidental injury in medicine. Banning most uses of the term 'accident' in 2001 the BMJ editors argued 'we believe that correct and consistent terminology will help improve understanding that injuries of all kinds – in homes, schools and workplaces, vehicles, and medical settings – are usually preventable. Such awareness, coupled with efforts to implement prevention strategies, will help reduce the incidence and severity of injuries'. See references 1–3.

[2] I am not concerned here with legal liability for medical harm, or with the regulatory response. There is a substantial literature on the regulatory response: see, for example, references 4–8.

[3] The text that has received most attention is Boyle et al. (reference 9); other leading texts are identified in references 10–12. See also references 13 and 14.

[4] There is a copious literature dealing with harm prevention, with seminal articles by Lucian Leape (see reference 15) and the landmark report of the Institute of Medicine *To Err is Human* (reference 16). A smaller literature deals with the response to harm once it has occurred. A seminal article in the field is identified in reference 17. A systematic review in 2004 noted that research on error disclosure had focused on the decision whether to disclose medical error at the expense of the process of disclosure and management of its effects (see reference 18).

That medical harm has not been more prominent in conceptions of the field may owe something to the origins of organizational ethics in the USA. Far fewer doctors there are employed by provider organizations, and the majority of doctors continue to give care to patients on a fee-for-service basis. Responsibility for addressing problems in professional performance has therefore remained more clearly a matter for the profession, and for local regulatory oversight, than for provider organizations and their lay managers.

Irrespective of whether their scholarship is viewed as organizational ethics, ethicists and clinicians in North America have nevertheless written compellingly about what must be done in the aftermath of medical harm [30–37]. There has as yet been little discussion of the responsibility that medical leaders (specifically) have, for promoting the processes of moral repair. In this chapter I explore two modes of leadership propriety central to moral repair. The first is inquisitorial propriety, conduct directed towards ascertaining the nature of the damage done to moral relationships. Inquisitorial propriety enables an objective record of morally relevant facts to be compiled, and is apparent in such action as temporarily suspending collegial bonds with colleagues under investigation, soliciting comprehensive testimony, investigating contrasting perspectives and demonstrating impartial judgement. The second is restorative propriety, conduct directed towards returning moral relationships to balance. Restorative propriety includes gestures such as attending to narratives of wrong, compiling narratives of witness, accepting anger or grief, tendering an apology and seeking or offering forgiveness.

The reparative proprieties are invoked in response to particular moral harms and moral needs. To comprehend the demands of moral repair in medical settings, we need to grasp the nature of medical harm, and the nature of the moral relationships the proprieties seek to restore. So before moving to a detailed examination of inquisitorial and restorative propriety, I describe the range of iatrogenic injury and the dynamics of trust in medical settings.

Understanding iatrogenic injury

Derived from the Greek word *iatros* meaning physician, 'iatrogenic injury' is commonly defined as 'physician-produced injury'. Defining medical harm as physician-produced, however, individualizes the problem. It does not make allowance for how contemporary medicine is embedded in organizational and institutional systems. Nor does it allow for the complex patterns of responsibility inherent in extended patient pathways and multi-professional team care, where injury might be as much a product of organizational omission as of medical or other health professional action. For this reason, Sharpe and Faden proposed a decade or so ago that the term 'iatrogenic' should be replaced. Drawing on the Greek word for care or attendance, *komein*, they suggested the neologism 'comiogenic', meaning 'care-produced' injuries [38(p117),39–41]. As the term has not been much adopted, my preference is to extend the meaning of iatrogenic beyond its etymological roots.

I use 'iatrogenic injury' to refer to any injury or adverse effect that appears to be the result of treatment, or that arises out of the way in which care is provided. To consider a salient example we learned in Chapter 2 of chronically ill patients who suffered serious complications because their primary care doctors failed to actively monitor their condition. The source of the problem was chaotic patient record systems. In the primary care setting the responsibility for patient records and management systems rested ultimately with the primary care practice partners, so these injuries could at least be said to be indirectly physician-produced. But in hospital settings, while clinicians update and manage the content in patient records, the care organization is ultimately responsible for their design, maintenance, and storage. According to my use of the term 'iatrogenic', harm to patients traceable to poor organizational systems in hospitals would still be iatrogenic injuries because they result from deficiencies in the organization of care.

There is an important moral distinction to be made between culpable and non-culpable acts leading to iatrogenic injury. We characteristically attach moral blame to unskilled, careless, mistaken or frankly misdirected treatment. We are more forgiving of what appear to be calamities that arise through chance constellations of events, chalking them up to accidents or 'Acts of God' [15].[5] But moral repair is required whatever the cause of the harm. For the most part in the discussion that follows, culpable and non-culpable injuries will be considered together.

Types of iatrogenic injury

In this study, iatrogenic injuries fell into five distinct groups: injuries that arose from the care setting; injuries that occurred as a side effect of treatment; injuries following more or less innocent medical error; injuries that arose from grossly negligent or intentional mistreatment; and moral injuries. I examine each of these in turn.

Iatrogenic injuries that arise from the care setting

The first group of iatrogenic injuries arises out of unforeseen or unmanaged hazards of hospital organization. Nosocomial (that is, hospital-acquired) infections such as MRSA or C. difficile,[6] where infection cannot always be traced to individual clinicians' agency, supply an obvious example. While careless hygiene practice by healthcare professionals has always been a significant contributory factor in nosocomial infection, so is the nature of the care environment in which professionals work. The task of treating a high volume of patients with compromised immunity in close proximity to each other imposes exceptional demands, demands to which individuals must adapt their behaviour in response. Care providers who work in environments with high infection risk and too little time to care for patients will find it more difficult to maintain adequate hand hygiene than care providers working with lower levels of infection risk and fewer patients. This is not to excuse poor hygiene practices, but to recognize how strategic decisions made at the level of health systems may carry ill-anticipated implications for professional conduct and patient management [42].[7]

The design of the care environment presents obvious risk to patients, risks again exacerbated through interaction with management practices and professional behaviours. Dr. Fox (The Three Spires Hospital) gave the example of a distressing episode in which a

---

[5] Leape memorably described how apparently accidental injuries arose through harm-prevention strategies whose flaws were disastrously aligned – somewhat like an unexpected line of holes in a Swiss cheese. Most of the time preventive actions are effective, but certain tragic circumstances arise because an error is able to 'pass through' the faults in each strategy.

[6] *Staphylococcus aureus* is a bacterium, some strains of which have become methicillin-resistant. It produces infections resistant to antibiotic treatment where immunity is compromised by medical condition or treatment. *Clostridium difficile* is a bacterium that causes severe or fatal colitis in patients receiving antibiotics.

[7] See, for example, reference 42.

confused patient attempted to leave their upper storey ward one night, by means of an unlocked window. The risk to that patient arose from a combination of poor building design, reduced staff at night and (possibly) a degree of inattention by those nurses who had been present. Rather differently, Dr. Kingsley (Cityside NHS Trust) had been obliged to inquire into the death of one patient who had killed themselves – whether deliberately or inadvertently never became clear – using an item commonly found in hospital wards, but which had never been thought to present any sort of risk even to patients intending self-harm.[8]

Iatrogenic injuries that arise from the care environment are only infrequently the result of overt actions or single failures. They often reveal hitherto unrecognized environmental risk. They also frequently emerge as the unintended consequence of well-intentioned routines (such as reliance on broad-spectrum antibiotics, which has facilitated the emergence of antibiotic-resistant bacteria) and organizational aims (such as achieving high bed-occupancy rates, which makes infection control more difficult).

There is a fuzzy boundary around this category of injury, a fuzziness that results from the kind of narrative that we produce in order to ascribe cause and responsibility. This in turn depends upon the normative expectations we hold. Is it an iatrogenic injury when a child dies in an ambulance on the way to a distant emergency department, because the local unit was closed? Only if we normatively expect a local 24 hour unit to be provided. And does it count as iatrogenic injury when a PCT will not pay for Herceptin, and a woman dies from breast cancer sooner than she had hoped? Only if we believe such drugs to be effective, and normatively expect them to be available.

Iatrogenic injuries that occur as a foreseeable risk of treatment

Side effects are an unavoidable peril of treatment. Ethical analysis of the moral injury that occurs if patients are not advised of risks, and are thereby denied the choice whether to undertake such risks, has been exhaustive. Indeed the issue of informed consent to research and treatment could be said to be the *sine qua non* of bioethics.

But whether a patient gives an informed consent to known risk cannot be our only concern when it materializes. Even if a patient does knowingly undertake a risk, if it arises there will be moral repair to be done. A beneficent act will have caused harm, albeit through no fault of any of the actors. The need will remain to rebuild patients' trust in the wake of negative outcomes, perhaps to attend to a family's grief, or to support a colleague in distress because they feel responsible for causing injury to a patient whom they intended to protect from harm.

The demands of practice, moreover, test the analytical difference between foreseeable side effects and unwarranted injuries. Anaesthesia carries a known risk of death. But how great a risk is it reasonable to offer a patient? Dr. Fox had had to lead colleagues at the Three Spires Hospital through deep disagreement over the risks to which a patient might properly consent. In the wake of one patient's post-operative death, Three Spires had carried out a full inquiry with the assistance of outside agencies. On one side of the dispute were anaesthetists who argued that their colleague was to be admired for taking on patients whom others judged to be too high risk for surgery. Their colleague was, in their view, the

---

[8] The highly unusual circumstances are not described for reasons of confidentiality.

only anaesthetist brave enough to offer one last desperate gamble to patients facing inevitable death or uncontrollable pain. On the other side was a group of anaesthetists who castigated their colleague for proceeding in the face of such risks, believing that an adverse outcome was so certain that to anaesthetize these patients was, in effect, to bring about their death. Death, in their view, was in these circumstances not a foreseeable side effect; rather it was so foreseeable an outcome that it was a direct effect. Dr. Fox granted that these patients had consented to the risk of death; but this did not obviate the need to consider whether it was proper to offer the risk in the first place, or what morally was owed to the family or colleagues as a result of death occurring.

I noted above that iatrogenic injury always necessitates moral repair, whether it was blameworthy or whether it was entirely innocent. But issues of fault and culpability are important in the course of doing moral repair, because they form an important part of personal and organizational moral narratives. We shall look below in some detail at Dr. Chalcraft's account of pursuing moral repair in the aftermath of a young patient dying in the course of complex surgery. In Chalcraft's case it was initially very unclear whether death was due to foreseeable but unavoidable risks, or whether it was due to avoidable errors. Iatrogenic injury that occurs during surgery, or during a course of treatment, frequently raises just that difficult question: is the realization of this foreseeable risk attributable to fate, or is it attributable to individual or organizational error? This brings us to the next category of injury; injury that arises as a consequence of error.

Iatrogenic injury as a consequence of medical error

It is medical error, whether owing to misfortune, misjudgement, incompetence or systemic failure, that has attracted most attention from ethicists concerned with moral repair [32,43].[9]

Paget's fine-grained phenomenological analysis of medical mistake has informed much subsequent discussion [44]. This is perhaps because she captured so compellingly three central features of error, features that warrant designating it a moral tragedy.

First, medical error is a well-intended action that has deviated from its purpose, an arrow benevolently aimed that hits a disastrously wrong mark.

Second, from the point of view of the actor, no act is a mistake at the very moment that it is made. Doctors who misdiagnose, amputate the wrong limb, prescribe the wrong medication, cut less skillfully, wrongly place a device, or otherwise misjudge what an occasion demands, realize only with hindsight the errors that they have committed.

Third, non-culpable medical error is intrinsic to medical practice. Medicine is a process of discovery, and it is intrinsic to a process of discovery that it sometimes reveals things to be other than they were first thought to be [45].[10] In Paget's words:

> medical work is discovered in action. Discovery is not like seeing or observing. Patients do not wear their illnesses as they wear apparel. One apprehends, one infers, one tests, one experiments, one tracks, one follows the course of events in order to disclose the nature of illness and affect it. [44(p19)]

---

[9] See, for example, references 32 and 43.

[10] Gorovitz and MacIntyre's well-known argument is that error is an artefact of any applied science arising from the cleavage between what is known in principle and what is known about individual cases. See reference 45.

As clinical time unfolds, and as diagnostic and treatment activities generate fresh clinical data, early hypotheses may come to be discounted, differential diagnoses can be refined, and inferential errors can be exposed. So long as the initial clinical hypotheses were reasonable, the treatment modalities were warranted and the clinical process did not culminate in serious injury, the errors intrinsic to discovery are not liable to be viewed as mistakes. They are best guesses discarded in light of further investigation that yields better evidence. It is only a medical mistake where a hypothesis, or the action or inaction that flowed from it, would have been judged wrong by skilled and knowledgeable practitioners at the time that it occurred [43,46–49].

The central facts with which moral repair of iatrogenic injury must grapple are thus that medical mistakes originate in a beneficent intent; that mistakes are integral to the practice of medicine; and that they are only evident in hindsight when time and actions cannot be reversed.

These inexorable features of error were captured in the case that Dr. Seddon described. In a devastating series of misjudgements, one of the consultants working at Saxonvale University Hospital Trust had systematically misdiagnosed and mistreated the symptoms of patients who had been referred to him over a period of several years. Once the facts had been established, there was little doubt that patients had been seriously harmed, that family who had cared for them had suffered great distress, and that the victims of this appalling series of errors were entitled to restitution. What remained a matter of dispute was who or what was to blame, whether it was right or just to forgive the error, and what measure of punishment would be fitting. For Dr. Seddon, the consultant had made very grave but ultimately innocent misjudgements. Theirs were mistakes that manifested Paget's conception of medical error as a benevolently aimed arrow that tragically misses its mark. Seddon recounted how the doctor had worked in relative isolation in a small specialty, and how the misdiagnoses flowed from their good intentions but outdated understanding.

> [Dr. X] was extraordinarily dedicated. [They] worked all hours – used to ring the patients up at 8 o'clock in the night and advise about drug treatments, and getting on, and doing this. Was absolutely dedicated to the job ... workaholic. And actually there were many patients would say, '[Dr. X] is wonderful, has just transformed our lives'. But [Dr. X] was off [the rails] .... Why did [they] get off the rails like that?

Dr. Seddon's answer to his rhetorical question was that a now outmoded perspective on diagnosis and treatment had prevailed during the early years of the consultant's career. Although their view of the clinical science had retained some adherents, most others in the field had rejected it. Until recently, some of those in the specialty would have endorsed the consultant's actions:

> but the [specialist] community had moved on and ... [Dr. X] didn't .... Partly because [Dr. X] had a personality which was terrier-like, like a dog with a bone. [Dr. X] was almost overbearing in [clinging to] opinions. But of course, we as doctors are taught to stick with our own thoughts.
> (Dr. Seddon, Saxonvale University Hospitals Trust)

Dr. Seddon's explanation makes clear that there are two senses in which error becomes error only with hindsight. One, specific conceptions of error are constructed by the community of practice. What would have been an acceptable medical hypothesis and intervention early in the consultant's career was, a decade later, regarded by many to be a culpable diagnostic and therapeutic mistake. But the consultant did not know this at the time that they were acting, with good intentions, as they did. Two, Dr. X, and many of Dr. X's patients and their families, believed at the time that the treatments were doing good for the patients. They interpreted the effects of the treatment as beneficial. It was only later, when a professional consensus determined that Dr. X was in error, that some began to see what had been done as having been harmful.

Iatrogenic injuries that arise from consciously negligent or deliberate wrongdoing

In his magisterial treatment of the profession of medicine, one of Freidson's central concerns was the quality of professional self-regulation. He noted the then prevalent belief among American medical professionals that doctors who descended to the level of 'butchers and moral lepers' [50] would be rapidly spotted and decisively controlled. He also observed 'almost all forms of deviance lie somewhere between the performance of the moral leper and that of the saint' [50]. What concerned Freidson was that it was the many doctors whose performance fell below required standards, but who were neither butchers nor lepers, that it was most difficult for other professionals to manage.

Freidson's anxieties were based in research that is now nearly half a century old. How closely do his findings match the situation I found among medical leaders in the UK in the early years of the twenty-first century? The picture is similar in some striking ways. It was leaders' oft-stated assumption that gross turpitude would be more tractable than 'middle ground' incompetence, and that butchers and lepers would be summarily dealt with. Where the picture I found appears different from the one that Freidson painted is in the level of concern that medical leaders had for deficient performance across the board. Freidson suggests that professionals in his studies did little more than wring their hands and deliver a stern 'talking-to' when confronted by poor performance they could no longer ignore. In this study leaders were prepared to go to considerable lengths to manage performance concerns, moving from initial 'talkings-to' and reprimand, through close supervision, restriction of practice and, ultimately, exclusion. Greater moral and managerial anxiety was elicited by marginal incompetence and careless error than by the prospect of gross malpractice and deliberate harm; and it was precisely in the middle ground that difficulties were encountered.

What of this view, however, that 'butchers' and 'lepers' are easy to identify and contain? Unfortunately, the evidence contradicts it. The catalogue of injuries caused by gynaecologists Ledward and Neale indicates that surgeon 'butchers' may practise unrestrained; while inquiries into the offences of Shipman, Ayling, Kerr and Haslam demonstrate that 'moral lepers' may not be easy to spot [51–57]. Indeed, all of those inquiries, alongside that into the Bristol Royal Infirmary and academic studies of the management of medical incompetence, have demonstrated how challenging the profession finds it to address failure either gross or subtle [58,59]. The introduction of mechanisms for managing performance 'in the middle ground' are discussed at the end of this section.

Iatrogenic injuries that are moral injuries

Certain iatrogenic injuries are not physical but moral: they harm the individual by doing injury to dignity, identity, trust or moral standing. That they do not result in lasting physical injury does not diminish their severity. Medical leaders recounted examples of sexual misconduct and 'boundary violations'; cases of treatment without informed consent;

breaches of confidentiality; infringement of privacy; and undignified care [60–63].[11] They also detailed failures of moral repair, where uncaring and inadequate responses to complaint had ended up heaping insult upon initial injury.

Moral injuries present their own challenge to moral repair. Moral injuries are frequently unseen and leave no visible trace. Dr. Dillon faced the difficulty, as did other participants in the study, of investigating allegations of sexual impropriety against doctors that doctors flatly denied. In Dr. Dillon's case there were no witnesses, no relevant history, and there was perhaps reason for an allegation to have been made out of ill will or confusion. To reject the allegation might do grave injustice to a patient; to uphold the allegation might do grave injustice to the physician. But Dr. Dillon could not decide nothing. He was compelled to decide something, on the unsatisfactory grounds of which story and what risks appeared the more compelling.

Some moral injuries outrage the victim while appearing reasonable, justifiable or downright trivial to the perpetrator. Dr. Chalcraft (The Royal Metropolitan Infirmary) described how a consultant continued to believe he had obtained a patient's fully informed consent to a difficult and dangerous surgical procedure, even though he had not explained that he would be absent from the hospital for a large part of it, leaving a qualified but less experienced colleague in charge. The surgeon defended his action on grounds that he had informed his patient of the risks, and obtained their signature on the standard NHS consent form, which noted a patient could not expect to be treated by a specific doctor. The impenitent surgeon regarded himself as compliant with the letter of hospital law; the patient and Dr. Chalcraft viewed his actions as wholly inconsistent with the spirit of informed consent.

Moral injuries also invite questions about the nature of the injury itself. Dr. Hutchinson (Evenlode Park NHS Trust) had decided to investigate when it was reported to him that an adult former patient had been observed apparently in a settled relationship with one of the doctors who had treated them. The patient flatly denied that any wrong had occurred, and protested that, in Hutchinson's words 'it wasn't any of our business'. While professional boundaries had, in the view of the professional who reported the incident, been violated, the episode raised awkward issues [60].[12] The subjective perception of the 'victim' was that no harm had been done and that they were not in any way vulnerable; one objective view of the circumstances (there are others) is that prohibitions on relationships with current and former patients serve to protect patients in general, because certain groups of patients are without doubt vulnerable. Where a subjective view of what is good for an individual patient differs from an objective view of what is good for patients, which should prevail?[13] Moreover, the conundrum of moral repair in this situation is not resolved simply by virtue of the rules regarding

---

[11] Boundary violations are abuses of the professional relationship between doctors and patients, which generally entail exploiting patients' vulnerability and trust in professional integrity. They are a breach of the fiduciary duty that doctors owe to patients. See references 60–63.

[12] Supplementary guidance was issued by the GMC in November 2006, and hence was not in effect at the date of this reported incident. Paragraph 5 stipulates: 'You must not pursue a sexual relationship with a former patient, where at the time of the professional relationship the patient was vulnerable, for example because of mental health problems, or because of their lack of maturity.' See reference 60.

[13] There is a more radical argument to be made. This is that any and all relationships with patients and former patients are inherently exploitative, and that patients who enjoy such relationships do not realize that they are based upon their vulnerability. In effect, the patient above suffered from a degree of 'false consciousness'. This view raises a host of difficult issues that cannot be pursued here.

conduct being clear. The 'victim' valued this relationship as a very significant benefit; how should the harm of the Trust being perceived to turn a blind eye to lax behaviour be weighed against the victim's self-identified good? Would pursuing the issue further itself do harm to this former patient; and if so, would that harm be justified in the overall interests of patients?

Finally, moral injuries may remain unhealed because complainants continue to feel that they have not been properly addressed. The reports of the English Parliamentary and Health Service Ombudsman evidence how this is true of continuing unhappiness about care that has gone wrong in the NHS [64,65]. Carelessness, callousness and failure to recognize the nature of wrongs all play a part in explaining why complainants remain unhappy for so long. Nearly three-quarters of complaints to the Ombudsman in 2009–2010 contained allegations that communication had been unhelpful or disrespectful, or that the response had been tardy; that patients had received a poor explanation of what had happened, an incomplete explanation, or a response containing factual errors; that there had been no acknowledgement of the mistake, that an inadequate apology was offered, or that recommendations on how to prevent future harm had not been been implemented. We should note, however, that opposing views on what ought to have been done in particular circumstances will sometimes remain irreconcilable. Where there is principled disagreement between differently situated actors holding different factual and moral perspectives on what happened, no explanation is likely to suffice.

Iatrogenic injury and the patient safety movement

We have noted that medical harm may arise from the actions or omissions of individuals, from the actions or omissions of organizations, and from the design of organizational settings. Earlier sociological studies of medical harm, such as Freidson's, tended to focus on individual error and professional responsibility. Latterly, the patient safety movement has drawn attention to how error arises from the nature of the systems that underpin individual practice, and to organizational-level responsibilities for minimizing harm. Systems-level approaches have implications for the organizational moral narratives that follow harm, and for the organizational narratives that prevent it.

For the patient safety movement, the first priority is to create organizational systems that work to minimize the possibility of individual error, and thus prevent harm from arising. As one of the seminal articles in this field has contended, 'the primary objective of *system* design for safety is to make it difficult for *individuals* to err' (emphasis added) [15]. One component of 'system design for safety' is organizational moral narratives that promote preventive action: from narratives that make it a collective responsibility to speak out and challenge action that appears untoward, to narratives that make it easier to report mistakes once they have happened.

It has been widely argued that a forward-looking restorative 'no-blame culture' will minimize error by encouraging clinicians to acknowledge their mistakes and near misses. This would, it has been argued, prove more conducive to patient welfare than a backward-looking retributive 'blame culture' that, to the extent that it exists to deter mistakes, hopes to do so by punishing lapses [16,66–69]. Recognizing, perhaps, that a forward-looking moral goal of error prevention needs to accommodate backward-looking moral goals of justice and restitution, a new rhetoric of 'fair blame' has emerged [70].

Returning to the case of Dr. X, the consultant at Saxonvale University Hospitals who systematically erred over a period of several years, Dr. X's medical director Dr. Seddon argued that the organization should shoulder its share of the blame. The organization had left Dr. X to work alone in a demanding specialty and had failed adequately to monitor Dr. X's work. Dr. Seddon's view of the organization's responsibility for error had as much to do with justice as error prevention. It was a moral narrative concerned with equitable apportionment of blame between the individual practitioner and the organization, an expectation that the organization be accountable for its own omissions in the past as well as in the future. The difficulty, as we saw in Chapter 2, is finding the right balance between the demands of justice and the demands of safety. The backward-looking narratives of blame and exculpation that consume medico-legal proceedings may be sharply at odds with forward-looking narratives of protection and prevention that consume those concerned with risk management.

Performance management in the middle ground

One consequence of past investigations into medical harm in the UK has been the introduction of a raft of statutory and administrative mechanisms designed to fill the lacunae found in professional self-regulation. One important aim of these has been to ensure that organizations that employ doctors, or commission primary care, take proper responsibility for managing poor performance. Professional self-regulation has thus been significantly augmented by additional managerial controls and structures of local bureaucratic accountability. These mechanisms are being further strengthened by the introduction of revalidation, the process through which doctors are required to renew periodically their basic licence to practise and – for those qualified in a specialty, as all NHS consultants must by law be – their specialty certification. Employing organizations will have a central role to play in this process, because quinquennial revalidation will be based on annual employer appraisal [71,72].[14]

The introduction of new management powers has made the middle ground newly problematic, for the very reason that it is more possible than it used to be to work it. It is in the middle ground that most deviance will be found. It is also in the middle ground that there is greatest uncertainty; it is here that judgements about causes of injury, about professional competence and about individual potential for improvement are all more finely balanced and contestable. It is in the middle ground, therefore, that the scope for injustice, to doctors or patients, is greatest. The middle ground troubles medical directors because it is here that the propriety of their investigations, and the propriety of proposed remedies, is most vulnerable to their own internal doubts and to external challenge.

Competing explanatory frameworks

Iatrogenic injury presents a profound challenge to the practice of medicine, to patients' and clinicians' capacity to make sense of what goes wrong, and to how we understand moral repair. We are not obliged, for the purposes of this study, to decide how iatrogenic injury may be best understood. Medical directors, however, cannot avoid doing so. In the process

---

[14] For the UK provisions see Appendix and 'Distancing Members from Community' in Chapter 2. At the time of writing, the view from the USA is that President Obama's health reforms are likely to promote greater clinical integration, rationalizing service provision and shifting signficant numbers of physicians from self-employment into hospital employment. Whether this will produce a similar shift from reliance on professional self-regulation to organizational managerial control is an interesting question for organizations and the profession.

of 'making things right', the practices of moral repair will inevitably confront different beliefs about 'what goes wrong'.

Chambers identified four different frameworks of explanation for how things go wrong, corresponding to some degree with the kind of wrong that has occurred. Sometimes fault is seen to lie with the doctor who miscalculates: a theory that treats the agent as fallible. Sometimes fault is seen to lie within the practice of medicine, a technically complex and intrinsically risky practice: this theory treats fallibility as a characteristic of the act not the actor. Sometimes fault is thought to lie neither with individuals nor systems alone but occurs where the two are disastrously misaligned: this is a theory of fallibility arising at the conjunction of actor and act. Finally, it is suggested that perhaps any sense of fault lies deep within impossible (normative) expectations of medicine, so that when we fail to control disease, master the body or conquer death we conclude that things have gone awry: this theory proposes that fallibility lies in the purposes that we assign to medicine [73].[15]

As we move on to consider the processes of moral repair in medicine, we should keep in mind that any attempt to put things to right must contend with any or all of those ways of making sense of what went so awfully amiss.

Understanding moral relations and moral repair

Moral philosophers following Immanuel Kant have often described ethics as answering the question 'What ought I to do?' This seems to imply a set of choices on a fresh page. One of our recurrent ethical tasks, however, is better suggested by the question 'What ought I – or, better, *we* – to do *now*?' after someone has blotted or torn the page by doing something wrong. [74(p6)]

Our understanding of the nature of moral relationships in medicine has significant implications for what needs to be done when moral relationships suffer damage. In this section I draw on philosopher Margaret Walker's work to review the particular bonds of confidence, trust and hope that practices of moral repair in medicine seek to restore.

Reliance and responsibility

We observed how normative expectations function in relation to fiduciary, bureaucratic and collegial propriety throughout Chapter 4.[16] In this chapter we will see how normative

---

[15] I replace Chambers' phrase 'fallible agency' with 'fallible conjunction'.

[16] Normative expectations were discussed in detail in Chapter 3. For readers who may encounter this chapter first, normative expectations fuse what we think ought to happen with what we think will actually happen. They are concerned with 'norms' in the sense that moral theorists use the word, referring to morally significant standards for behaviour. 'Respect patient autonomy' is a norm familiar to doctors. The existence of norms elicits expectations from those with an interest in them. So 'respect patient autonomy' elicits expectations from healthcare professionals, as well as from patients, carers, regulators and others. Such expectations are 'expectations' in two senses. First we 'expect' others to adhere to certain standards, taking the view that they ought to respect these standards because the standards embody values important to us. Second we 'expect' that much of the time others will observe these standards, because they have demonstrated a willingness to abide by them or because they have expressed sentiments suggesting they support them. So we expect (in a moral sense) doctors to respect patient autonomy, and we expect that (in a predictive sense) doctors will for the most part try to do so.

expectations underpin trust-based moral relationships between doctors, patients and organizations; and how practices of moral repair after harm serve to shore up such normative expectations. Walker has argued that the practice of morality

> consists in trust-based relations anchored on our expectations of one another that require us to take responsibility for what we do or fail to do, and that allow us to call others to account for what they do or fail to do. [74(p23)]

Our capacity to take responsibility for what we do or fail to do, and to call others to account for what they do or fail to do, rests to a significant degree upon attitudes of confidence, trust and hope. Our normative expectations are founded in our confidence that we share certain moral standards with others; in our trust that others will observe shared moral standards; and in confidence, trust and hope that when important norms are breached others will join us to take action against the offender. It is *standards* in which we repose our confidence, our conviction that we have general agreement about what it is alright to do; and it is *people* in whom we place our trust, our belief that they will generally want to do what it is all right to do. Our confidence and our trust mean we can live in hopefulness, imagining futures and pursuing life projects that we believe to be reasonable according to our shared understandings.

When normative expectations are disappointed, confidence, trust and hope are what empower us to object, to negotiate, to 'forgive and forget', to reprove, or to rally a response and seek a way of insisting that others live up to them. But when confidence or trust or hope is undermined, it becomes more difficult to make moral sense of situations. We may not know what to expect, what we have a right to demand, who to hold responsible, whether or how to hold them to account. We are at risk of losing our capacity to locate ourselves, and our value as moral agents, in relation to others, and their moral agency. These are the circumstances in which moral repair is required. In helping to recapture attitudes of confidence, trust and hope, moral repair helps to maintain or if necessary restore the functionality in our normative expectations.[17]

What medical injury threatens first is the confidence that patients repose in the authority of the moral norms governing medical care. How could they have come to harm in a system truly committed to protecting them [75]?[18] Is the system a danger to others too? Will anyone be called to account? Do norms of beneficence, non-maleficence and justice not govern medicine after all? Iatrogenic injury also has the potential to destroy trust. Do doctors not care enough about their patients to make them safe? Are they not properly trained and fully competent? Do they not consider themselves accountable? Do they not regret what they have done? Are their patients merely objects to them? Are patients not worthy of respect? Do they not deserve compassion?

Confidence in standards and trust in persons are concepts frequently conflated. When we take care to distinguish them, as Walker does, we see more clearly what moral repair must accomplish, and the difficulties with which it must contend. How, for example, can

---

[17] Walker notes an important complicating factor here: if the normative expectations arise out of an unjust social order, moral repair either restores relationships that are morally questionable or may be directed towards changing them.

[18] Using the term protection echoes bioethicist Soren Holm's notion of protective responsibility, which fits well with Walker's account of trust as reliance linked to responsibility. See reference 75.

damage to confidence in the authority of standards be repaired when it is impossible to agree what went wrong? How can confidence in standards be rebuilt if organizations decline to review or restate them? How is confidence to be restored unless organizations openly declare what they will do to prevent similar harm to others? Rather differently, how can trust be repaired when doctors exploit medico-legal procedures to deny responsibility? How can trust be reconstituted if the person who broke it does not acknowledge they have done so? How can trust be reinstated unless someone who has done harm demonstrates they can change their behaviour?

Trust is so central to the relationship between medical directors and the doctors they lead, as well as to the relationship between doctors and the patients the serve, that it bears some further comment. Walker has observed that the challenge for philosophical conceptions of trust lies in accommodating the full range of trusting relationships [74(p74ff)]. This is particularly true of conceptions of trust in medicine. It seems that a single concept must explain the trust that a medical director reposes in her consultant staff; the trust of clinicians in lay managers and vice-versa; the trust of a parent, who knows their child's disability intimately, in clinicians who understand neither this child nor this particular disability; the trust of a chronically ill patient, expert about her own illness, in a doctor who owns both a different perspective on disease and the key to resources such as prescription drugs; and the trust of a patient undergoing elective surgery in the hands of surgeon they have deliberately chosen on grounds of outcome data.

Seminal analyses, such as those by philosophers Annette Baier and Philip Pettit, have proven useful and have found a place in the medical-ethical literature. They do not, however, quite satisfy this requirement to explain of all of the variants [76–78].[19]

Baier, for instance, argues that trust entails reliance upon the good will and competence of others to take care of whatever we entrust to them. One this account, when we trust, we voluntarily accept that we are vulnerable to others' decisions about how to use their discretion in discharging that trust. But the emphasis Baier places on both the good will of the practitioner and the voluntary act of entrusting excludes common features of trust in medical settings. In relation to good will, doctors are expected to treat patients well, whether they feel good will or not; indeed, the true test of a doctor's professionalism is what he does when he fails to feel any good will towards the patient whatsoever. And in relation to voluntarism, trust may be necessary when one has absolutely no choice but to entrust what we care about to the care of others, as in patients entrusting themselves to emergency treatment or a medical leader entrusting patients to his consultant colleagues.

Walker has usefully proposed a more parsimonious definition: trust is a basic mechanism that links reliance on others to their responsibility for meeting certain needs. When we rely upon the people that we trust to fulfil our normative expectations, we believe we are entitled to hold them responsible if they let us down.

Treating trust as reliance upon others to fulfil normative expectations for which they may be held responsible expresses the basic dynamics of trust across a wide range of medical circumstances. It encompasses the trust medical leaders place in their clinical staff to treat patients effectively and with respect; the distressed husband who has no choice but to entrust his confused wife to the care of a junior doctor in the emergency department; the

---

[19] E.g. Beauchamp and Childress cite Baier and Pettit without qualification.

trust of the expert medical consumer who has selected an elite specialist doctor. It captures, especially, the reliance that patients have on clinicians to fulfil our normative expectation that they will protect us from harm.

Responsibility and medical harm

Walker's analysis invites us to consider two salient aspects of reliance and responsibility in relation to medical harm. Patients rely upon others to carry out both forward-looking and backward-looking responsibilities; and they place their reliance in both collective bodies and individual professionals.

Patients rely upon doctors both to protect them from the risk of iatrogenic injury and to acknowledge harm when it has occurred. The prospective aspect is intimately tied to the goals of risk reduction that we associated earlier in this chapter with the patient safety movement. In the discourse of the patient safety movement, the prospective dimension has come to be closely associated with organizational responsibilities for coordinating preventive action. The preventive approach includes eschewing blame and punishment in the interests of openness, developing organizational strategies to avert future injury, developing checklists, protocols and other practice standards that enhance predictability, and so on. The retrospective aspect is intimately tied to requirements of accountability and justice. In the discourse of medical law, retrospective analysis has tended to track individual responsibility, fault and blame. Activities thus include identifying what went wrong, accounting for why it went wrong, understanding the nature and quality of harm, and determining whether any one or any thing is at fault.

It is noticeable that in what is still a rather scant corpus of ethical analysis of medical mistake, the focus has been less on prospective, protective and organizational responsibilities than on retrospective, restitutive and individual responsibilities [38,79,80].[20] This discussion shares with other ethical analysis a concern for how past wrongs are righted; but moves beyond the individual to consider the responsibilities of the organization.

The distinction between individual and collective responsibility is of real significance to medical leadership of moral repair. Medical leaders need to understand who or what patients, carers and colleagues have trusted; and therefore who or what is capable of discharging the responsibility for moral restitution. Those adversely affected by iatrogenic injury include, as well as the patients who suffer it, the carers who behold it and the doctors who were involved in inflicting it. In most cases those involved will have trusted both individuals (the professionals in the team providing care) and organizations (the care setting, and those responsible for ensuring the competence of the professionals providing care). It follows from this that moral repair work must be the responsibility of both the trusted individuals and the trusted organizations. Ideally, both will do whatever is necessary to restore trust. Unfortunately, one or other may not. Can moral repair be achieved in such circumstances?

American legal theorist Joel Feinberg made the influential observation that legal liability can be separated from moral fault; but while legal liability can be passed on to another to discharge, fault and the guilt that goes with it remains with the person who committed the wrong [81]. We see this very clearly in those medical negligence claims where injury is attributable to an individual doctor's acts or omissions. In the UK, the

---

[20] Cf. references 38, 79 and 80.

National Health Service Litigation Authority accepts the burden of legal liability. But fault, guilt, shame, reprobation and reproof belong to the doctor whose behaviour caused the harm.

We can trace a similar pattern in the relationship of legal restitution to moral repair. The cost of legal restitution can be passed on, but the burden of moral repair remains with the person who committed the wrong. In civil law it makes sense to separate liability from moral fault and pin liability onto an organization capable of meeting the claim, because civil law is concerned with financial restitution. Money is a universal mode of exchange, and if money is what is needed to compensate for injury then it does not matter where it comes from. But trust is not a universal currency. Trust is placed in particular persons, and if trust is betrayed it is particular persons who betray it. A relationship of trust, once it arises, comprises a moral bond that an individual cannot unilaterally deny. In consequence, an individual's responsibility for restoring moral relations can be shared with another, but it cannot, it would seem, be discarded.

Imagine first the situation where a doctor is clearly at fault for making an error, but she denies responsibility. The organization issues an apology. Will it suffice; does the organization have the moral standing to issue an apology that will effect moral repair? However fulsome the organizational apology, it is unlikely to suffice as a gesture of repair unless it indicates how the doctor has been called to account. An essential ethical task remains undone and either the doctor must do it, or the organization must find a means to make the doctor do it.

Now imagine the opposite circumstance. Organizational systems have failed in such a way as to expose patients to harm; a serious outbreak of *C. difficile* perhaps. The organizational leaders deny that the organization bears any responsibility, as an organization. Again, a well-intended apology from a faultless, or only partially faulty, medical professional on his own behalf does not correspond to the wrong. Moral repair requires the organization, in the person of its leaders, to acknowledge its fault and remedy the situation.

Medical leaders therefore have multiple responsibilities in relation to moral repair following medical harm. They are responsible for what they personally do; and they are symbolically responsible for what the organization as a whole does. The medical leader has a moral responsibility for holding individual doctors accountable to the organization; a moral responsibility for holding individual doctors accountable to individual patients; a moral responsibility to doctors to hold them to account fairly; and a moral responsibility to stand as a symbol of the organization's accountability to patients and other stakeholders.

Morally managing iatrogenic injury: organizational narratives of acknowledgement

The prominence given to morally managing iatrogenic injury in my account of organizational ethics is consistent with the nature and scope of the narratives that participants recounted. But medical directors rarely portrayed the events included in this chapter as moral management of medical harm. Rather, they couched the issue as the thorny problem of 'performance managing' errant colleagues. The decision to treat moral repair as central to the enactment of organizational ethics places a particular construction upon those data.

A superficial and instrumental interpretation, one that reflects medical directors' responsibilities and accountabilities, would be that the behaviour of errant colleagues gives them cause for moral concern because they are answerable for the quality of care. Medical directors are responsible for managing clinical performance problems, and ultimately responsible for their organizations' responses to complaints about medical treatment. In light of their role responsibilities, it is therefore hardly surprising that the majority of participants referred to managing clinical performance problems as a major source of moral anxiety.

A deeper, less instrumental interpretation is that medical leaders' narratives reveal an intense appreciation of the moral significance of iatrogenic injury, and the moral significance of the processes that follow in its wake. Their concerns were more than merely role-related. Managing iatrogenic injury, and managing the colleagues who might cause it, brought to the surface concerns about what was morally right and proper: concerns about trust and confidence, reliance and responsibility, care and commitment. These concerns were sometimes less choate than their more instrumental worries, but they were no less present and no less significant.

The starting point for my analysis of moral repair is that it is a fundamentally narrative practice. It is grounded in acknowledging how the fabric of confidence, trust and hope has been rent asunder; and in acknowledging what must be undertaken if these are to be restored. Inquisitorial and restorative propriety underpin this narrative practice. They are the ways in which medical leaders work to orchestrate an organizational narrative of acknowledgement. Walker, Smith and Berlinger have all offered philosophical analyses that help us to understand what it is that has to be acknowledged in order for moral repair to succeed; as might be expected each of their accounts differs somewhat [32,74,82]. Medical leaders' narratives of moral repair shared in common with those analyses the following seven critical acts of acknowledgement:

(i)   acknowledging an injured party as a moral interlocutor;
(ii) acknowledging the authority of shared norms;
(iii) acknowledging injury;
(iv) acknowledging responsibility;
(v)   acknowledging that remedy is due, and that the injured party may define what is owed;
(vi) acknowledging righteous anger, or other negative feelings, in those who have been injured; and
(vii) acknowledging that in injuring another, we should experience sorrow and regret.

However well they address the sense of injury, such acts of acknowledgement cannot reverse time, nor can they undo moral or physical harm. They can, however, help to redress the pervasive feelings of loss of control that injury brings in its wake. When we harm another, even unintentionally, we inflict upon them a new and unwanted reality, a new present and future, a new life narrative that, like it or not, they are obliged to live. We compound the injury if we go on to deny the harm, disregard the wrong, and impose our own definition of what is morally acceptable. In the face of injury, practices of acknowledgement serve to reiterate the moral authority of a community, to demonstrate its willingness to hold members to account, to symbolize the (possibly innocent) offender's deference to collective appraisal, and to reinstate the moral position of the injured party. Practices of acknowledgement take from those who may have inflicted injury their power to define good and bad, right and wrong, what and who counts, and what and who does not; and they reinvest that power in the community and in the injured party.

A worked example of moral repair

In this part of the chapter my aim is to analyse the practices of acknowledgement that come to be expressed in a single narrative of moral repair. Following this, I move on to explore how the inquisitorial and restorative proprieties contribute to orchestrating many more such moral narratives.

The Royal Metropolitan Infirmary is a venerable teaching hospital with a highly qualified consultant body, a diverse patient population, a high proportion of tertiary referrals and a significant research base. The Infirmary's Medical Director is Dr. Christopher Chalcraft, a well-known and widely admired medical leader who has probably enjoyed rather more than his fair share of high-profile successes and setbacks. Our story starts several years ago, not long after Chalcraft arrived at the Infirmary. The hospital had for some time been providing care for a patient with several challenging medical conditions. Eventually a delicate and demanding surgical procedure was proposed, and with some qualms it was agreed that the operation should go ahead. Sadly, the patient died shortly afterwards. The patient's family was distraught. They felt that the people to whom they had entrusted the care of their loved one had not lived up to their expectations.

In the extended – and very little edited – interview extract that follows, Chalcraft supplies a cogent and almost complete description of doing moral repair.[21] We see how moral repair is an intrinsically narrative process, in which the demands of moral relationship are fully acknowledged through practices of propriety. I have left Dr. Chalcraft's account intact because it so vividly exemplifies how the integrity and effectiveness of moral repair rests upon its components being sutured into a coherent whole. The narrative has been broken into sections below, but it was delivered unbroken in the interview itself.

> §1. Let's take as an example a complaint that I got more involved in than I usually do. A local GP wrote to me as an advocate for a family whose disabled relative had died in the hospital. The GP was concerned, because although we had responded to a written complaint the family was unable to understand what had gone wrong. They had met the consultant involved, and they still didn't understand the sequence of events that had led to this death. So the complaints team and I looked at the issues and we responded a second time. But the family was no more satisfied than they had been the first time, so I decided to do an internal investigation in much greater depth.

Dr. Chalcraft started by recounting the family's standing as moral interlocutors; that is, he acknowledged their entitlement to hold others to account. We should note three features. The family did not achieve the position of moral interlocutors alone. They were supported by their GP, who asserted a claim to Dr. Chalcraft's attention through an exercise in fiduciary propriety, advocating on behalf of the deceased patient and the family. Moreover, Dr. Chalcraft was not himself the perpetrator of the injury. The family had already sought out individual 'offenders' through the complaints procedures, and had met the consultant concerned. How, then, could Chalcraft engage with them as a

---

[21] The transcript has been sparsely edited where necessary, with the aim of retaining the tone of Dr. Chalcraft's account while preserving confidentiality.

moral interlocutor? Importantly, he did so as a representative of the moral agency, and hence the moral accountability, of the organization. Finally, Dr. Chalcraft's exercise of organizational moral agency was in significant respects voluntary. Bureaucratic procedures had been implemented, not once but twice. The family could have complained to a higher authority, and Dr. Chalcraft could have left them to get on with it. But something about their plight exerted a claim on his attention. We are entitled to view his decision to act, I think, as a moral response to the normative expectations that the GP made clear.

The substance of their GP's argument had also not only been that the family ought to be acknowledged as moral interlocutors. The GP asserted the authority of community norms. Later in the interview, Dr. Chalcraft described the GP's influence on his decision to take further action: 'This family had got a very good advocate in their GP who was saying "I'm not going to let you off the hook, and this troubles me. As an outside observer with medical knowledge, I see no reason, from what I know, that this relative should have died. I accept that they had complex problems and the treatment was difficult to do but I still don't see why they died. The answers that your organization have given don't satisfy me, so I have some sympathy with these [people]. . ."

§2. I suggested to the GP that I met the family and try to get from them what the issues were. They weren't keen to do that, so I worked through the GP. We held a sort of panel of inquiry. The death had been about two years previously, so quite a lot of the staff at a training level had moved off to other hospitals. We set up a process to call them back in, and like any inquiry of that sort people couldn't remember what had happened. It was quite a tortuous, long-winded process: trying to get to the bottom of how decisions were made, whether people worked to the right standards, whether they handed over issues of care and responsibility in appropriate ways, whether the team was working at a medical level that was appropriate, at a nursing level that was appropriate, what the leadership of the Consultant was like. A lot of quite testy things being discussed. We recorded all of that evidence, produced notes, and fed that back to the relatives as it went along . . . . Then I did a big review myself of the patient's record, used all this evidence, and wrote a report of what I thought had happened, what I thought had gone wrong. At each point where I thought something had gone wrong, I made an analysis of that, and a recommendation for action.

As he recalled the course of the investigation Dr. Chalcraft recounted more of how shared norms came to be stated, applied, interpreted, and their authority acknowledged. His investigation articulated not only norms of medical treatment and nursing care, but also norms of medical responsibility, of professional accountability, and, as we consider later, norms of inquisitorial propriety.

§3. I think that's only been partially successful . . . . One of the things for me, having made a report containing a lot of recommendations for change, is that the team doesn't accept that their standards didn't hit the button that day and therefore might not hit the button every day . . . . Secondly, we'd agreed that we would issue this report to the bereaved relatives as part of good practice, sharing an analysis of where things had gone wrong and what we were going to do about it. They were quite pleased in some ways because the report acknowledged what had gone wrong. Up until that point the responses were a bit 'Sorry, the outcome wasn't that great. But frankly, what else could you expect?' This was a much more detailed response saying 'On *that* day at 8.33 a decision was made which wasn't the best one. Five hours later it was compounded by another error. Then maybe the recognition of things going wrong was too slow.

When you add all of these things together, in a very complex case patients can die. That's bad practice, and we need to do some things about it'. So the relatives liked that bit of it. What they didn't like was that I didn't recommend that individuals should be singled out and punished. They took on, if you like, the punishment aspect, by reporting the nursing staff to the Nursing and Midwifery Council and the medical staff to the GMC. In the end, that's of course their choice.

When he finally set out and reported the conclusions of his inquiry to the family, Dr. Chalcraft acknowledged the injury that had been done and acknowledged the responsibility of the organization. From his description of the effects of the report, it is not clear whether Dr. Chalcraft appreciated from the outset the moral significance of a full and detailed narrative of events and his recommendations for change. As he explains in §4 however, instrumental aims made it important to review the quality of care with an exactitude that would protect future patients from harm. But Dr. Chalcraft also movingly describes in §5 how his meticulous account helped the family to understand what had happened, and how, in and of itself, this had helped to repair some of the damage that had been done.

Giving an undertaking to change injurious practices gives substance to the acknowledgement of responsibility, and is one of the most significant ways of acknowledging that remedy is due. To the extent that Dr. Chalcraft's recommendations constituted a promise to the family it was, however, a promise that could prove difficult to fulfil. The remedy that he acknowledged was due and the changes in practice that he recommended were not his to execute. They lay within the power of a team that, as he reported here, did not accept or wish to implement them.

> §4. There are some really big challenges about how at an individual level you get a change in mindset, and therefore how you get changes in the whole system. It's really challenging work, to find ways of reviewing care which don't just put people off, or make them feel that they're being punished, or that it's just demoralizing because you did your best and then everybody criticizes you afterwards because your best wasn't good enough on that day.

The practice of acknowledging that remedy is due contains a second element, acknowledging that the injured party has a legitimate view about what the remedy should be. For the family, Dr. Chalcraft's recommendations for change were not, in themselves, sufficient remedy. They sought punishment of the individuals concerned. In these circumstances Dr. Chalcraft had no option other than to accept their choice, and it is unclear how far he acknowledged directly to them that they possessed the right of those who have been wronged to make their choice of remedy. The remedy that the family sought seemed to Dr. Chalcraft to run counter to the interests of other significant moral actors: to some extent those of the professionals involved, and more importantly those of future patients. Bonds of collegiality may have been in part what dissuaded Dr. Chalcraft from pursuing punitive action, but so too was an interest in building a 'fair blame' culture that worked in favour of greater patient safety.

> §5. The team that I have to help me do clinical governance, I think were impressed with the outcome and the nature of the report and the depth with which it went into medical matters. In keeping with many hospitals and organizations, there's a bit of a view that doctors don't take this very seriously – they just assume they're very good – and nobody ever gets down to the bottom of what doctors do. So I think there was a bit of improved 'street-cred' for me with that group. It did help the bereaved family to move on a bit. Part of the reason they were so limpet-like was that they

had looked after their relative for over a decade, and were fantastically expert at it. Then they suddenly saw a team who *claimed* to be expert, not very good at providing the care . . . . At least the report helped them to understand what had happened and it eased some of that for them. It allowed them to use the route which they'd wanted to do, which was to get at one or two staff and say 'We don't think you're any good'. I'm disturbed by that, because although I understand the human motive the potential for demoralizing clinical staff is very high and very destructive.

Dr. Chalcraft's reflection on the impact of the investigation on the clinical governance team, speaks eloquently of the heterogeneity of 'community' moral norms in healthcare organizations. This was an organizational 'community' divided over the meaning and value of clinical governance to the various 'sub-communities' within it. Dr. Chalcraft's inquiry served to reinforce the authority of the moral norms upon which clinical governance activities were based.

Going further into the emotional dimension of moral repair, Dr. Chalcraft's account suggests in §1, §2 as well as here in §5 a genuine readiness to countenance the family's distress and righteous anger. But he also sought to deflect it from the clinical staff involved, seeing it as potentially destructive. It is part of the tragedy of iatrogenic injury that a moment of inattention, a habitual practice acceptable in all situations but one, or a series of plausible but less than optimal decisions can have devastating consequences. It is clearly morally right to acknowledge the harm that has been done to a person who suffers injury. Ought we also to acknowledge the harm to the person who commits the error? On the one hand, to articulate the pain of the professional responsible for the injury may be to imply that their suffering is in some way morally equivalent to the suffering of the injured patient. On the other hand, not to do so may imply that the error is of no consequence to the person who made it, and that they do not suffer genuine remorse [32].[22]

Remorse and regret are close cousins, which brings us to the final requirement of moral repair: acknowledgement that injury demands unconditional regret. Dr. Chalcraft tells us rather little about whether or how he expressed regret to the family. But to the extent that Dr. Chalcraft himself did so, it may not have been sufficient. The fact is that Dr. Chalcraft was not the agent who made the mistake and was not, therefore, the agent whose regret would most count.

Dr. Chalcraft's account of his investigation into this patient's death has shown very clearly how moral repair is a narrative process grounded in acknowledgement. Meaningful acknowledgement – acknowledging what did actually happen, and acknowledging the moral significance of what actually happened – rests, in turn, upon inquisitorial and restorative proprieties. In the next two sections, we shall examine how inquisitorial propriety enables fitting moral narratives to emerge, and how restorative propriety uses narrative devices to effect moral repair.

Inquisitorial propriety

The most challenging issues countenanced by medical leaders investigating iatrogenic harm are determining how harm has arisen, and protecting the moral interests of all of the different parties concerned as they do so. Inquisitorial propriety is, of all the proprieties, the

---

[22] See Ch. 3 in reference 63.

one that is most closely associated with the process of organizational sense-making that we considered in Chapter 2. I argued there that sense-making requires us to settle both matters that are uncertain, and which may be amenable to resolution when more information has been collected, and matters that are equivocal or values-based, where information-gathering is of little use because the issue is only amenable to principled reasoning. For the most part, those investigating medical injury are dealing with uncertainty, and they do so by gathering data. But some questions, such as what constitutes an acceptable way to behave, may remain equivocal.

As well as determining how harm has arisen, investigators must manage the fraught circumstances surrounding medical harm. Managing an investigation and its surrounding circumstances entails balancing legal, moral and emotional commitments owed to patients, to families, to colleagues, and to others. In this section, my focus is on how inquisitorial propriety enables this delicate balance to be achieved. Extensive legal and administrative principles, rules and requirements comprise a significant backdrop to the accounts that follow.[23] The legal principles that endeavour to ensure that natural justice is seen to be done, and the principles that protect individual interests through imposing requirements of due process, are of substantial moral as well as legal significance. But medical leaders are not lawyers, and my purpose here is to explore how propriety is actually expressed in their thinking and in their actions. Natural justice and due process in their legal guise are undoubtedly informing their approach, but the organizational narratives through which these principles are expressed are organizational *moral* narratives. This discussion of inquisitorial propriety could thus be treated as evidence of how the law pervades non-legal action.

In the discussion that follows I am largely concerned with the conduct that propriety demands of medical leaders themselves. But propriety is a relational practice in which those with authority define normative expectations of others. Medical directors held definite views about the modes of conduct befitting doctors under investigation. These have important implications for doctors, whose conduct during an investigation may exert significant influence over the extent to which medical directors continue to repose their trust in them. I therefore conclude my discussion of inquisitorial propriety on the part of medical leaders by considering the reciprocal expectations that apply in turn to doctors.

The centrality of procedure to inquisitorial propriety

I have a maxim which is 'If you've got a process, use it'. . . . By and large most eventualities are covered by set procedures or protocols, either local to the organization or national statutory . . . . I'm not beyond scrutiny and certainly not above scrutiny, but if scrutinized, then what I've done is appropriate. (Dr. Rosenberg, St. Frideswide Hospitals NHS Trust)

One of the first questions to confront medical directors countenancing a possible episode of iatrogenic harm is a backward-looking one: what exactly has happened? The next is forward-looking: are patients at risk of future harm? The question that naturally follows

---

[23] For discussion of the procedures in place in the NHS for managing performance concerns see Appendix 3 and also the section 'Negotiating conditions for community membership' in Chapter 2.

is procedural: how can these questions be answered in an effective and fair way [83]?[24] This is the realm of inquisitorial propriety. Inquisitorial propriety refers to the practices involved in assembling a just narrative of events. But investigating moral harm and restoring moral balance are activities not neatly separable. A sincere inquiry into the causes of harm is a significant part of the restitution that many victims seek, and there is much that may be done at the inquisitorial stage to ameliorate the sense of moral injury that victims of iatrogenic harm experience.

In many situations where fair assessments of fault have to be made, there is no independent yardstick by which the outcome can be judged. How can we be sure we have arrived at the correct answer? We cannot. Instead, we rely heavily upon following the correct procedures, believing that by doing so we will find our way to a 'good enough' narrative of what happened and who is responsible.[25] Procedures serve to guide action in such circumstances; they help to render actions consistent with the normative expectations that arise on every side, and in accord with the demands of accountability. Compliance with practices of procedural fairness, such as eliciting the testimony of those who have been harmed, underpins the validity of adjudication. They assist those who are interested in the proceedings to accept the outcome, even where it is one that goes against them [84].

Dr. Rosenberg pointed to the association between inquisitorial propriety and the demands of administrative and legal processes that transcend individuals and their organizations:

> the need at all times to make sure that I'm following due process, because clearly one gets into the area of litigation, employment law, vulnerabilities, organizational responsibilities, data protection, freedom of information, a huge raft of statutes that you have to abide by.
>
> (Dr. Rosenberg, St. Frideswide Hospitals NHS Trust)

I have noted that legal principles demanding that natural justice be observed and due process be applied when individuals are under investigation are a critical factor shaping inquisitorial propriety. But while legal and administrative requirements help to structure reparative action, they are generalized and abstract prescriptions. They cannot precisely specify what must be done in this situation right now, and however exhaustive the advice a leader receives it is still down to them to perform whatever must be done. So legal and administrative requirements are significant, but they are not exhaustive of ethical enactment. A truly moral practice demands far more nuanced and considerate behaviour than merely dutiful or even enthusiastic compliance with rules. Rosenberg went on to hint at the interpersonal demands that invariably accompany acting in accordance with procedures; at the delicate balance involved in 'holding the line' on due process while enacting compassion towards individuals in distress:

---

[24] Where moral repair generally attends to a torn moral fabric, inquisitorial propriety prompts the 'stitch in time' that sometimes saves it. Throughout the discussion of inquisitorial propriety, I draw on medical directors' accounts of managing the risks of prospective iatrogenic injury as well as managing reported iatrogenic injury. Although the focus of this chapter is moral repair, inquisitorial propriety is important as a response to harm that has been avoided but which remains a possibility.

[25] A common-sense expression of 'pure procedural justice': 'there is a correct or fair procedure such that the outcome is likewise correct or fair, whatever it is, provided that the procedure has been properly followed'. See reference 83.

and therefore the need for me, as a fairly disorganized person … to make sure that everything is done properly. That we're fair and equitable in dealings with the individual practitioner, in dealings with the legal representatives, in dealings with patients' representatives. That there's no bias, that there's no disadvantage, that's there's no prejudice on my part expressed in either direction …. It's particularly difficult when you're face-to-face with somebody who is suffering as a consequence [of medical injury] whether it's patient or whether it's practitioner.

(Dr. Rosenberg, St. Frideswide Hospitals NHS Trust)

If compliance with natural justice and due process is thus, in most situations, a necessary ingredient in moral repair, it is not in any way sufficient. Narratives of moral repair have to contend with three difficulties that inquisitorial propriety assists in resolving, and that we shall examine in turn. First, they must affirm or reinstate the moral worth of individuals, and their standing in the eyes of others. This is assisted through providing an arena for hearing the voice of those who have been injured, and through overt demonstrations of impartiality that emphasize no party's voice will carry greater weight than any others. Second, they have to affirm the authority of shared norms, demonstrating how they shape reasonable expectations and bind all members of the community. Inquisitorial propriety addresses this difficulty through careful interpretation of standards. Third, they must recognize the experience of a 'broken world', a world in which moral harm has been done. Inquisitorial propriety endeavours to acknowledge injury without necessarily accepting that all statements are true.

Inquisitorial propriety as 'hearing the other side'

Seeking to understand the varying perspectives on events, and accepting that each might legitimately be held, is a basic requirement of inquisitorial propriety. It is the ethical expression of a principle that is 'as old as the law, and is of universal justice, that no one shall be personally bound until he has had his day in court' [85]. This is so venerable and familiar a principle that we rarely consider its moral basis.

Briefly, hearing the views of differently situated actors is morally valuable for at least three reasons. It respects the dignity of the parties involved through recognizing each as a moral interlocutor. It enhances accuracy in decision-making by ensuring that differently situated actors have each described events, as they understand them. And open hearings or circulation of findings to interested parties both impose constraints on partiality, because those subject to a decision have, in principle, access to the same information as the adjudicator [86]. These considerations are as relevant to quasi-legal or informal inquiries as they are to legal proceedings. It is reasonable to view them as the concerns that ground our normative expectations in respect of inquiries and adjudications.

To fail to invite those interested to state their case would thus be an egregious breach of inquisitorial propriety. Those entitled to attend may demur, as did the carers in Dr. Chalcraft's inquiry. But those summoned to be present are bound by strong normative expectations that they will attend and honestly answer awkward questions, as Chalcraft expected junior doctors to do. Furthermore, doctors who attempt to deflect accountability through medico-legal obfuscation may (as did Dr. Lister's colleague, encountered in Chapter 2) succeed in winning the argument, but only at the cost of losing their colleagues' trust and respect.

Inquisitorial propriety as impartiality

The worst problems that I have are the effects of when things are going, or perceived to be going, wrong, and the modern requirement for blame. And trying to protect my colleagues from that, and certainly from unfairness .... The difficulty is that I have to be very careful ... I don't [want to] overstep a boundary, protecting [colleagues]. Because you can step over, and then you'll start protecting people when actually it's wrong.

(Dr. Samuel Seddon, Saxonvale University Hospitals Trust)

A central requirement of moral repair is to reaffirm the equal moral worth of individuals. The apparent impediment to this is the natural partiality we show to one another in social relationships. In the context of iatrogenic harm, the partiality that threatens fair judgement is the collegial propriety that we examined in the last chapter. Inquisitorial propriety offers overt demonstrations of impartiality by way of a solution. Procedural fairness must not only be done, it must be seen, and indeed felt, to be done. Collegial propriety sustains normative expectations of mutuality, tolerance, charity and forgiveness. If partiality is not to lead to injustice, then these expectations must temporarily be suspended.

Recalling the experience of dealing with allegations against a colleague, as well as (unrelated) allegations against himself, Dr. Hutchinson depicted these temporary suspensions of collegiality as 'proper' but nevertheless painful.

We're a very proper organization, so you're always left a bit – people don't sidle up to you and say 'Oh don't worry, whatever comes out you'll be okay'. The Chief Executive ... he's the most upright, proper – so you just don't [express support] no matter how much you want to be supportive of somebody. You wouldn't. So ... there will be times when you will be left to dig down, to get your own resources to support yourself through something. I had friends who knew about [allegations against me], but they didn't quite understand [that professional relationships would not protect me]. They thought it was all sort of cut and dried. (Dr. Hutchinson, Evenlode Park NHS Trust)

When partiality is suspended, all of the parties become equally entitled to a share of impartial empathy. So while Dr. Hutchinson accentuated the importance of being 'proper' he also stressed the importance of conducting oneself in such a way as to make it plain that:

at the centre of every case there's a human being, even though they might have done something you don't approve of.

Mentally extricating themselves from ties of community enables medical leaders to avert the twin risks of unjustly favouring colleagues because they were part of the community of practice; or of unjustly condemning them for fear that their alleged actions would bring disgrace to the community of practitioners.

What sentiments replace the bonds of collegiality that are thus temporarily suspended? Interestingly, there is a tendency to draw analogies between investigating colleagues and treating patients. There are some informative similarities, as Dr. Rosenberg shows below. But there is more at stake here, I think. Placing possibly errant colleagues in the category of 'cases for treatment' makes it possible to withdraw the privileges of collegial partiality while protecting colleagues from the status degradation associated with the category of 'malefactors'. Investigating iatrogenic injury is, then:

> a test of one's impartiality. I think [impartiality is] something that you learn as a clinician when you're dealing with your patients. It's this old thing that doctors mustn't get too involved with their patients. You obviously have to empathize, you obviously have to approach them holistically, you have to recognize their problems, you have to understand the wider implications of an illness and its manifestations. But at the end of the day you're required to stand to one side and to make judgements and decisions . . . . If you become too involved, emotionally involved, then it actually gets in the way of effective practice . . . . In the same way, as a medical director you have to stand to one side and allow this process to inform you and so you mustn't allow yourself to get emotionally involved and to say 'I don't trust this man, he's a rogue and he's an awful practitioner'. You've got to say the evidence demonstrates that he is capable of doing this and if the evidence tells me, that's what the evidence tells me and you've got to accept that objectively rather than subjectively in the context . . . . So it's a little bit like clinical decision-making in, in that sense.
>
> (Dr. Rosenberg, St. Frideswide Hospitals NHS Trust)

The complex bonds of collegiality tug in several different directions, however. Far from being a threat to impartiality, collegial propriety may summon a supply of objective guidance. It is standard practice to bolster impartiality by bringing in knowledgeable and dispassionate outsiders who are members of an extended collegial network.[26] These are frequently specialist assessors trained for the role by their respective medical Royal Colleges, but in small specialties may be an influential member of the College. While this strategy holds out the prospect of impartial assessment, it cannot guarantee it, and neither can it dispense with the need for independent judgement. Thus Dr. Seddon, for example, wondered whether his reliance on an external expert had introduced a different source of bias.

> I got someone very good who was my rock, really. He enabled me to go through that very difficult process, and was able to give me an external and fairly impartial opinion on, not just the actual events of what had happened, but also about how it had developed into that. He gave me a lot of perspective and a lot of the words to use in trying to portray to both the public and the management exactly what had happened and how it had got to that . . . . The difficulty was that I came to rely on him so much . . . . You need someone external to be able to act as a sounding board, and make sure you're getting it right. But you can get too cosy with that person and actually I think in retrospect I probably should have tried to spread the net a little bit further. I did spread it actually, we did have other people involved, but it was very difficult to get a really objective opinion; very difficult.
>
> (Dr. Seddon, Saxonvale University Hospitals Trust)

Hearing a range of perspectives, and seeking objective and impartial opinions, generates information. It helps to resolve uncertainties about what has actually happened. But to make moral sense out of 'what has actually happened', information has to be viewed from the standpoint of an authoritative norm. Information turns into evidence when it is used to test whether or not a norm has been breached. Testing whether or not a norm

---

[26] The role of various bodies in assisting with the management of injury or performance concerns is reviewed in Appendix 3 and in 'Negotiating conditions for community membership' in Chapter 2.

has been breached requires both that the norm is tolerably clear, and that it is tolerably clear in application. The problems that arise in the course of applying a norm can only multiply when norms of practice are varied and contestable, as they are in medical practice, and when norms of behaviour are subject to interpretation, as they are in any walk of life. The negotiation of standards is thus an inescapable function of inquisitorial propriety.

Inquisitorial propriety and the interpretation of standards

> I've got enough information before me now to have concerns about this person operating on my mother ... (Dr. Evans, Brickvale Hospital NHS Trust)

So far, we have been dealing with matters that are uncertain and which are amenable to being answered through careful data-gathering. (In real life, data-gathering does not always generate clear findings; but the principle holds true.) We now move to matters more equivocal, matters that call not for data-gathering but for the negotiation of moral responsibility.

Ultimately, setting a standard is a matter of judgement; of deciding where to draw the moral line. All jurisdictions have, of course, formal legal definitions of negligent or non-negligent medical care [46–49,87,88].[27] In the UK they are found in a series of judicial pronouncements that all stem from the decision in the *Bolam* case in 1957. These common law legal principles are lent greater specificity by later reported cases, by good practice protocols promulgated by the National Institute for Health and Clinical Excellence, through specialty standards set by committees of the medical Royal Colleges, and by local organizational protocols. All of these are impersonal standards, in the sense that they assume an abstract doctor-patient relationship and stipulate how a universal doctor should treat a universal patient. The standard that many medical leaders favour is, however, strikingly personal: 'given what I suspect, would I allow this practitioner to treat a member of my family'? They replace the abstract patient with 'a person for whom I have a special affection and personal responsibility'. There are echoes here of fiduciary propriety. Faced with the question whether a doctor was good enough, medical leaders asked whether the doctor was good enough to treat a person who depended upon them: my granny, my mother, my child, my spouse. Their verdict on this 'family treatment test' served to summarize their justification for more (or less) active intervention.

For Dr. Evans, the 'family treatment test' marked the turning point (what narrative theorists call the *peripateia*) in a byzantine narrative of misbehaviour, mistrust, mounting doubt, and misadventure:

> I've got enough information before me now to have concerns about this person operating on my mother .... So the investigation takes place, it clearly says that on these two occasions he didn't properly consult and alongside it there's [additional concerns about] other cases. At that point I meet him and his representatives and say 'Well look, I'm going to restrict you from all clinical practice at the moment until we can bottom this out. The way to bottom this out is to

---

[27] In a line of cases following *Bolam v. Friern Hospital Management Committee* [1957] 2 All ER 118: 'The test is the standard of the ordinary skilled man exercising and professing to have that special skill .... A doctor is not guilty of negligence if he has acted in accordance with a practice accepted as proper by a responsible body of medical men skilled in that particular art.' McNair J, at pp. 121, 122.

ask for the Royal College to come in and do a proper review'. What I'm really trying to do, I'm trying to be fair to him, and there's some morals and ethics there. Ultimately [my priority is] patients being safe and not putting them at excess risk so that's the overriding moral and ethical issue that runs here. (Dr Evans, Brickvale Hospital NHS Trust)

If the 'family treatment' test is widely favoured, however, there was at least one dissenter from it in the study. Dr. Rosenberg's maxim, it will be recalled, is 'If you've got a process, use it'. Consistent with this conscientious regard for proceduralism, Dr. Rosenberg emphatically endorsed the principle of impartiality, disapproving of the common rule of thumb as subjective and improper.

> You've got to say, 'The evidence demonstrates that he is capable of doing this'. If the evidence tells me, that's what the evidence tells me. And you've got to accept that, objectively rather than subjectively .... If somebody presented me with a question of 'Would you let your wife or daughter or child be operated on by this man?' then maybe that's when the emotional tie-in gets too great. I wouldn't ever ask myself that question. The question is 'Would you let a patient of this organization be operated on by this man?' not 'your wife or your mother or your child?'
> (Dr. Rosenberg, St. Frideswide Hospitals NHS Trust)

Here we return to the problem of evidence. Intuition, practitioner gossip, private conversations, troublesome behaviour, 'near misses' and worrying outcomes short of demonstrable harm to patients can all contribute to doubts about whether a practitioner would pass the 'family treatment' test. Dr. Jonathan Jay sketched a portrait of one of his problem practitioners that typified many others in the study: the type of practitioner that, so I was told from the very first interview onwards, every medical director knows to be at work in their hospital.

> His clinical work is okay. It's hard to say that he's incompetent, because he's not incompetent; but sometimes you would question his lack of judgement and his attention to detail. He does on occasion appear a bit slap-dash and occasionally a bit cavalier, although I can't put my hand on my heart and say that audit has shown that his results are any worse than anybody else's. But if one of my kin had a condition that needed that sort of attention, he would not be the surgeon I'd want to do it, which is usually a fair indicator. (Dr. Jay, The Charter NHS Trust)

Fiduciary propriety and inquisitorial propriety appear to be pulling in different directions here. Fiduciary propriety, in the form of the 'family treatment test', implies a high threshold of satisfactory performance. Consistent with legal requirements of natural justice and due process, inquisitorial propriety and institutional procedures designed to ensure fairness necessitate that hard evidence be produced before steps are taken to constrain a clinician's sphere of activity. Without fact of iatrogenic injury, without data to support a rebuttable belief that harm might occur, without clear indication of a lack of probity, restrictions on practice are difficult to justify. But fact, data and clear indications may be hardest to come by on the fuzzy margins of 'almost good enough' clinical work.

To recall Freidson, it is in this 'middle ground', between the standards of the butcher and the standards of the saint, that battles over interpretations of behaviour and proper normative expectations are fought. From a medical leaders' perspective the apparently troublesome behaviour of a doctor with performance difficulties might fairly raise doubts about his skill and judgement, and suggest that he lacks insight. From the perspective of the doctor in difficulty it might seem that he is the victim of unfair criticism, arbitrary standards, or discriminatory treatment on grounds of ethnicity, sex, religious affiliation or place of training. Poor practice rarely presents as *res ipsa loquitur*, that is, a situation in which facts speak clearly for themselves. A measure of interpretation is invariably required.

Much that is valuable about medical practice has seemed to resist being reduced to quantifiable outcomes [89–97].[28] A valid and accurate assessment of clinical practice has long been, and to some extent remains, a stubbornly qualitative exercise in judging clinical artistry. The problem with judgements of artistry, of course, is that they are open to contestation. It is hardly surprising, then, that those charged with making such contested judgements have sought out less contestable measures of performance. In the absence of valid instruments for measuring the medical artistry of doctors in primary care, Dr. Thirtle, along with other primary care medical directors, had come to depend upon a range of 'proxy' indicators. These offered more objective grounds for questioning whether the normative expectations they held on behalf of patients were being met, even if they did not quite capture the finer points of clinical practice.

The Quality and Outcomes Framework (QOF) that has been used to commission primary care has required clinical performance to be assessed against primarily quantitative values, and has entailed judging not artistry but management processes and numerical targets. Does a practice have an adequate clinical records system? What are its procedures for monitoring diabetic patients? How many cervical smears has it carried out relative to the eligible population? Making the assumption that a well-organized practice was likely to be a safe and sound practice, QOF performance indicators supplied Dr. Thirtle and his management colleagues with an attractively procedural substitute for more debatable clinical judgements.

Proxy measures have their limits, though. To consistently apply and enforce normative expectations of professional practice still demands conscientious reflection, a willingness to ruminate on and defend one's judgement of practice standards. Dr. Woodhouse was the medical director of Meadborough Primary Care Trust, whose primary care doctors spanned the age range and ethnic diversity of the inner-city area in which they worked. As a relatively youthful, white British medical director, he regularly asked himself:

> how much are my internal prejudices influencing my decision-making? I think that is apparent around the older GPs in particular. The decision is about whether they're just practising in a slightly old-fashioned way that may not be ideal but it's alright and safe; or whether it's actually on the unsafe side of the fence so that we need to do something much tougher. I often spend time reflecting myself about how much I might be influenced by ethnicity, by culture, by language, by the fact that people can't write English clearly, making those kind of judgements where it's the borderline cases.

In the acute sector, the proliferation of clinical protocols intended to guide clinical judgement seems not yet to have subsumed assessments of clinical artistry. There thus remains pressing need to negotiate and compare standards across the community of practice. Where contentious judgements are to be made, a methodical review by an outside authority such as a Royal College 'rapid response team' (see earlier) satisfies two requirements. It is a

---

[28] For an excellent overview of the difficulties surrounding valid and reliable measurement of clinical performance, including Patient Reported Outcome Measures (PROMs), surveys of patient satisfaction and surveys of patient experience read reference 89. For further discussion see references 90–97.

convincing demonstration of impartiality; and it signifies deference to the normative expectations of the community of practice.

The hard question, then, for medical directors, is what to do if they conscientiously disagree with the findings of an impartial investigation carried out by respected members of the community of practice. I shall return to discuss this difficult situation after we have considered the propriety invoked in managing information.

Inquisitorial propriety in normative expectations regarding use of information

I noted earlier that the reparative aim of recognizing a victim's experience of moral harm frequently confronted the problem of our imperfect knowledge of the world. Inquisitorial propriety must contend not only with uncertainty but also with normative expectations about what information it is proper to use when inquiring into iatrogenic harm. The difficulty lies in deciding whether and how to use sensitive information that comes to the attention of those with inquisitorial responsibilities. Here again, formal principles of due process that might commend themselves to a legalistic mindset (for example, setting aside anecdotal evidence) may appear to run counter to the aim of protecting patients from possible harm. In the next paragraphs I discuss two such cases, but am obliged to do so in sparse detail. This itself reflects how information about iatrogenic injury is sensitive, and hedged about by considerations of propriety. The two cases have had to be heavily veiled to preserve anonymity, and the reader may find some of the unavoidable imprecision frustrating. If the resulting argument seems unconvincing, however, it is at least further evidence of the bind that Dr. Vaisey described in the previous chapter. It is the detail in a narrative that persuades us to place trust in the narrator and the narrator's judgement; but it is sometimes just such detail that moral narrative must do without.

The omnipresent obligation of confidentiality poses particular problems for inquisitorial propriety. Consider the situation in which a patient reveals during a clinical consultation that another practitioner has made sexual advances, but the patient does not themselves wish to make a complaint. Looking at the goal of moral repair from the victim's point of view, the opportunity to voice their account to another professional able to validate the perception that this was indeed a moral wrong may be all that is desired. Further investigation may be the very last thing the victim wants. Looking at moral repair from an organizational perspective, however, the trust of other patients and trust in the organization are at risk. There are therefore strong prudential reasons for instigating further inquiry [60–63,98–108].[29]

---

[29] The development of practices of 'adult safeguarding' (protecting vulnerable adults from abuse by professional, paid or unpaid caregivers) seems to have impacted on professional conceptions of adult autonomy and vulnerability, and modified views on the situations that adults are expected to manage for themselves. Professionals may justify uninvited intervention in adult abuse situations on grounds that abuse takes place because victims are afraid to challenge it for fear of losing the support of caregivers; and also that healthcare professionals who violate boundaries with one patient are likely to do it to others. See references 98–102 for Department of Health guidance and 60–63 and 103–108 for further discussion.

It is clear that where patients are at risk of harm, a breach of confidentiality may be justifiable. At the outset, however, propriety suggests that confidentiality should be respected where possible. Thus, if a patient wishes to remain anonymous, inquisitorial propriety implies considerable circumspection. Care will be required to determine how the circumstances are described and to whom, and how a party accused is informed of the allegations in order that facts can be admitted or rebutted.

Information may be hedged about with normative expectations for reasons other than clinical confidentiality. It is characteristic of communities of professional practice that members come into possession of information, reliable and unreliable, about each others' professional competence. Rumours concerning clinician performance circulate and recirculate throughout all specialty communities, and are abroad in all provider organizations. It it their very abundance that gives rise to problems, because the question that naturally arises is to what gossip medical leaders ought to pay attention. There is of course a professional obligation to act upon serious concerns about fitness to practice, either by mobilizing organizational channels or by referring doctors to the GMC. But the informal knowledge that comes the way of medical leaders is frequently opaque, and it may also be subject to considerations of procedural rectitude.

Dr. Anne Archer (The Royal City Hospital NHS Trust) had already harboured her own doubts about one doctor in her organization; let us call him Dr. Y. Having encountered him outside the hospital in private practice, she had scant regard for his clinical abilities. But she had no convincing reason at that stage to believe that Dr. Y's practice was so poor that he was putting patients in danger. She also knew that Y been through internal disciplinary proceedings during his employment in the NHS. There too, hard evidence had not been forthcoming. Those proceedings had failed to establish that there was wrongdoing sufficient to warrant a penalty, and the file had been closed. Archer summarized what she had thought at the time:

> I knew this chap was of doubtful clinical ability. I knew he was a liar. I knew he was a
> bully. I knew he was dishonest in a number of ways. But you can't sack a man because you
> don't like him.

Dr. Y subsequently became the focus of an internal investigation after a cluster of iatrogenic injuries had been found in patients for whom he was responsible. As an investigator, what ought Archer to do with her informal, unsubstantiated 'knowledge' of past events?

Dr. Archer felt suspended between competing responsibilities and their attendant proprieties. She continued to lack proof of her suspicions, and inquisitorial propriety implied it would be improper to rely upon uncorroborated opinion or on unproven (and unprovable) allegations. On the other hand, as a doctor she was in possession of information that suggested to her that patients could be placed at risk. Fiduciary considerations required her to act on that unconfirmed but worrying information. Finally, as the hospital's agent Archer felt morally and legally bound to act within the scope of employment law and the protections it offered Dr. Y. How could she properly reconcile the aims of procedural fairness with prevention of medical harm and with the protection afforded by employment law? Dr. Archer eventually concluded that the best way forward would have been to comply with her fiduciary obligations, and breach other modes of propriety. To her considerable relief, in the end the situation resolved itself when her colleague elected to resign his post. This course of events itself raises further questions, however, about the obligations that might be owed to potential future employers and patients in other organizations.

The inescapability of judgement

Dr. Evans, medical director of Brickvale Hospital Trust, orchestrated an eventful narrative over a period of two long and demanding years. In a difficult investigation of a series of suspected injuries, Dr. Evans confronted both counter-allegations against him and an exculpatory report on the doctor's performance by a Royal College. With some trepidation, Dr. Evans rejected the external report, believing that its conclusions were unsound. After he had reached the end of his story, I invited Dr. Evans to reflect upon what had been the most difficult moral aspect of the entire two year process.

> *What for you has really been the core, most difficult, moral aspect of it; the absolutely central concern for you?*
>
> The most difficult bit was the challenge, to say to the College 'Look, this isn't appropriate, you've not done this properly' .... I was quite fair, [the doctor] got a copy of the College report and a copy of my letter to the College saying how I didn't think the report was specific or had gone into enough detail. And of course ... [the doctor] said if you read the [College] report, it could be interpreted as there's a bit of victimization going on here.
>
> It's about – it's about what's the right thing to do. An external body has come in and investigated them. They didn't do it well.

Dr. Evan's answer is all the more striking, I suspect, when it concludes the long and complex narrative that has gone before. Several features made the twist in his tale truly morally difficult. Dr. Evans was convinced that the College's investigative procedure was flawed, and that they had ignored crucial evidence. He continued to believe that the doctor's patients had suffered injury and would do so in future. But he was also beginning to worry that the clinical director who had brought the initial problem to his attention might be on something of a moral crusade. He began to wonder if he had correctly answered the question of where the line might fairly be drawn. When Evans set aside the College's report, it exposed him to allegations that he was acting inappropriately by continuing proceedings against the doctor. Ultimately, rejecting the College report meant Dr. Evans elevating his own judgement above that of his peers. But in the end, he had to persist in trusting his own moral sense of what he was called upon to do as a fiduciary for patients.

> Somewhere within all of this, I have to interpret what I'm hearing, what I'm feeling, and where I feel with this position. And I didn't feel that the position was safe with this doctor. Until I was sure we could make it safe, from what I was seeing I was going to have to challenge everything.
>
> (Dr. Evans, Brickvale Hospital NHS Trust)

It was, in fact, just such situations that Dr. Hutchinson had had in mind when I asked him what he had felt were the most troubling aspects of the medical director role:

> The bits which I suppose are most difficult, are the bits which leave you feeling most alone.
>
> (Dr. Hutchinson, Evenlode Park NHS Trust)

Inquisitorial propriety and reciprocal expectations

The reciprocal nature of inquisitorial propriety is a matter of considerable importance, because it is in failing to accommodate these reciprocal expectations that doctors' behaviour becomes liable to be viewed as improper. The picture that emerges of the 'proper' response to allegations of injury is clear and consistent, and it bears a close resemblance to Bosk's account of the expectations surrounding error in surgical training [109].[30] Dr. Evans spoke for many of his colleagues when he told me:

> Doctors make mistakes: some people try and be a little bit over optimistic about their abilities, get caught out and then they get reined in .... I come from a position of having very strong beliefs about fair play and honesty .... If somebody made a huge, huge cock-up and came to me and said 'I made a huge, huge cock-up', [I'd say] 'Okay, fine we'll work through it. Yes you may have to get some flack over this but right, remorse [is good] let's move on'. If somebody lies to me, even about a small thing, my hackles get raised. Because if I can't trust consultant colleagues then it is very, very, very difficult to do my job ....
> The consultants in this Trust ... have a huge amount of power and responsibility over patient care, and could do some very nasty and stupid things, and cause lots of harm. If I can't trust – ... Where people are dishonest or try and cover up their mistakes or try and blame other people when they've made a mistake, that I find really, really difficult.
>
> (Dr. Evans, Brickvale Hospital NHS Trust)

Relationships of trust in medicine appear to rest on a set of normative expectations that are clear, if not to all doctors, at least to many medical leaders. Medical leaders expect that the proper behaviour they enact will be reciprocated by the doctors they lead. What follows is a synopsis of their expectations.

Doctors should demonstrate they wholeheartedly accept the principles and practices of accountability as they apply to them. Because every doctor has a duty, to patients and the profession, to report injuries, mishaps, near misses, errors and inappropriate behaviour, 'proper' doctors accept that others must and will report anxieties about them. They will not treat such reports, or the action that follows such reports, as inflammatory or persecutory. They will defer to temporary restrictions on their practice, pending an inquiry. Moreover, they will honour any informal bargains, such as agreements to refrain from aspects of practice, notwithstanding the absence of formalities.

Doctors ought to accept inquisitors' need to distance themselves from those who are the subject of inquiry, and 'really proper' doctors will indeed politely initiate a temporary suspension of collegial expectations. They will make an open disclosure of all their mistakes. They will not contact witnesses, either patients or colleagues, or endeavour to influence others working on the inquiry. They will not pursue an excessively medico-legal defence of their own actions, especially where this impedes the objective of managing risk to patients. They will restrain their representatives from excessive advocacy on their behalf.

When they have been deemed to be responsible for injury to patients, 'proper' doctors will accept the judgement with good grace. They will not make excuses for their conduct, but will demonstrate insight into their actions. They will acknowledge any wrongdoing. They will exhibit contrition. They will show proper (measured) remorse.

'Proper' doctors will accept responsibility for attending to their own health and welfare where that is the cause of the problem. They will identify educational needs or changes in their practice so as to prevent similar harm. They will support organizational initiatives to change professional practices that have been found to be deficient. They will not retaliate with malicious gossip, hostility, counter-allegations or vexatious grievance complaints.

---

[30] Normative expectations surrounding inquisitorial propriety are thus close cousins to (but less categorical than) the normative and quasi-normative errors included in Bosk's typology. See reference 109.

Finally, 'proper doctors' will willingly meet with patients and carers, and graciously accept any righteous (or unrighteous) anger or chastisement directed at them. [110–115][31]

It would be wrong to suggest that violating these principles, either singly or severally, immediately invokes a penalty. Egregious offences, such as endeavouring to persuade complainants to withdraw their complaint, are likely to be treated very seriously. But more generally, acting beyond the bounds of propriety elicits negative judgements of doctors' trustworthiness. It indicates that doctors do not share medical leaders' normative expectations regarding standards of practice; and the view that they are not trustworthy members of the community of practice may have significant repercussions. What they will be depends upon the circumstances. In this study the repercussions ranged from mild ostracism (justifying withdrawal of collegial support) to outright exclusion (comprising a contributory factor in dismissal from the organization or referral to a regulatory body).

Restorative propriety

Earlier in my discussion of the 'reparative proprieties', I proposed that moral repair turned upon seven critical acts of acknowledgement: (i) acknowledging an injured party as a moral interlocutor; (ii) acknowledging the authority of shared norms; (iii) acknowledging injury; (iv) acknowledging responsibility; (v) acknowledging that remedy is due, and that the injured party may define what is owed to them; (vi) acknowledging righteous anger, or other negative feelings, in those who have been injured; and (vii) acknowledging that in injuring another, we should experience sorrow and regret.

The term moral repair refers both to inquiring into moral harm, and to restoring moral balance. It is through acknowledging and inquiring into harm that the process of moral repair begins. It is through activities aimed at restoring moral balance that moral repair is completed. Through inquiry, the fundamentals of an organizational moral narrative emerge. Through behaviours of moral repair, this moral narrative is given fuller expression. It is to restoring moral balance that we now turn our attention.

The central feature of restorative propriety in this account is a focus on the victim and their needs. Much that is done in the process of an inquiry, such as being invited to recount perceptions of injury, will begin to remedy harm. But some aspects of an inquiry, such as impartial treatment of an alleged wrongdoer, may well aggravate the victim's sense of injury. Furthermore, there are some tasks, like issuing a 'categorical apology', that can only be done following an inquiry [82,116,117].[32] This is because a 'categorical apology' requires more than just acknowledgement that harm has occurred; if a culpable error has been made the situation requires a frank admission of wrong. So restorative and inquisitorial propriety certainly shade into one another, but equally certainly are not coterminous.

---

[31] Written guidance produced by the NHS Patient Safety Agency on meetings with patients following adverse incidents stresses the importance of openness and accurate information but unsurprisingly does not provide detailed instruction on how clinicians should comport themselves. See reference 110 and 111–115 for further discussion.

[32] Smith's 'categorical apology' encompasses eleven elements: a corroborated factual record; acceptance of blame; identification of harm; identification of the moral principles underlying each harm; endorsement of the moral principles underlying each harm; recognition of the victim as a moral interlocutor; categorical regret; performance of the apology; redress; appropriate intent; and appropriate emotion. See reference 82, and 116 and 117 for further discussion.

By comparison with inquisitorial propriety, medical directors had rather less to say about restorative propriety. This is, in part, an artefact of the research. There were few occasions when I pressed medical directors to explain how they had worked with patients. This was a blind spot on my part. Because my focus was on medical management I did not, at the time, appreciate how medical leaders' ethical comportment could be expressed in interactions with patients. In addition, while it is clear that iatrogenic injury can also have devastating consequences for the healthcare professionals responsible for it, these effects were infrequently discussed. Because they too suffer, healthcare professionals are also, or ought also to be, beneficiaries of moral repair. But medical directors' responsibility for holding doctors accountable, maybe a sense that fiduciary concerns should be voiced in the research interview, and perhaps a reluctance to be seen to identify too closely with other professionals, oriented our discussion of their moral concerns towards the harm done to patients.

The analysis that follows is thus in no way complete. But it explores two expressive elements that emerged as central to restorative propriety: attending to narratives of harm, and representing narratives of harm.

The remedy of attention

Although they are two sides of what often turns out to be the same coin, the concepts of 'complaint' and 'apology' seem to invoke very different responses. 'Apology' has recently been elevated to the status of a fit subject for moral philosophy and thus the higher echelons of the ivory tower; 'complaints management' remains a bureaucratic, instrumental, and frankly rather lowly activity [32,82].[33] Symbolizing this difference, apology has been analysed as a quintessentially moral act, the cardinal ritual of moral repair; complaints management, on the other hand, is depicted as a quintessentially instrumental good, serving to supply a source of feedback and opportunities to rebuild 'customer relations' [118–122].[34] Inevitably, this stark dichotomy is blurred in practice. But it nevertheless expresses an important variation in current perceptions of the two activities, and the different values that are formally assigned to them.

It might be thought unwise to start a discussion of restorative propriety through examining complaints management in the NHS, which has been the object of robust criticism, anxious self-examination and reformist attention in recent years [53,123–128]. And I hesitate to offer Dr. McGregor's narrative, which follows shortly, as an exemplary account of the enactment of 'complaint ethics'. But McGregor conveyed an appreciation of the moral dimension of complaints that, if it is present in the official literature, tends to remain concealed. At the same time, however, his capacity to do so appeared constrained both by the impoverished moral discourse surrounding complaints and by the burden of instrumentalist reasoning in health management.

---

[33] Smith and Berlinger (references 32 and 82) refer to a burgeoning literature on the philosophy of apology.

[34] Reference 118, Principle 1, 'Getting it right', stresses the benefits of complaints management to the National Health Service. Principle 2, 'Being customer focused', includes several components of Smith's 'categorical apology' without any hint of a moral dimension to apology. For an interesting reflection on the limitations of managerial complaints discourse see reference 119, and 120–122 for further discussion.

Dr. McGregor's reflection on responding to complaints followed his account of the adverse effects of a relentless and uninhibited drive to raise clinical productivity. In Remembrance Hospitals Trust this had resulted in considerable pressure on bed space such that although 'technical' standards of care were maintained, the 'moral' standard of care had suffered.

> And we got some fairly distressing complaints from patients saying 'This is really rather unpleasant to be in this ward, because you aren't protecting [privacy or dignity] . . . . And we realized that we had got that wrong.

There had been something in Dr. McGregor's tone of voice when he first referred to these complaints: a genuine sense of regret, a trace of mortification, perhaps, that is not present in the transcript. I pressed him to tell me a little more about how he experienced such complaints.

> *I got the impression (and tell me if I'm wrong about this), that the nature of the complaints which came forward and the way in which they were couched were quite compelling for you?*

> Oh yes, absolutely. Well, they were compelling in the sense of, 'This is not the service we want to produce. And it is clear that we have gone below the standard we wanted to here'. And so it isn't as though we just look at the complaints and say, 'Oh well, it's a bit unfortunate'. It's actually, 'No, this is not what we want to do' . . . . So dealing with it is not a matter of, 'Oh, we must deal with it in case they go to the newspapers'. We must deal with this because it's unacceptable. We would not want to be in that position ourselves. We wouldn't want our relatives to be in that position. We do not want our patients to be in that position.
>
> (Dr. McGregor, Remembrance Hospitals Trust)

Pushed to describe his reaction to complaints, Dr. McGregor's first recourse had been to an instrumental discourse of standards and service improvement. But his emphatic rejection of the idea that responding to complaints was a defensive activity moved him towards more overtly moral ground. Enacting ethics is, at a very basic level, an expression of understanding, empathy and responsiveness to the moral perspectives of others. This was what lingered in his talk of things deemed unacceptable to 'ourselves', 'our' family, and 'our' patients. Hinting at a richer moral conception of complaints than is encapsulated in the term 'customer focus' he invokes the significance of the normative expectations, and concomitant responsibilities, that create moral community.

Dr. McGregor had an ample team to respond to complaints on his behalf. But he treated it as of singular importance to read for himself all of the letters of complaint that related to clinical care: not a report, not a synopsis, not a table of complaints analysed by department or doctor, not a summary of actions in response, but each of the individual letters, one by one. He did this not, I think, because he distrusted his complaints managers. Rather, he seemed to have perceived reading patients' accounts of their experience to be of almost sacramental importance. Those letters testified to patients' experience, and their testimony was worthy of his consideration.

The remedy of attention applied, too, to meeting patients who remained distressed about their treatment or about how their complaint had been handled. Patients' own words captured the richness of the clinical encounter in all of its complex intersubjectivity, with its hoped-for satisfactions and sometimes lasting sorrows:

> if that patient didn't feel they've been treated in a dignified way or felt their privacy was invaded, that's true. You can't argue with that. You can't say, 'Oh no, it wasn't.' Because that's their perception, and their perception is ultimately [what counts].

Sometimes you feel 'We've really let down a patient'.... You know as a doctor ... [that] not everything always goes well. You get lots of thank you letters; but occasionally you just know that 'this' is not what you wanted to happen .... Seeing that in complaints [about other doctors], I understand that things don't always go well. But equally you feel that you have let patients down, and we as an organization should have done better, even if individuals have done their best.

(Dr. McGregor, Remembrance Hospitals Trust)

Whether it is underpinned by a moral or instrumental orientation, the process of complaining and of addressing complaint is manifestly a narrative one. At its centre is a narrative that demands to be heard. That is its essence: a complaint is a narrative petition for attention to a perceived wrong. The seeds of moral repair are thus sown in paying attention, in showing a complainant that they have been heard (either literally or metaphorically) as a moral interlocutor. Enacting ethics begins, and may indeed end, in the simple but demanding task of attending to narrative. This is emphatically not the same as answering a narrative.

The remedy of acceptance

To answer a narrative of complaint is to attempt to alter the narrative's direction, to head it away from anger and resentment towards acceptance and forgiveness. This is the case even where the answer is a frank acknowledgement of wrongdoing together with a fervent promise to change. As the complainant, to accede to an answer is to change one's narrative of complaint, to modify its content and embrace it in its altered form. There is a sense in which to accede to an answer is a form of submission. As Dr. McGregor recognized, therefore, an answer may be wanted but not accepted.

Sometimes it's difficult, because sometimes patients are so angry that it's actually very difficult to – and they need to get their anger out of their system; and you can't – whatever you say to them, they won't ... You have to accept you can't always send everyone away happy I'm afraid .... Sometimes you have a discussion with patients or relatives, and you think at the end of it, you've really moved on. But I think quite often you feel actually, they have let out some of their anger or whatever, but they haven't really moved on. They're still going away from it angry.

(Dr. McGregor, Remembrance Hospitals Trust)

It is a common desire to want to answer a narrative of complaint with a narrative of one's own: an alternative account, a tale of exculpation, a justification, an excuse, a suggestion of remedy or an apology. If paying attention to a complaint is to acknowledge the complainant as a moral interlocutor, then formulating a response seems to be to engage in moral interlocution.

But moral repair is a matter of restoring moral balance, redressing an enduring sense of moral disregard. Returning relationships to moral balance may require more in the way of unconditional acceptance (that is, attentive listening) than a worked response (that is, responsible answering).

Just as Dr. McGregor did, Dr. Seddon was obliged to accept the burden of others' anger as part of the process of repair. Dr. Seddon's inquiry, which we encountered earlier in this chapter, concerned allegations of years of misdiagnosis and misguided treatment by a single consultant. Dr. Seddon accepted that the consultant had always acted with good intent, and now experienced deep remorse and regret. But the task of acknowledging the righteous anger of those who had been injured, whether directly as patients or indirectly as carers, fell to Dr. Seddon. He had thought that what was wanted was a response; his voice. But he found that what was needed was attention; his presence.

> I had a very big meeting with the [patients and families] which was probably the most uncomfortable thing I've ever done in my life. It was a big room full of people. And trying to put the viewpoint over, with people not just heckling but basically saying they had no confidence in what I was doing, shouting and screaming actually, for an evening and in a very unprotected environment – it was a very very unpleasant thing to do. And I did find that hard . . . . And I'm very much into a no-blame culture; people call it 'just and fair' now, but I like the phrase 'no blame' . . . . I cannot tell you how vindictive these [patients and families] were – hanging, drawing and quartering would have been too good for them. They were absolutely 'hell hath no fury'.
>
> (Dr. Seddon, Saxonvale University Hospitals Trust)

It is of course distressing to be the foil for other people's anger, whether the anger is directed towards oneself or what one represents. And it is natural, perhaps, to attempt to 'draw the sting' by explaining it away as unjustified or vindictive. That granted, one aspect of Dr. Seddon's discomfort was, I believe, the disjuncture between complainants' need to rehearse narratives of hurt and disregard, and his sense that it was his role to provide a reparative answer. It was, after all, his duty to repair the situation; and yet nothing he could offer by way of a response turned out to be adequate or acceptable.

Both Dr. McGregor and Dr. Seddon reported feeling that their reparative efforts in the face of unresolved anger were futile. Dr. Hutchinson too gave an example of the difficulty in facing righteous anger. On this occasion, however, he had experienced the restorative force in simply attending to a narrative of distress.

> [The general manager said] 'We've had a complaint about a patient from a patient's brother. The patient has died. Would you meet with us to help resolve it?' It turns out that the brother [was a daunting authority figure who] wanted to have his say. I was there for about an hour and a half, with the manager. And actually we did a lot of grief work in the meeting. [129,130][35]
>
> (Dr. Hutchinson, Evenlode Park NHS Trust)

The remedy of public testimony

We are finally approaching the end of my exploration of propriety, and of the role propriety plays in orchestrating organizational moral narrative. So it seems especially fitting to conclude with an extract about the moral significance of narrative.

Dr. Katie Kingsley (Cityside NHS Trust) is a clinical academic as well as a former medical director, and she brought a distinctive framework to bear on her account of moral leadership. She thought of healthcare organizations as systems of communication, channelling knowledge through structures and hierarchies and containing it within either legitimate or questionable boundaries. Knowledge became the property of some; it fell into the possession of others; it was rightly closely guarded by a few; and it was circulated by the many. Because Dr. Kingsley saw the organization as a communication system, she also saw

---

[35] For an excellent sociological review of theories of grief see reference 129. Charmaz argues that the concept of grief as work, which can be traced through the work of Worden (reference 130) and others from the 1990s onwards, has its roots in a dominant American Protestant ethic. In my own experience as a bereavement counsellor, however, I have witnessed the profound emotional effort that grief sometimes, at least, demands; and the sheer exhaustion that sometimes, at least, it generates,

that it was vulnerable to corruption by shameful secrets, concealments, obfuscation, wilful obtuseness, unwitting ignorance and wrongful disclosure. Determining when, how and to whom awkward truths should be told, and when, how or from whom information should be withheld, were therefore matters of ethical import.

Dr. Kingsley was present throughout a confidential internal inquiry into the death of a patient who was killed in a bizarre accident.[36] During the inquiry she had listened with ever deepening discomfort to carers' accounts of the patient's distressing experiences in her hospital. This testimony was morally important, a narrative of witness, as much as it was instrumentally important, a source of 'feedback'. How then, ought it to be treated?

The proper use of testimony is critical to remedying the moral wrongs perpetrated by organizations. Where an individual has done wrong, an individual may remedy it. In a purely dyadic relationship between a wrongdoer and an injured party, for the wrongdoer to acknowledge the wrong directly may be enough. But where organizations have done wrong, or where organizational systems have failed, individuals alone cannot remedy it. The normative expectations that have been breached transcend individuals. A proper record of the wrong must therefore be made, and it must be pressed upon the attention of those who ought properly to know of it.

This chapter closes with Dr. Kingsley's account of the testimonial dimension of restorative propriety. This testimonial dimension contributes towards the restoration of moral balance by authenticating sufferers' narratives of wrongdoing, and offering them as essential 'truth to power' [131].[37]

> [A relative and a friend of the patient] came along and talked at enormous length about how awful the ward was physically. They talked about the lack of facilities on the ward, the terrible food, the just terribly impoverished furnishings, the lack of morale . . . . They spoke on, and on, about just how awful it was to come and see the patient in this awful, awful place.

> The report that was written – by the person who looked after the transcript, but it was checked, I think, by one of the executive directors – hardly mentioned anything about what was described by [the carers]. And for me, this was the thing that made me feel embarrassed and terrible. It was not so much the death of [the patient], which I really think was unavoidable. I don't think that the staff had mismanaged it in any way. But it was the terrible experience that this [relative] had had of their [loved one] being in hospital. It was heartrending. It was awful. And that would not be communicated.

> It was a bland account of this inquiry . . . . I wrote back saying that my memory was that we were all terribly shocked and embarrassed about the way in which the relative described the patient's experience and that this should be reflected in the report . . . . We've made a promise to this relative that we are looking into this in order to understand it; and if things need to be changed, to change them. Or else, their loved one's death becomes meaningless. How do you cope with the death of a [relative] in their twenties? You need to find that some good will come from it; it's terribly important isn't it?

> And if important lessons from this death are not heard, or played down, then that is a betrayal.
> (Dr. Kingsley, Cityside NHS Trust)

---

[36] I have used the term accident carefully here. It seemed that no reasonable preventive measures could have been taken to protect the patient from sustaining a fatal injury from an apparently innocent item.

[37] The phrase derives from a Cold War Quaker pamphlet; see reference 131.

Further reading

Walker MU. *Moral Repair: Reconstructing Moral Relations after Wrongdoing.* Cambridge: Cambridge University Press; 2006.

Paget MA. *The Unity of Mistakes; A Phenomenological Interpretation of Medical Work.* Philadelphia: Temple University Press; 1988.

Berlinger N. *After Harm: Medical Error and the Ethics of Forgiveness.* Baltimore: The Johns Hopkins University Press; 2005.

Smith N. *I Was Wrong: The Meanings of Apologies.* New York: Cambridge University Press; 2008.

Clarke S, Oakley J, eds. *Informed Consent and Clinician Accountability: The Ethics of Report Cards on Surgeon Performance.* Cambridge: Cambridge University Press; 2007.

References

1. BMJ bans 'accidents': 'Accidents are not unpredictable'. *BMJ.* 2001;**322** (7298):1320–1.

2. Doege T. An injury is no accident. *N Engl J Med.* 1978;**298**:509–51.

3. Evans L. Medical accidents: no such thing? *BMJ.* 1993;**307**:1438–9.

4. Rosenthal M. *Dealing with Medical Malpractice: The British and Swedish Experience.* Durham, NC: Duke University Press; 1988.

5. Walshe K. *Regulating Healthcare: A Prescription for Improvement?* Maidenhead: Open University Press; 2003.

6. Moran M. *Governing the Health Care State: A Comparative Study of the United Kingdom, the United States, and Germany.* Manchester: Manchester University Press; 1999.

7. Jost TS. *Regulation of the Healthcare Professions.* Chicago: Health Administration Press; 1997.

8. Gray A, Harrison S, eds. *Governing Medicine: Theory and Practice.* Maidenhead: Open University Press; 2004.

9. Boyle PJ, DuBose ER, Ellingson SJ, Guinn DE, McCurdy DB. *Organizational Ethics in Health Care: Principles, Cases, and Practical Solutions.* San Francisco, CA: Jossey-Bass and AHA Press; 2000.

10. Hall RT. *An Introduction to Healthcare Organizational Ethics.* New York: Oxford University Press; 2000.

11. Smith Iltis A, ed. *Institutional Integrity in Health Care.* Dordrecht: Kluwer Academic; 2003.

12. Spencer EM, Mills AE, Rorty MV, Werhane PH. *Organization Ethics in Health Care.* New York: Oxford University Press; 2000.

13. Morrison EE, Monagle JF. Part III - Critical issues for healthcare organizations. *Health Care Ethics: Critical Issues for the 21st Century.* Sudbury, MA: Jones and Bartlett; 2008.

14. Dudzinski DM. Review of organizational ethics in health care: principles, cases, and practical solutions. *Cambridge Quarterly of Healthcare Ethics.* 2005;**14**:464–7.

15. Leape LL. Special communication: error in medicine. *JAMA.* 1994;**272**(23):1851–7.

16. Kohn LT, et al., eds. *To Err is Human: Building a Safer Health System.* Washington DC: Institute of Medicine: National Academy Press; 2000.

17. Vincent C. Understanding and responding to adverse events. *New England Journal of Medicine.* 2003;**348**(11):1051–6.

18. Mazor KM, Simon SR, Gurwitz JH. Communicating with patients about medical errors. A review of the literature. *Archives of Internal Medicine.* 2004;**164**:1690–7.

19. Cantor MD, Barach P, Derse A, Maklan CW, Wlody GS, Fox E. Disclosing adverse events to patients. *Joint Commission Journal on Quality and Patient Safety.* 2005;**31**(1):5–12.

20. Lander LI, Connor JA, Shah RK, Kentala E, Healy GB, Roberson DW. Otolaryngologists' responses to errors and adverse events. *The Laryngoscope.* 2006; **116**(7):1114–20.

21. Leape LL. Ethical issues in patient safety. *Thoracic Surgery Clinics*. 2005; **15**(4):493–501.

22. Clark AP. Taking the high road: what should you do when an adverse event occurs? Part I. *Clinical Nurse Specialist*. 2004;**18**(3):118–9.

23. Volker DL, Clark AP. Taking the high road: what should you do when an adverse event occurs? Part II. *Clinical Nurse Specialist*. 2004;**18**(4):180–2.

24. Kirby RS. Learning the lessons from medical errors. *BJU International*. 2003;**92** (1):4–5.

25. Sorensen R, Iedema R, Piper D, Manias E, Williams A, Tuckett A. Disclosing clinical adverse events to patients: can practice inform policy? *Health Expectations*. 2010;**13**(2):148–59.

26. Berwick DM. Errors today and errors tomorrow. *New England Journal of Medicine*. 2003; **348**(25):2570–2.

27. Palmieri PA, DeLucia PR, Peterson LT, Ott TE, Green A. The anatomy and physiology of error in adverse health care events. *Advances in Health Care Management*. 2008(7): 33–68.

28. Vincent CA. Analysis of clinical incidents: a window on the system not a search for root causes. *Quality and Safety in Health Care*. 2004 August 1, 2004;**13** (4):242–3.

29. Buchanan A. Intending death: the structure of the problem and proposed solutions In: Beauchamp T, ed. *Intending Death: The Ethics of Assisted Suicide and Euthanasia*. Upper Saddle River, NJ: Prentice-Hall; 1996, pp. 23–41.

30. Berlinger N. Avoiding cheap grace. Medical harm, patient safety, and the culture(s) of forgiveness. *Hastings Center Report*. 2003;**33**(6):28–36.

31. Berlinger N. Missing the mark: medical error, forgiveness and justice. In: Sharpe VA, ed. *Accountability: Patient Safety and Policy Reform*. Washington: Georgetown University Press; 2004.

32. Berlinger N. *After Harm: Medical Error and the Ethics of Forgiveness*. Baltimore: The Johns Hopkins University Press; 2005.

33. Zientek D. Medical error, malpractice and complications: a moral geography. *HEC Forum*. 2010;**22**(2):145–57.

34. Gallagher TH, Denham CR, Leape LL, Amori G, Levinson W. Disclosing unanticipated outcomes to patients: the art and practice. *Journal of Patient Safety*. 2007;**3**(3):158–65. 10.1097/ pts.0b013e3181451606.

35. Robbennolt J. Apologies and medical error. *Clinical Orthopaedics and Related Research*. 2009;**467**(2):376–82.

36. Kaldjian L, Jones E, Wu B, Forman-Hoffman V, Levi B, Rosenthal G. Disclosing medical errors to patients: attitudes and practices of physicians and trainees. *Journal of General Internal Medicine*. 2007;**22**(7):988–96.

37. Cox W. The five a's: What do patients want after an adverse event? *Journal of Healthcare Risk Management*. 2007;**27** (3):25–9.

38. Sharpe VA, Faden AI. *Medical Harm: Historical, Conceptual, and Ethical Dimensions of Iatrogenic Illness*. Cambridge: Cambridge University Press; 1998.

39. Sharpe VA. Promoting patient safety. An ethical basis for policy deliberation. *Hastings Center Report*. 2003;**33**(5): S3–18.

40. Leape LL, Fromson JA. Problem doctors: is there a system-level solution? *Annals of Internal Medicine*. 2006;**144**(2): 107–15.

41. Milligan F. *Defining Medicine and the Nature of Iatrogenic Harm*: Cambridge: Blackwell Science; 2008.

42. Grol R, Grimshaw J. From best evidence to best practice: effective implementation of change in patients' care. *The Lancet*. 2003;**362**:1225–30.

43. Smith ML, Forster HP. Morally managing medical mistakes. *Cambridge Quarterly of Healthcare Ethics*. 2000;**9** (1):38–53.

44. Paget MA. *The Unity of Mistakes; A Phenomenological Interpretation of Medical Work.* Philadelphia: Temple University Press; 1988.

45. Gorovitz S, MacIntyre A. Toward a theory of medical fallibility. *Journal of Medicine and Philosophy.* 1976;**1**(1):51.

46. Bolam v Friern Hospital Management Committee. 1 WLR 5821957.

47. Bolitho v City and Hackney HA. 1998 AC 2321998.

48. Hucks v Cole. 1993 4 Med L R 3931993.

49. Marriott v West Midlands Health Authority. *Lloyd's Rep Med* **23** 1999.

50. Freidson E. *Profession of Medicine: A Study in the Sociology of Applied Knowledge.* Chicago: University of Chicago Press; 1970, p. 152.

51. An inquiry into quality and practice within the National Health Service arising from the actions of Rodney Ledward. Department of Health; 2000.

52. Independent investigation into how the N.H.S handled allegations about the conduct of Richard Neale *Cm* 6315; 2004.

53. Shipman Inquiry. Safeguarding patients: lessons from the past – proposals for the future. *Cm* 6394; 2004.

54. Independent investigation into how the NHS handled allegations about the conduct of Clifford Ayling. *Cm* 6298; 2004.

55. Independent investigation into how the NHS handled allegations about the conduct of William Kerr and Michael Haslam. *Cm* 6640; 2005.

56. Allsop J. Regaining trust in medicine. *Current Sociology.* 2006;**54**(4):621–36.

57. Samanta A, Samanta J. Safer patients and good doctors: medical regulation in the 21st century. *Clinical Risk.* 2007;**13**(4): 138–42.

58. Learning from Bristol: the report of the public inquiry into Children's Heart Surgery at the Bristol Royal Infirmary. *Cm* 5207; 2001.

59. Rosenthal M. *The Incompetent Doctor.* Buckingham: Open University Press; 1995.

60. Maintaining Boundaries: Guidance for Doctors2006: Available from: http://www.gmc-uk.org/guidance/ethical_guidance/maintaining_boundaries.asp; http://www.gmc-uk.org/static/documents/content/Maintaining_Boundaries.pdf. Paragraph 5.

61. Subotsky F, Bewley S, Crowe M, eds. *Abuse of the Doctor-Patient Relationship.* London: Royal College of Psychiatrists Publications; 2010.

62. *Vulnerable Patients, Vulnerable Doctors.* London: Royal College of Psychiatrists; 2002.

63. *Vulnerable Patients, Safe Doctors: Good Practice In Our Clinical Relationships 2007.* Available from: http://www.rcpsych.ac.uk/files/pdfversion/CR146x.pdf.

64. Thompson DF. *Restoring Responsibility: Ethics in Government, Business, and Healthcare.* Cambridge: Cambridge University Press; 2005.

65. *Listening and Learning: the Ombudsman's review of complaint handling by the NHS in England 2009–2010*: Available from: http://nhsreport.ombudsman.org.uk/assets/files/downloads/Listening_and_Learning_HC482-PHSO-0110.pdf.

66. Reason J. *Managing the Risks of Organizational Accidents.* Aldershot: Ashgate; 1999.

67. Barach P, Small S. Reporting and preventing medical mishaps: lessons from non-medical near-miss reporting. *BMJ.* 2000;**320**:563–79.

68. West E. Organisational sources of safety and danger: sociological contributions to the study of adverse events. *Quality & Safety in Health Care.* 2000;**9**(2):120–6.

69. Helmreich R, Merrit A. *Culture at Work in Aviation and Medicine.* Aldershot: Ashgate; 2001.

70. McDonald R, Waring J, Harrison S. 'Balancing risk, that is my life': the politics of risk in a hospital operating theatre department. *Health, Risk & Society.* 2005;**7**(4):397–411.

71. Shaw K MacKillop L, Armitage M. Revalidation, appraisal and clinical governance. *Clinical Governance: An International Journal* 2007;**12**(3):170–7.

72. Shaw K, Cassel CK, Black C, Levinson W. Shared medical regulation in a time of increasing calls for accountability and transparency. *JAMA.* 2009;**302** (18):2008–14.

73. Chambers T. Framing our mistakes. In: Rubin SB, Zoloth L, eds. *Margins of Error: The Ethics of Mistakes in the Practice of Medicine.* Hagerstown, MD: University Publishing Group; 2000, pp. 13–24.

74. Walker MU. *Moral Repair: Reconstructing Moral Relations after Wrongdoing.* Cambridge: Cambridge University Press; 2006.

75. Holm S. *Ethical Problems in Clinical Practice: The Ethical Reasoning of Healthcare Professionals.* Manchester: Manchester University Press; 1997.

76. Beauchamp TL, Childress JF. *Principles of Biomedical Ethics.* 5th edn. Oxford: Oxford University Press; 2001.

77. Baier A. *Moral Prejudices.* Cambridge, MA: Harvard University Press; 1994.

78. Pettit P. The cunning of trust. *Philosophy & Public Affairs.* 1995;**24**:202–25.

79. Sharpe VA. Taking responsibility for medical mistakes. In: Rubin SB, Zoloth L, eds. *Margin of Error: The Ethics of Mistakes in the Practice of Medicine.* Hagerstown, MD: University Publishing Group; 2000, pp. 183–94.

80. Sharpe VA. Behind closed doors: accountability and responsibility in patient care. *Journal of Medicine and Philosophy.* 2000;**25**(1):28–47.

81. Feinberg J. Collective responsibility. In: Lanham MD, ed. *Collective Responsibility: Five Decades of Debates in Theoretical and Applied Ethics.* Lanham, MD: Rowman and Littlefield; 1991.

82. Smith N. *I Was Wrong: The Meanings of Apologies.* New York: Cambridge University Press; 2008.

83. Rawls J. *A Theory of Justice.* Revised edn. Cambridge, MA: Harvard University Press; 1999, p. 86.

84. Solum L. Procedural justice. *78 Southern California Law Review.* 2004;**181**.

85. Mason v. Eldred. 73 US (6 Wall) 1867.

86. Kaplow L, Shavell S. *Fairness Versus Welfare.* Cambridge, MA: Harvard University Press; 2002.

87. Mulheron R. Trumping Bolam: a critical legal analysis of Bolitho's 'gloss'. *Cambridge Law Journal.* 2010;**69**(3):609–38.

88. Harrington J. Law's faith in medicine. *Medical Law International.* 2008;**9**(4): 357–74.

89. Coulter A, Fitzpatrick R, Cornwell J. *Measures of patients' experience in hospital: Purpose, methods and uses.* London: King's Fund; 2009.

90. Marshall S, Haywood K, Fitzpatrick R. Impact of patient-reported outcome measures on routine practice: a structured review. *Journal of Evaluation in Clinical Practice.* 2006;**12**(5): 559–68.

91. Frost MH, Reeve BB, Liepa AM, Stauffer JW, Hays RD, the Mayo FDAP-ROCMG. What is sufficient evidence for the reliability and validity of patient-reported outcome measures? *Value in Health.* 2007;**10**:S94–S105.

92. Valderas J, Kotzeva A, Espallargues M, Guyatt G, Ferrans C, Halyard M, *et al.* The impact of measuring patient-reported outcomes in clinical practice: a systematic review of the literature. *Quality of Life Research.* 2008; **17**(2):179–93.

93. Rothman ML, Beltran P, Cappelleri JC, Lipscomb J, Teschendorf B, the Mayo FDAP-ROCMG. Patient-reported outcomes: *conceptual issues. Value in Health.* 2007;**10**:S66–S75.

94. Marquis P, Arnould B, Acquadro C, Roberts W M. Patient-reported outcomes and health-related quality of life in effectiveness studies: pros and cons. *Drug Development Research.* 2006;**67** (3):193–201.

95. Greenhalgh J. The applications of PROs in clinical practice: what are they, do they work, and why? *Quality of Life Research.* 2009;**18**(1):115–23.

96. McClimans L. A theoretical framework for patient-reported outcome measures. *Theoretical Medicine and Bioethics.* 2010;**31**(3):225–40.

97. Street A. Future of quality measurement in the National Health Service: 'Are NHS patients more likely than their more consumer-conscious counterparts in the USA to consider a hospital's star rating when exercising choice?' *Expert Review of Pharmacoeconomics and Outcomes Research.* 2006;**6**(3):245–8.

98. *No Secrets: guidance on developing and implementing multi-agency policies and procedures to protect vulnerable adults from abuse.* Department of Health; 2000.

99. *Safeguarding Adults: report on the consultation on the review of 'No Secrets'.* Department of Health; 2009.

100. *Making Safeguarding Everybody's Business: a post-Bichard vetting scheme: analysis of the responses to the consultation.* Department of Health; 2005.

101. *Safeguarding Adults: the role of health service managers and their boards.* Department of Health; 2011.

102. *Safeguarding Adults: the role of health service practitioners.* Department of Health; 2011.

103. Mathew D, Brown H, Kingston P, McCreadie C, Askham J. The response to No Secrets. *The Journal of Adult Protection.* 2009;**4**(1):4–14.

104. Sumner K. Social services' progress in implementing No Secrets – an analysis of codes of practice. *The Journal of Adult Protection.* 2009;**6**(1):4–11.

105. McCreadie C. No Secrets: guidance in England for the protection of vulnerable adults from abuse. *The Journal of Adult Protection.* 2009;**2**(3):4–16.

106. Gutheil TG, Brodsky A. *Preventing Boundary Violations in Clinical Practice*: New York: Guilford Press; 2008.

107. Feeney LJ. There is more to post-termination boundary violations than sex. *Advances in Psychiatric Treatment.* 2009;**15**(4):318–

108. Fischer HR, Houchen BJ, Ferguson-Ramos L. Professional boundaries violations: case studies from a regulatory perspective. *Nursing Administration Quarterly.* 2008;**32**(4):317–23. 10.1097/01.NAQ.0000336730.57254.b1.

109. Bosk CL. *Forgive and Remember: Managing Medical Failure.* 2nd edn. Chicago: University of Chicago Press; 2003.

110. *Being open: communicating patient safety incidents with patients, their families and carers2009*: Available from: http://www.nrls.npsa.nhs.uk/resources/all-settings-specialties/?entryid45=83726.

111. Aasland OG, Forde R. Impact of feeling responsible for adverse events on doctors' personal and professional lives: the importance of being open to criticism from colleagues. *Quality & Safety in Health Care.* 2005;**14**(1):13–7.

112. Sorensen R, Iedema R, Piper D, Manias E, Williams A, Tuckett A. Health care professionals' views of implementing a policy of open disclosure of errors. *Journal of Health Services Research & Policy.* 2008;**13**(4):227–32.

113. Whitehouse S. Being open when things go wrong. *InnovAiT.* 2010;**3**(1):57–8.

114. Feinmann J. You can say sorry. *BMJ.* 2009;**339**:b3057

115. Ottewill M, Vaughan C. Being open with patients about medical error: challenges in practice. *Clinical Ethics.* 2010;**5**(3):159–63.

116. Boyer AR. *In a 'sorry' state: the ethics of institutional apologies in response to medical errors 2009.* Available from: http://challenger.library.pitt.edu/ETD/available/etd-04202009-132523/unrestricted/Boyer_ETD2009.pdf.

117. Wittig J. Why it is unethical to apologize: an examination of apology and regret. . 2009;**36**:80–91.

118. *Principles for Remedy 2007*: Available from: http://www.ombudsman.org.uk/_data/ assets/pdf_file/0009/1035/Principles-for-Remedy.pdf.

119. Allsop J, Jones K. Withering the citizen, managing the consumer: *Complaints in Healthcare Settings. Social Policy and Society.* 2008;7:233–43.

120. Allsop J, Mulcahy L. Maintaining professional identities: doctors' responses to complaints. *Sociology of Health and Illness.* 1998; 20(6):802–24.

121. Jain A, Ogden J. General practitioners' experiences of patients' complaints: qualitative study. *BMJ.* 1999 June 12, 1999;318(7198):1596–9.

122. Nettleton S, Burrows R, Watt I. How do you feel doctor? An analysis of emotional aspects of routine professional medical work. *Social Theory & Health.* 2008;6 (1):18–36.

123. *Making things better?* Health Service Ombudsman; 2005.

124. *Spotlight on Complaints.* Healthcare Commission; 2007.

125. Annual Report: Parliamentary and Healthcare Ombudsman; 2007.

126. Annual Report: Parliamentary and Health Service Ombudsman; 2008.

127. *Consultation Document: Making Experiences Count.* Department of Health; 2007.

128. *Feeding back? Learning from complaints handling in health and social care.* HC 853: National Audit Office; 2008.

129. Charmaz K, Milligan MJ. Grief. In: Stets JE, Turner JA, eds. *Handbook of the Sociology of Emotions.* New York: Springer; 2006, pp. 516–43.

130. Worden WJ. *Grief Counselling and Grief Therapy: A Handbook for the Mental Health Practitioner.* Oxford: Routledge; 1991.

131. *Speak Truth to Power.* American Friends Service Committee; 1955.

Epilogue to Chapters 4 and 5

The concept of the 'proprieties' is one of the most novel aspects of my account of moral leadership. Gratifyingly, my account of the proprieties has rung true with the healthcare leaders with whom I work. They have found it a useful tool for understanding some of the tensions they experience in their role; for guiding their deliberations; and for developing expressive ethical performance. Practitioners readily grasp the general idea, and propriety seems to be evident to them in their own practice. As a novel concept, however, it requires some further specification. In this epilogue I consider briefly some of the theoretical and practical issues it raises.

How does my ethical analysis relate to actual practices of propriety?

Throughout Chapters 4 and 5 I introduced the proprieties by reference to normative argument from a number of fields, and then went on to describe how propriety appeared to be performed in practice. So fiduciary propriety was introduced by reference to normative claims about fiduciary obligations in medical ethics and law; bureaucratic propriety was introduced by way of discussion of the benefits of bureaucracy; reparative propriety was introduced after discussion of philosophical claims about the nature of trust; and so on. This approach might elicit three questions from readers. First, was propriety evident in the interview data because the study used a preconceived framework of fiduciary, bureaucratic, collegial, inquisitorial and restorative norms? Second, what is the nature of the association between medical leaders' behaviour and the norms I have discussed? Third, if medical leaders are not consciously acting according to moral principle, is their behaviour really 'moral' behaviour?

Were interview data fitted into a preconceived framework?

There is an important point to reiterate here about the nature of the study and the status of the study data. As I commented in the prologue to these chapters, it might at first glance appear that I use medical leaders' descriptions of their moral activity merely to illustrate an a priori conceptual framework. This is not the case. The proprieties emerged from the interview data through an iterative, interpretative process. Formal conceptions of fiduciary responsibility, bureaucracy and collegiality are discussed here because in their interviews medical directors gave informal accounts of fiduciary, bureaucratic and collegial propriety.

My meetings with medical leaders supplied loosely structured, narrative-style interviews. Analysis of the interview data started with development of categories and concepts according to how medical leaders described to me what they did. Later, the categories and

concepts that had emerged from the data were further investigated by referring to normative frameworks. This allowed me to give greater weight to some issues that I might
otherwise have passed over, and to refine the analysis. My claims about the nature of moral
leadership are therefore data-led, but they are not theoretically uninformed.

The research strategy I used was an 'abductive' one, which social theorist Blaikie
describes as follows.

> The starting-point is the social world of the social actors being investigated: their construction
> of reality, their way of conceptualizing, and giving meaning to their social world, their tacit
> knowledge .... The task is then to redescribe these motives and actions, and the situations in
> which they occur ... [S]ocial scientific typifications provide an *understanding* [1(p75),2][1] of the
> activities, and may then become the ingredients in more systematic explanatory accounts. [1(p25)]

As a method abduction has 'two stages: describing social actors' activities and meanings;
and deriving categories and concepts that can form the basis of an understanding or an
explanation of the problem at hand' [1(p117)].

The key feature distinguishing deductive, inductive and abductive research strategies
from one another is the relationship between concepts and data. A deductive strategy draws
on concepts and definitions in order to formulate a hypothesis, and then uses them to guide
data collection and analysis. An inductive strategy does the opposite, so that data are
collected first and concepts are developed that are capable of accounting for the data.
In an absolutely pure form, induction would have to eschew the use of any pre-existing
concepts. But as Blaikie observes, 'presuppositionless [sic] data collection is impossible'
[1(p104)] so that inductive strategies are obliged to draw upon some existing concepts and
their definitions. The abductive strategy shares with the inductive the aspiration to derive
knowledge concepts directly from data. In the case of abductive research the data consist
specifically of other actors' descriptions and conceptions of everyday life. As with the
inductive strategy some presuppositions are required in order to know what is worth
researching and to guide data collection, and these presuppositions inevitably permeate
data analysis.

What contribution did preconceived concepts make to the specification of the proprieties? Concepts and categories were initially derived from the data through processes that
practitioners of grounded theory refer to as micro-analysis, constant comparison and open
and axial coding. I would describe it as reading and re-reading the interviews; drawing
elaborate data maps with different-coloured pens; and staring at extracts of data until an
elusive sense that something connected them resulted in a proposition that could be
articulated. This process generated the concept of propriety, five dimensions of which were
originally extrapolated from the data. These dimensions came eventually, following some
theoretical reflection, to be conceptualized as fiduciary, bureaucratic, collegial, inquisitorial
and restorative propriety. When I started to write about the five proprieties I began to draw

---

[1] The distinction between 'explanation' and 'understanding' originated in the critique of positivism
offered by nineteenth-century sociologists, including Weber and Simmel. '*Explanations* identify
causes of events or regularities, the factors or mechanisms that produced them, and *understanding* is
provided by the reasons or accounts social actors give for their actions .... *Explanations* are
produced by researchers who look at a phenomenon from the 'outside' while *understanding* is based
on an 'inside' view in which researchers grasp the subjective consciousness, the interpretations, of
social actors involved in the conduct' (see reference 1, p. 75). See also reference 2.

on theoretical literatures to describe more clearly what was hinted at in the interview data. I also sought to justify how these proprieties could be treated as moral goods; I say more about this in my discussion of the relationship between practice and normativity below.

Each of the literatures to which I have referred has thus assisted and informed a process of analysis that was led by and grounded in the interview data. The relationship between the data and the theoretical literatures has been an iterative one. Provisional concepts emerged from the study data. These data-led concepts were compared with those in existing analytical frameworks, and the data were re-examined. Aspects of the theoretical accounts were questioned or rejected; aspects of the data-led concepts were revisited and refined. The aim of this iterative process was emphatically not to fit the study data to externally derived theories or concepts. It was to examine what the data and the theories had in common, or where they differed; and it was to import normative analysis into an account of norm-oriented action.

Are medical leaders consciously shaping their behaviour to comply with moral norms?

> I think this is one of the really tricky bits actually about being a Medical Director . . . . You do learn by experience, there's no doubt about that, you get better at it. However, the knowledge you acquire is not easy to apply to the next situation you come across – because of course, no situation is the same. I do think it is quite difficult to say 'Ah, well, there's the the the nugget, the grain of truth about this; if I just do X every time that'll sort it' so . . . .
>
> (Dr. Chalcraft, Royal Metropolitan Infirmary)

It should be remembered that morally capable medical leaders will practise each of the five proprieties as occasion demands, and will more or less effectively be managing the tensions between them. The question of how and where medical leaders develop this capacity to practise the proprieties is an intriguing one.

There is clearly some association between the normative arguments I have set out in my analysis of the proprieties and the practices that medical leaders described. It is surely not mere chance that medical leaders' behaviour in core areas of medical leadership activity is consistent with moral norms applicable to that domain. But what exactly is the nature of this association? The difficulty in seeing a causal association is that the moral norms are not very explicit. How can medical leaders be shaping their behaviour to comply with moral norms of which they are not consciously aware?

One answer might lie with the nature of normative expectations. We have noted that normative expectations are a combination of norms in the behavioural sense (this is what people will do) with norms in the moral sense (this is what they ought to do). So normative expectations contribute an understanding that X *will* be done, as well as contributing an understanding that X *ought* to be done. Could it be that medical leaders are shaping their behaviour to comply with norms in the sense of anticipated behaviours, as well as or instead of norms in the sense of moral standards? On this account, the practices of propriety are a little like shaking hands or removing one's shoes when entering a mosque. Observing such actions to be the normal way of behaving, one mimics them. When pressed, a knowedgeable social actor would describe how shaking hands and removing one's shoes express important values, so that it is right to comply with the governing principles of the practice.

This answer is only partially satisfactory. Propriety is not as simple as knowing when to shake hands or take off one's shoes. It is a sophisticated expertise with many different components and, as Chalcraft observed, it calls for a different response on every occasion to an infinite variety of situations. Unlike practices and principles of respectfully removing one's shoes, the permutations are limitless. In addition, the relevant moral norms are themselves both subtle and contestable. Fiduciary norms are perhaps those most likely to be voiced by practitioners, albeit under the rubric of the GMC's principles of Good Medical Practice or Beauchamp and Childress's four principles. So fiduciary norms could, conceivably, be serving as some sort of guide to action. But the norms of bureaucratic, collegial, inquisitorial and restorative propriety are hardly easily explicable or readily to hand. In fact, medical leaders are not unlikely to voice suspicion of bureaucracy, worry that they will be accused of being too collegial, and profess ignorance of inquisitorial or restorative norms. Finally, medical leaders have very few role models whose behaviour they might emulate. It is hard to see how they could learn such sophisticated behaviours, or such subtle moral norms, from so few exemplars.

A more satisfactory answer might be derived from drawing upon activity theory [3–5].[2] Activity theory posits that humans learn how to comport themselves, settle what the 'rules of the game' should be, and become conscious of what the 'rules of the game' are, through interacting with each other over repeated cycles of activity. What this suggests is that the practices and principles of propriety emerge dynamically from the activities in which they are most relevant. They are collaboratively developed, initially only tacitly understood, and learned in social interaction. As fields of activity mature, what was initially tacitly understood becomes more explicit. It can then be made available for scrutiny, debate and conscious teaching and learning. On this account, the proprieties of moral medical leadership are being shaped primarily by the activity in which medical leaders are engaging. During this process, medical leaders are drawing on whatever suitable cultural norms are readily to hand, and inventing or re-inventing norms in response to circumstances.

The leaders I interviewed appear to have mobilized each of the five proprieties when occasion called for it, adapting their behaviour to what they sensed was fitting. It would seem that we can develop, negotiate and orientate ourselves towards morally reasonable normative expectations without being able to state the underlying relevant norms. This is not to say that medical leaders did not think about what they were doing, nor that developing a capacity for performing with propriety was done without effort. It seems to me that practising with propriety requires considerable effort, subtle interaction, collaborative learning, perspicacious analysis and real self-discipline. For this reason I am content to view propriety as moral action.

If medical leaders are only tacitly aware of underlying moral norms, is propriety truly a practice of morality?

It is surprisingly unfashionable in ethics to think about moral responsibility for things that we do not deliberate about or to think about actions that may seem automatic, everyday, picayune, or mundane. Habitual actions such as where we stand when we talk to a patient, whether we make eye contact, how long we pause to listen for answers to our questions, whether we allow ourselves to feel what the patient is feeling and to hear what the patient is saying contribute much of the meaning to doctors' behaviour ... [T]hese are precisely the actions that form the fabric of moral life. [6]

---

[2] Contemporary activity theory draws on the work of psychologist and learning theorist Lev Vygotsky; leading proponents are Engestrom and Cole. See references 3–5.

It is two decades since Dreyfus and Dreyfus (leading theorists of skilled performance and famous for their theory of expertise) argued that true moral expertise was evident in spontaneous and habitual activity as well as in deliberation over difficult matters. And it is a decade since bioethicist John Lantos made the observation above, that bioethics tended to give undue prominence to deliberation and deliberative action. The field has changed little in the intervening period. It is still dominated by what Margaret Urban Walker identifies as a 'theoretical-juridical model' of morality, in which moral deliberation is king and moral action is a lowly serf.

I discuss Walker's characterization of the theoretical-juridical approach in Chapter 6, but two aspects are worth noting here. The theoretical-juridical model takes as its starting point that real moral knowledge is propositional in form: that is, it can be stated and tested for its truth value. It proceeds from here to make a further assumption, that true moral action makes use of propositional moral knowledge. To act morally, people must first deliberate over the moral norms applicable, and then act on their conclusions.

In my discussion of propriety I have suggested, however, that medical leaders' moral knowledge is deeply embedded in activity. In that case, medical leaders' moral *awareness* does not necessarily derive from mastery of propositional moral knowledge, and neither are their *actions* always based on propositional moral knowledge. So: either medical leaders are not 'doing' morality; or the theoretical-juridical model is wrong about what morality is. I prefer the latter conclusion.

Dreyfus and Dreyfus built on philosopher John Dewey's distinction between 'knowing that' and 'knowing how' in order to develop their model of expertise. They argued that novices in a new sphere of activity clung anxiously to rules and plans, had only a crude perception of the situations they found themselves in, and rarely exercised discretionary judgement. Experts, on the other hand, had an intuitive grasp of situations that was based on deep tacit understanding, used analytic approaches only for novel situations or when problems arose, and held a vision of the possible. Applying this model to moral activity, they argued that ethical experts would have an intuitive grasp of situations based on deep tacit understanding, and would deliberate only over new or difficult problems. Their moral expertise was to be found in their 'ethical comportment' not their propositional moral knowledge [7,8].

The Dreyfuses' conception of 'ethical comportment' is an interesting response to prevalent assumptions about the deliberative nature of ethical action. But it is not a satisfactory account of the kind of moral expertise that I observed. The problem is that in the Dreyfus model, ethical expertise is still dependent on moral rules because it results from mastery over them. The Dreyfuses view 'ethical comportment' as an outcome of assiduous practice of moral deliberation. As normative reasoning is mastered, consideration of moral norms comes to be superseded by 'spontanous ethical coping'. Only rare problems call for a return to deliberation. But we have already noted that propriety comes to be expressed in circumstances where the 'rules of the game' are very opaque. In the case of propriety it is not that the rules of the game have been learned and superseded, it is that it appears possible to play the game without anyone being able to articulate the rules. Propriety and ethical comportment are thus rather different.

There is a far closer fit between the findings of the study and the 'expressive-collaborative model' that Walker proposed as an alternative to the theoretical-juridical model. The expressive-collaborative model has tacit negotiation of normative expectations at its heart, and it is consistent with the activity theory to which I referred above. I discuss the expressive-collaborative model further in Chapters 6 and 7 too.

How can practices of moral leadership help others to know what they *ought* to do?

In Chapters 4 and 5 I have described what medical leaders do when they are confronted by certain kinds of problem. I have then labelled this behaviour propriety, clearly implying that it has a positive moral value. In fact, I have gone further and argued that this is genuinely moral action. Evidently, I hope that moral leaders in medicine will adopt some of these practices. Have I succumbed to the fallacy that Hume famously identified, of confounding 'is' with 'ought' [9]?[3] I have several grounds for maintaining that I have resisted it.

The most straightforward ground is that I have endeavoured to justify why I have assigned a positive moral value to each of the proprieties. Hume's argument was not that states of affairs and normative propositions should be decoupled from one another: it was that because ought, or ought not 'expresses some new relation or affirmation, *'tis necessary that it shou'd be observ'd and explain'd*; and at the same time that a reason should be given' (emphasis added) [9]. So I have reasoned that fiduciary propriety is valuable because the fiduciary obligation is protective of patient interests; bureaucratic propriety is valuable because bureaucracy protects the interests of the collective; collegial propriety is valuable because collegiality promotes the interests of both colleagues and patients; inquisitorial propriety is valuable because it promotes just adjudication; and restorative propriety is valuable because it reinstates parity in moral relationships.

There is also a more subtle argument to be made: pure social description and pure abstract reason are impossible. All social description is 'contaminated' by value judgements, and moral reasoning proceeds on the basis of described states of affairs.

To start with, the notion that the social researcher is a neutral observer with a 'view from nowhere' is simply not tenable. Contemporary (post-positivist) social research assumes that all social description is inescapably value-laden. It is impossible to describe a state of human affairs without importing value-based assumptions into the research. What the investigator decides is worth studying (I thought moral leadership was important); who she talks to (my view of organizational ethics is shaped for good or ill by my decision to speak to medical directors, not directors of nursing or finance); what she asks about (I asked what 'troubled' medical directors, and perhaps they should have been troubled by other things) [10];[4] what meaning she assigns to it (I concluded that some concerns were less morally weighty than others); all of these are value-laden activities.

Similarly, the expectation that moral theorizing might find a universal 'view from nowhere' is unsustainable. Moral reasoning reflects our socially situated and subjective

---

[3] 'In every system of morality, which I have hitherto met with, I have always remark'd, that the author proceeds for some time in the ordinary ways of reasoning, and establishes the being of a God, or makes observations concerning human affairs; when all of a sudden I am surpriz'd to find, that instead of the usual copulations of propositions, is, and is not, I meet with no proposition that is not connected with an *ought*, or an *ought not*. This change is imperceptible; but is however, of the last consequence. For as this *ought*, or *ought not*, expresses some new relation or affirmation, 'tis necessary that it shou'd be observ'd and explain'd; and at the same time that a reason should be given; for what seems altogether inconceivable, how this new relation can be a deduction from others, which are entirely different from it'. See reference 9.

[4] As I write, the Parliamentary and Health Service Ombudsman has just issued a report into poor care of the elderly in the NHS (see reference 10). None of my interviewees raised care of the elderly as a concern.

understanding of social realities: it proceeds on certain understandings about wants, needs, aspirations and activities in those areas of life of which we are aware, and about how we should think about them. New paradigms such as 'care ethics' or 'narrative ethics' have been animated by recognition that established ethical theories had overlooked aspects of experience that are now thought to be important. In the case of care ethics, it was recognizing that womens' experiences and the values that emerged from them had been missing, that supplied the initial impulse to develop new approaches [11,12]. In the case of narrative ethics it was recognizing the narrative underpinnings of everyday life that prompted new developments [13,14].

The upshot of this is that worthwhile ethical inquiry proceeds through an exchange of meanings embedded in empirical description, and meanings found in normative frameworks [15]. If too much weight is placed on empirical description, we either end up asking 'so what?'; or we end up confounding what is normally done with what it would be good to do, treating preferences as if they were moral norms [15–17]. Conversely, if too much weight is placed on abstract normative analysis, we end up confounding what philosophers think is important with what others among us understand to be morally compelling demands. As Walker pointed out, without 'empirically saturated reflective analysis of what is going on in actual moral orders ... ethics has nothing to reflect on but moral philosophers' own assumptions and experiences' [18].

My intention in this study has been to achieve theoretical equilibrium by integrating analysis of the moral troubles that research participants experienced, with reasoned consideration of the norms that appear to be associated with them.

How is the notion of propriety different from virtue?

At first glance it might appear that notions of propriety and notions of virtue have something in common. Neither rests upon an assumption that morality can be equated with rule-following; both seem to direct attention to how practitioners behave. The key difference, however, is that virtue is a disposition or feature of one's character; whereas propriety is an expressive performance that need bear no relationship to preferences or characteristics.

Adopting MacIntyre's argument, many contemporary commentators agree that if we want to know what is virtuous, we should look at what needs to be done to achieve the goods 'internal' to a practice [19]. In the practice of medicine, 'internal' goods are, for example, prevention of ill health; cure; alleviation of pain; and alleviation of anxiety. The 'external' goods are such benefits as professional recognition and a good standard of living. Following this course of reasoning, the virtues most often associated with medicine have been those of compassion, discernment, trustworthiness, integrity and conscientiousness [20]. US bioethicist Pellegrino has argued that medicine demands seven primary virtues: fidelity to trust and promise; benevolence; intellectual honesty; compassion and caring; prudence; justice; and effacement of self-interest (putting the patient before your bill). Behaviour that is prompted by virtue and behaviour that expresses propriety would thus appear to have some significant commonalities: trustworthiness, compassion and conscientiousness have all been discussed in Chapters 4 and 5.

My claim is that – at least so far as the proprieties I have observed are concerned – such behaviours are a response to situations, not a manifestation of deep character [21,22].[5] In

---

[5] This renders propriety consistent with John Doris's situationist ethics; see references 21 and 22.

order to practise virtue, one works to develop a virtuous temperament. Indeed, the development of a virtuous temperament proceeds in a manner somewhat analogous to the development of Dreyfus's notion of ethical comportment; one practises. The difference is that to learn virtue one practises doing what a virtuous person would do, until it becomes part of one's character; to learn ethical comportment one practises deliberation on moral rules, until moral judgement becomes habitual.

But to learn propriety does not mean to internalize it to the extent that it becomes a part of one's personality or self-identity. All that is required is that propriety is sincerely performed on the appropriate occasions. The stolid comportment of the good bureaucrat might plausibly be adopted as a persona for moral purposes by medical leaders who are in their personal lives partisan, opinionated, chaotic and disorganized. We noted in Chapter 4, in fact, that some medical leaders who had played the role of good bureaucrat with considerable flair felt it to be quite at odds with their true character.

How useful is an understanding of 'propriety' to medical leaders?

My analysis of medical leadership has identified that at its heart are some insoluble contradictions. Each propriety claims priority for its object of concern. Fiduciary propriety puts individual patients and their interests first. Bureaucratic propriety puts patients as a group and the organization first. Collegial propriety puts fellowship with colleagues first. Inquisitorial propriety puts dispassionate compliance with procedure first. Restorative propriety puts compassionate acknowledgement of harm first. Evidently, these priorities will sometimes conflict with one another.

Understanding that the proprieties make contradictory demands on leadership behaviour, and that they will inevitably do so, makes managing the tension very much easier. Inability to resolve the tension ceases to be a personal or organizational failure.

I have suggested that switching between the 'proprieties' as required is, perhaps, even more demanding than choosing between moral norms. This is because the proprieties are not, we have seen, founded on explicit rules; nor are they yet consciously recognized forms of behaviour. The knowledge that medical leaders have of the 'proprieties' is largely tacit. This means that they may experience a strong pull towards a particular response, without being fully aware of the basis for this decisional bias. And the 'proprieties' are a form of habitual behaviour. This means that habit may take hold of the situation before there is any conscious decision about how best to proceed.

Greater awareness of the demands of propriety has the same effect as greater awareness of the inevitable tensions between different proprieties. It potentially makes them easier to manage. Understanding the proprieties also opens up the prospect of further developing 'proper' behaviour, consciously shaping action to even better fit the aim of building ethical healthcare organizations.

References

1. Blaikie N. *Designing Social Research: The Logic of Anticipation.* Cambridge: Polity Press; 2000.

2. Schwandt TA. Three epistemological stances for qualitative inquiry. In: Denzin NK, Lincoln YS, eds. *Handbook of Qualitative Research.* 2nd edn. London: Sage; 2000.

3. Engeström Y. Innovative learning in work teams: analysing cycles of knowledge creation in practice. In: Engeström Y, Mieyyinen R, eds. *Perspectives on Activity Theory.* Cambridge: Cambridge University Press; 1999, pp. 377–406.

4. Engeström Y. *Learning by Expanding: An Activity-Theoretical Approach to Developmental Research.* Helsinki: Orienta-Konsultit; 1987.

5. Cole M, Engeström Y. A cultural-historical approach to distributed cognition. In: Salomon G, ed. *Distributed Cognitions: Psychological and Educational Considerations.* New York: Cambridge University Press; 1993, pp. 1–46.

6. Lantos JD. Reconsidering action; day-to-day ethics in the work of medicine. In: Charon R, Montello M, eds. *Stories Matter: The Role of Narrative in Medical Ethics.* New York: Routledge; 2002, p. 154–9.

7. Dreyfus HL, Dreyfus SE. What is moral maturity? A phenomenological account of the development of ethical expertise. In: Rasmussen D, ed. *Universalism v Communitarianism: Contemporary Debates in Ethics.* Cambridge: MIT Press; 1990, pp. 237–63.

8. Varela FJ. *Ethical Know-How: Action, Wisdom, and Cognition.* Stanford: Stanford University Press; 1992.

9. Hume D. *A Treatise of Human Nature.* 1739, Book III, part I, section I.

10. Abraham A. *Care and Compassion: Report of the Health Service Ombudsman on ten investigations into NHS care of older people.* Parliamentary and Health Service Ombudsman. 2011.

11. Held V. *The Ethics of Care: Personal, Political and Global.* Oxford: Oxford University Press; 2007.

12. Slote M. *The Ethics of Care and Empathy.* New York: Routledge; 2007.

13. Brody H. 'My story is broken; can you help me fix it?' Medical ethics and the joint construction of narrative. *Literature and Medicine.* 1994;13(1):79–92.

14. Arras JD. Nice story, but so what? Narrative and justification in ethics. In: Nelson H, ed. *Stories and Their Limits: Narrative Approaches to Bioethics.* New York: Routledge; 1997.

15. Borry P, Schotsman P, Dierickx K. What is the role of empirical research in bioethical reflection and decision-making? An ethical analysis. *Medicine, Health Care and Philosophy.* 2004;7:41–53.

16. Goldenberg M. Evidence-based ethics? On evidence-based practice and the 'empirical turn' from normative bioethics. *BMC Medical Ethics.* 2005;6.

17. Hoeyer K. Ethics wars: reflections on the antagonism between bioethicists and social science observers of biodmedicine. *Human Studies.* 2006;29:203–27.

18. Walker MU. *Moral Understandings: A Feminist Study in Ethics.* 2nd edn. New York: Oxford University Press; 2007, p. 11.

19. MacIntyre A. *After Virtue.* 3rd edn. London: Duckworth; 2007, p. 187ff.

20. Beauchamp TL, Childress JF. *Principles of Biomedical Ethics.* 5th edn. Oxford: Oxford University Press; 2001.

21. Doris JM. *Lack of Character: Personality and Moral Behaviour.* New York: Cambridge University Press; 2002.

22. Doris JM. Persons, situations, and virtue ethics. *Nous.* 1998;32(4):504–30.

Understanding organizational moral narrative

[A] man is always a teller of tales, he lives
surrounded by his stories and the stories of
others, he sees everything that happens to him
through them; and he tries to live his own life
as if he were telling a story [1].

Jean Paul Sartre's words above are often quoted in narrative social research, perhaps implying that such research carries Sartre's imprimatur or is at least consistent with his views. Interestingly, in the passage quoted the narrator continues with the observation 'But you have to choose: live or tell'. Do we really need to make such a choice? Perhaps we must in some areas of life. But not, I think, where the purpose is moral leadership in medicine; then, the living of the story and the telling of the story are both equally vital. In this chapter I explore what, exactly, the terms 'narrative', 'shared narrative' and 'moral narrative' mean and I discuss in greater detail how organizational narratives appear to work. This chapter is one of the more theoretical in the book, and it is aimed at those readers with an interest in further exploring the conceptions of narrative that underpin my account of medical leadership.

Before proceeding to my detailed examination of narrative, it is worth recalling some of the implications of treating moral leadership as a process of orchestrating organizational efforts to produce a fitting moral narrative. First, conceptualizing moral leadership as production of organizational narrative implies that a leaderly response to moral trouble entails facilitating many morally important decisions, rather than making just one; and that moral leadership is a continuous process of coordinating organizational responsiveness rather than a single action. Second, it invites us to focus on understanding the processes that might lead to credible, compelling, collective, moral narratives coming into existence. We begin to see that morally good outcomes, or moral failure, are produced through multiple social interactions in which normative expectations, reactive attitudes and the promptings of propriety play an important part. The upshot of the first two findings is that, third, we are obliged to revise common notions of moral or ethical expertise. Viewing moral or ethical leadership as skilful orchestration of a shared narrative, we see that the necessary expertise is as likely to reside in interpersonal knowledge and dexterity as it is in personal moral wisdom; and that moral expertise is as likely to reside in the dynamic systems that drive group behaviour as it is in the cognitive sophistication of individuals.

While we are examining narrative in the next section, we should keep in mind that we have conceived of moral leadership as a continuing negotiation of normative expectations and responsibilities, a process that harnesses the knowledge and wisdom of groups.

Conceptualizing moral narrative

In this section, I outline how narrative manifests social meanings; where narrative is located in time and social space; and what is distinctive about moral narrative as a genre. There is a vast literature on the nature of narrative: on its forms, structures, content, functions, uses and interpretation. There is also a substantial literature on narrative medicine, narrative ethics and the languages and forms of talk in medical practice. I have drawn upon only a tiny fraction of that scholarship in order to understand moral leadership, and even less of it to explain the notion of narrative that I use here. There is very much more that could be said, but this chapter deals only with a few key questions.

Narrative manifests social meanings

I use the term narrative to refer both to a product (a report, story, policy or other narrative genre) that seeks to account for the past and perhaps anticipate the future, and also to a process (collaborating to create narrative) that takes place in the present.

The first of those meanings is very well established, and narrative-as-product is almost invariably what we think of when we think of narrative. We have little difficulty conceptualizing narrative in this form. Few would contest that narrative is central to human life, and that humans live surrounded by narrative artefacts. There is a vast corpus of theory helping us to understand this aspect of narrative.

The second meaning is rather less well established, and the notion of narrative-as-living-process is more speculative. We have far less knowledge of the role that narrative plays in structuring perception and shaping behaviour, and there are many theories of mind and action to compete with it. Narrative-as-living-process is a concept worth considering, although it cannot be claimed that the evidence for it is incontrovertible. In any event, even if the concept fails to convince readers my other arguments about the nature of moral leadership are capable of standing alone. Cognitive scientist Mark Johnson captures the notion of narrative-as-living-process in this convenient précis:

> Narrative ... is not merely linguistic and textual ... *narrative characterizes the synthetic character of our very experience* and it is prefigured in our daily activities and projects .... There is a narrative (or, at least, protonarrative [*sic*]) structure to experience, to our identity, and to action, which is the basis for our concern with verbal narratives that constitute the most pervasive mode of rational explanation we have. [2(p163–164)] (emphasis in original)

Thus narrative is how we experience interactions with the world. It orders our lived interactions because it is how we comprehend moral, political, cultural and other norms. And it is how we represent our interactions with the world. If all of this is true for narrative in general, so too would it be for shared moral narrative in particular. It is how we experience morally significant interactions with others. It is to be found ordering interactions in groups and organizations because it is how we comprehend moral responsibilities. And it is the means by which the morally significant experience of groups and organizations is transmitted.

The conception of narrative that I use in this research falls towards the 'broad' end of a definitional spectrum noted by the leading narrative researcher Catherine Kohler Riessman.

> There is considerable disagreement about the precise definition of narrative. Among one group the definition is so overly broad to include just about anything. In the clinical literature, for example, there is reference to illness narratives, life stories, and narration in psychotherapy about the past . . . . The definition of narrative has been quite restrictive among another group. Labov, in particular, assumes all narratives are stories about a specific past event, and they have common properties. [2–19][1]

Although my conception of narrative is broad, it nevertheless possesses a clear meaning. It is as follows.

Narrative does not need writing or speech

Barthes supplied a useful thumbnail portrait of narrative, one that helps us to understand both what it presupposes and what it does not.

> In the first place the word narrative covers an enormous variety of genres which are themselves divided up between different subjects as if any material was suitable for the composition of the narrative; the narrative may incorporate articulate language, spoken or written; pictures, still and moving; gestures and the ordered arrangement of all of the ingredients: it is present in myth, legend, fable, short story, epic, history, tragedy, comedy, pantomime, painting, stained glass windows, cinema, comic strips, journalism, conversation. In addition, under the almost infinite number of forms, the narrative is present at all times, in all places, in all societies. [20]

First of all, the concept of narrative does not presuppose written or spoken words. Barthes's inclusion of the stained glass window in his description of narrative brings a significant claim to the fore. It is that narrative may be inferred from what actors see, even though they may need to understand arcane cultural conventions in order to comprehend the narrative that is present. For those who can 'read' the signs, ecclesiastical architecture imparts a series of complex narratives; to those who understand the conventions, a stained glass window represents far more than an aesthetic ordering of colour or form. It supplies characters, each of which occupies a certain place in a known moral universe.

This points us towards the first aspect of moral narrative. A meaningful moral narrative may be present even where it is captured neither in writing nor in speech.

Narrative does not need a narrator

Moreover, although the notion of narrating would seem to suggest that narrative needs a narrator, narrative does not presuppose a teller who reports events. Direct telling may even be the least effective narrative form. Tragic plays, feature films, television sitcoms and pantomime are all narratives, even though the first rule of dramaturgy in each of those different media is 'show, don't tell'. Narrative is most thrillingly expressed in dialogue and gesture flowing back and forth between people. We infer narrative when we observe how others act and react, and when we glean the ostensible meanings of their actions and reactions.

---

[1] On the narrative turn see, for example, references 5–7. On narrative theory see references 2 and 9. On illness narratives see references 10–13. On narrative in clinical practice see references 14–16. On narrative bioethics see references 17–19.

This points towards the second aspect of moral narrative. Moral narrative comes into being in interpersonal interaction, and it may emerge from the exchange of inexplicit expectations and inferences as much as explicit accounts of moral value. Thus the actions that moral leaders are seen to perform are at least as potent a source of moral narrative as anything they have to say. Indeed their actions may, to coin an old cliché, speak far louder than words.

Narrative is an 'ordered arrangement of . . . ingredients'

If the existence of narrative depends neither upon language nor a narrator, what does define it? The way in which I intend to use the term is summed up in Barthes's rather obscure, but ultimately helpful, notion of an 'ordered arrangement of all of the ingredients'. Narrative-as-product is what we end up with when we have rendered things comprehensible. Narrative-as-living-process renders things intelligible at every present moment, anchoring our actions in our beliefs about the past and the future.

Narrative orders and arranges its ingredients according to the principle of 'first this, then that'. In the best narratives, we understand that it is 'because of this, then that'. Narrative can be predominantly backward-looking, the narrative mode favoured in the 'medico-legal' paradigm. Alternatively, narrative can be predominantly forward-looking, the narrative mode that grounds the 'risk-reduction' paradigm. (We noted both of these paradigms in Chapter 2.) Either way, narratives arrange a sequential pattern of relationships between events and between actors.

Narrative-as-product – that is, tales that we could tell if we wished – ascribes meaning to the past, anticipates future possibilities and enables decisions in the here and now to take account of preceding and anticipated events. Narrative-as-living-process – that is, perceiving narrative-wise what we are doing right now, and proceeding narrative-wise to what we do next – creates order and meaning all of the time. The internal structure of narrative, then, orders the world.

Narratives produce private life and social life

Arguing that the virtuous life is realized by reference to a personal moral narrative, Alasdair MacIntyre introduced to virtue ethics Barbara Hardy's claim that 'we dream in narrative, day-dream in narrative, remember, anticipate, hope, despair, believe, doubt, plan, revise, criticize, construct, gossip, learn, hate and love by narrative' [21(p211),22].

When Hardy wrote that people 'plan, revise, criticize, construct, gossip, learn, hate and love by narrative' she turned the focus of her inventory outward from the individual and towards the constructs of social life. When we act in intelligible ways, narrative is exteriorized. It elicits recognition, and frequently a response from others. To Hardy's list of narrative activities, we might add coordinating group action through narrative, allocating resources through narrative, including individuals in social groups or excluding them from society through narrative, winning friends and allies and making enemies through narrative, and waging war to impose narrative. In producing shared narratives, people produce social life. Shared narratives determine who may do what to whom when, and with what consequences [23].

It might be objected that my concept of narrative is so all-encompassing that it explains everything and nothing. My project, though, is not to develop a theory of narrative, but to produce an account of enacted ethics that is 'good to think with'. The criterion by which it should be judged is whether thinking about moral leadership as the production of shared moral narrative enables us to better understand the institutions – the tangible institutions such as hospitals, and the intangible institutions such as ethical medicine – within which we live.

Narrative within the expressive-collaborative model of morality

The account of moral leadership that I have developed in this book aims to capture the key features of moral experience as medical leaders described that moral experience to me. At a theoretical level, one striking feature of their descriptions is how closely they accord with Margaret Walker's expressive-collaborative model of morality. What makes this particularly striking is that while Walker's model has its roots in the feminist scholarship that also grounds care ethics, members of a managerial elite largely consisting of white middle-aged males supplied my research data. Care ethics has already transcended the gender concerns associated with its feminist origins, to offer a more widely applicable theory of the nature of moral life [24].[2] In a similar way the feminist-inspired expressive-collaborative model seems better able to account for moral life as it is lived by both men and women than more traditional (whisper it) male-dominated theoretical-juridical moral theories.

The theoretical-juridical model was first introduced in the epilogue to Chapters 4 and 5. It needs to be further examined here, because the expressive-collaborative model cannot be fully appreciated without understanding what it aims to displace: which is precisely that theoretical-juridical model.

The theoretical-juridical model

For many moral philosophers the theoretical-juridical model (TJM) represents, Walker observes, simply what moral philosophy, and thus ethics, is. But Walker argues the TJM has distorted our understanding of moral life. Walker argued that three strong constraints are central to the TJM:

(TJM1) Restriction of morality to knowledge: the task of moral philosophy is to discover and validate the knowledge in which moral capacity or the justification of its results (essentially) consists.

(TJM2) Restriction of moral knowledge to moral theory: moral knowledge consists in a completely general theory, which explains (the derivations of) and so justifies all true moral judgements.

(TJM3) Restriction of moral theory to the 'scientific' model: an adequate moral theory will be structurally and functionally similar (or analogous) to a 'scientific' one. [25(p44)]

Walker locates these constraints in Sidgwick's ambition to establish a 'scientific' ethics of general principle: abstract, universal and predicated upon presumptively neutral logico-deductive reasoning. According to Walker, it was Sidgwick's quintessentially nineteenth-century intellectual aspiration that supplied the template for twentieth century Anglo-American moral philosophy [26(p75)].[3]

Walker has argued that five other significant assumptions are implied in the TJM. The first is the codifiability assumption, the view that all essential moral knowledge will

---

[2] Slote has offered a strong argument that care ethics justifies public political rights and obligations as well as private ones (see reference 24).
[3] Others refer to Moore's *Principia Ethica*, such as reference 26 (p. 75).

be propositional in form, capable of being stated and taught. The nomological assumption is that such propositional knowledge will consist in law-like generalizations that correspond with the actual moral judgements about what to do in particular situations. According to the logical priority assumption, these law-like generalizations are where essential moral knowledge resides; and not, for example, among the concrete processes of living a moral life. The assumption of systematic unity creates the expectation that all relevant moral knowledge will be reducible to a very few, non-contradictory and internally consistent general rules. An assumption of impersonality expects that the one uniform and codified morality will, if true, be true for everyone.

These rules and assumptions, Walker concludes:

> define code-like theory building, testing, and fine-tuning, with standard appeal to 'intuitions' and vulnerability to intuition-based counter-examples, as the premier genre of, and perhaps simply as 'what to do', in ethics. [25(p50–1)]

The growing field of narrative medical ethics is in many respects a reaction against the constraints inherent in this theoretical-juridical model. I return to narrative ethics again at the end of this chapter to locate my study in relation to that field.

The expressive-collaborative model

In Walker's expressive-collaborative model, as in my own account of moral leadership for ethical enactment, narrative is central. She summarizes her model as follows:

> An expressive-collaborative model looks at moral life as a continuing negotiation among people, a practice of mutually allotting, assuming, or deflecting responsibilities of important kinds, and understanding the implications of doing so. As a philosophical model, this representation of morality functions both descriptively and normatively. Descriptively, it aims to reveal what morality 'is' – what kinds of interactions go on that can be recognized as moral ones. Normatively, it aims to suggest some important things morality is 'for' – what in human lives depends on there being such practices, and how these practices can go better or worse. [25(p67)]

The central practice of morality is, according to this model, the continuing mutual negotiation of responsibility within moral community. Narrative is the key to moral negotiation, but we should look first at the significance of moral community.

Moral community is what creates the conditions for mutual intelligibility; and continued attempts at mutual intelligibility are what create the conditions for moral community. Morality demands that we negotiate responsibilities through recurring rounds of interpersonal interaction. The ceaseless flow of interaction generates and sustains mutually recognized values. Engaging in moral practice in this way, we are made responsible to ourselves, and we are responsible to others, for the moral sense we make with our lives. Accordingly, to be enacting moral life is to be engaging in:

> a social negotiation in real time, where members of a community of roughly or largely shared moral beliefs try to refine understanding, extend consensus, and eliminate conflict among themselves. [25(p71)]

What emerges from successive rounds of negotiation is moral equilibrium in Walker's sense: knowledge of what to expect morally of others, and knowledge of what others expect morally of us. Walker identifies narrative as one of the central modes of moral engagement. Narrative, she argues, is the form in which it is possible to represent past experience, map new situations and project future possibilities. It is the form in which moral problems are represented.

Walker proposes that three kinds of narrative are central to moral negotiations. Narratives of relationship are those that express expectations, understandings, responsibilities and bonds between those joined, however tenuously, in the flow of negotiation. She appears to be most centrally concerned with relationships and expectations that we assume in a more or less voluntary way, relationships based primarily in trust and integrity. Narratives of moral identity record the values that a person has exhibited in the ways that they act and in what they care for over time. Narratives of value connect narratives of relationship and of identity by expressing shared understandings of what is morally important to a group or moral community. It is in the coherence of such narratives, and in the way that they are brought into relationship with one another, that we create and identify the distinctive shape of a moral life.

Those interested in a fuller account of Walker's expressive-collaborative model will find it discussed again in Chapter 7, in the context of its contribution to healthcare organizational ethics as a field. For the moment, it is Walker's conception of narrative that is of interest. Her notion of narrative functions, it seems to me, at a higher level of abstraction than my own. The narratives that I discuss below – what we might think of as the 'narrative in hand' – are all composed out of fragments of larger narratives of relationship, larger narratives of identity, and larger narratives of value. The 'narrative in hand' draws down whatever components it requires from the larger stock of narrative resources that are available.

Importantly, because 'narratives in hand' deal with concrete problems, and concrete solutions, they all possess one crucial feature that seems to be absent from Walker's description of morally relevant narratives: they identify morally relevant events, causes and consequences. So we may add a fourth narrative to Walker's three narratives of relationship, identity and value central to moral negotiations: the fourth is narratives of morally significant fact.

I turn now to look at the so-called 'narratives in hand'. We return to more abstract concerns at the end of the chapter when I locate this study in the context of other approaches to narrative in social research and ethics.

Co-creating narrative: the example of planning for pandemic influenza

The question that this section addresses is what the 'being' of a shared moral narrative is. Where and how does a shared moral narrative exist? I use the metaphor of an expanding circle to describe narrative emerging in activity over time. In the example that follows, I illustrate the several different 'perimeters' of a 'narrative circle'. The circle is inscribed in interactions between people:

(i)   through discussion between colleagues;
(ii)   through initial actions;
(iii)   in meanings ascribed to others' statements and actions;
(iv)   in actors' espousing or modifying others' narratives;
(v)   in interactive enactment of decisions;
(vi)   across the social arena of a moral issue; and
(vii)   in the awareness of peripheral players.

The expanding circle of narrative action is clearly apparent in the way that planning for pandemic influenza took place at Remembrance Hospitals Trust around 2007.

Located in the heart of a major city, the Remembrance Hospitals Trust is a symbol of the state of healthcare in Britain. Hosting both a large medical school and a prodigious range of clinical research activities, Remembrance Hospitals care for people living dramatically different lives in terms of culture, wealth and health. Specialist tertiary and secondary care services receive patients from all over the world, as well as just around the corner. In the corridors and clinics, homeless refugees cross paths with the business elite, middle-class retirees wait next to migrant workers, members of the city's white working class sit alongside the small-scale entrepreneurs who arrived in Britain from her former colonies. The Trust's buildings exemplify the successive eras of healthcare and hospital architecture, from the artful curlicues of Victorian baroque through brutalist post-war modernism to clean, clear, cold, twenty-first-century glass plate. The Portakabins that never leave its car parks, however, stand witness to the vagaries of planning and to the elasticity of healthcare supply and demand. Walking into Remembrance Hospitals, we are reminded that ill health is the great leveller, that major British cities are now global cities, and that however hard we try healthcare needs will never be fully met.

All of this is germane to the emerging narrative that its medical director, Dr. Matthew McGregor, instigated. As I did in Chapter 3, I present the medical leader's account as a third-person narrative. I do so in order to back away from the familiar misconception that narrative is limited to what that gets said; and in order to make evident that the narrative we are analysing is not the interview text itself but the organizational moral narrative to which the interviewee referred. This is a report on a moral narrative that is in being elsewhere, and it is the narrative in being elsewhere that claims our attention.[4]

> A working group on pandemic influenza been convened to plan and prepare ethical and practical guidance for staff in the event of an outbreak of pandemic influenza. These needed to be put in place in advance so that staff could respond in a consistent and predictable way, so that the Trust knew resources would be being used to best effect, and so that it could defend its staffs' decisions retrospectively.

> An outbreak of pandemic flu seemed almost inevitable and would present hospitals with difficult ethical decisions. An obvious one would be having limited resources and enormous demand. They expected that about a quarter of staff would be off sick, they would have a huge patient load, there would be limited supplies of treatment and they would soon be affected by what other hospitals were doing. Patients and carers would be distressed if they thought treatment was being allocated unfairly or irrationally. Until they knew what peoples' needs would be, and what resources they would have available, they could not say who should get priority for what. The circumstances would be difficult for the doctors and nurses looking after patients, and worse if they had to make hard decisions about access to treatment without any guidance.

> Dr. McGregor acknowledged they needed to do more thinking about the position of staff in the event of a pandemic. But there is a moral bargain that healthcare professionals have made, which is that they have agreed to put patients' interests before their own. His colleagues' response to major incidents in the past proves that they are very committed to that principle. But he and they would also have families to care for, which puts them in a difficult position.

---

[4] There are some difficulties in treating interview narrative as faithful reports on something that exists independently and outside the interview setting. I discuss these difficulties in my reflections on method.

Leaders like him would have to demonstrate commitment to patient care, and expect frontline staff to follow their example.

As employers the Trust would have to do everything it can to protect staff and their families, although it may not be possible to offer realistic protection. If some staff absented themselves from work, that would have to be challenged. It is difficult to know how, until you know the exact circumstances. Disciplining absentee staff may encourage others or it may be counter-productive. Ultimately, the test of what to do regarding staff would be what worked out best for patients.

(Dr. McGregor, Remembrance Hospitals Trust)

It is intriguing, in light of events, to look back on this narrative as it stood at the time of our interview. Dr. McGregor and his team were planning to avert a public health disaster, with projections that ranged from 'bad' to 'catastrophic' [27–40].[5] When the anticipated new strain of influenza broke out in Mexico City in 2009, however, it was the H1N1 virus. Despite careful forward planning at the Department of Health and in many NHS hospitals, the virus took everyone by surprise: H1N1 influenza was far less threatening than epidemiology had led public health experts to fear. In the event, the decisions which had to be made were somewhat unexpected: for example, whether the cost of antivirals was justified in view of the mildness of the symptoms, or whether to recommend vaccination when the vaccine was potentially more debilitating than the disease itself [41–49].[6]

Explaining how he and his colleagues were approaching the task of preparing for pandemic influenza, McGregor suggested seven avenues through which moral narrative was coming into being. Dr. McGregor's reflections were prompted by his responsibility for ensuring that Remembrance Hospitals were fully equipped to cope with the coming crisis, so I will start my analysis with McGregor's own place in the narrative.

(i) The seeds of moral narrative emerging among colleagues

Dr. McGregor observed that in his experience doctors rarely talked directly about their values. Rather, they assumed them, because values were expressed in what they did. However, much of what clinicians 'do' together is talk [50,51]. Moral narrative is assembled in that talk, even though moral values may not be voiced directly or overtly or in the language of morality.

We noted in Chapter 2 a vivid example of moral proclamation that was devoid of the verbiage of value but redolent of moral judgement nevertheless: it was Dr Usborne's declarations to colleagues and others that one of failing practices in her area (Churchland Primary Care Trust) was 'supervising the premature death of hundreds of people'. The example makes apparent how a sophisticated moral proposition can be encapsulated in very sparse terms when it is expressed within a community of practitioners.

Similarly terse statements summarized Remembrance Hospitals' values. Dr. McGregor recalled that one of the first comments his clinician colleagues offered was that 'there's no point in just having an ethical system [here] if other hospitals nearby don't have a similar system. Because, there are patients with pandemic flu, you'd soon know which hospital, treats what!'

---

[5] So too were the ethicists. The SARS outbreak was perhaps the template to which people were working. See references 27–34 for articles discussing ethical issues in pandemic planning and references 35–40 for analyses of the SARS outbreak.

[6] See reference 41 for a response from WHO about the H1N1 pandemic, 42 and 43 for Department of Health analyses, and 44–49 for further academic commentary on ethics and pandemics published after the outbreak.

Embedded in that reminder were assumptions about the importance of fairly sharing healthcare goods among a given population, and about maintaining the integrity not of a single organization but of a whole health economy. In the event of pandemic influenza, a reasonable decision by one organization to not treat a certain class of patients could overwhelm others, were the response not coordinated. It is not just that a decision to treat or not treat would impact on other organizations. It is that inequity would arise between patients, according to the arbitrary criterion of which organization they presented themselves at. That such inequity is in fact an everyday aspect of NHS care does not render irrelevant the general principle of equity.

(ii)   Moral narrative developing through overt actions

Moral narrative is expressed in, and may be inferred from, social action. The actions that concern us here are two of the basic processes of moral leadership: involving others in ethical sense-making, and engaging others in enacting a vision of what is good or what is right. Within these two processes, actors engage with the moral narrative in slightly different ways.

Involving others in ethical sense-making, actors adopt as their primary focus the figuring out of moral narrative. Actions are therefore oriented towards the resolution of ambiguities and uncertainties. But from the outset, actions also begin to express an unfolding moral narrative. When Dr. McGregor acted to convene a working group of colleagues, he signalled that preparing to deal with a pandemic was an ethical issue that deserved to be given some priority and warranted the attention of organizational leaders. When Dr. McGregor's colleagues came together to discuss how they would prepare for a pandemic, their discussion prompted collaborations – such as coordinating their work with other healthcare organizations – that extended and embedded the moral narrative.

(iii)   Moral narrative subsisting in ascribed meanings

As a moral narrative begins to meet with acceptance it begins to achieve a nascent existence. Narrative subsists in relationships of meaning, but meaning is fluid and approximate. A moral narrative exists as a shared narrative in the minds and actions of a group, but what one person knows might only approximate what any others truly understand. Human endeavour proceeds willy nilly through misunderstanding and misinterpretation, as much as comprehension and correct inference.

Although Dr. McGregor and his colleagues were engaged in collaborative sense-making, it is unlikely that any one of them achieved a perfect understanding of what each other truly thought or felt. Nor is it likely that any of them would possess a perfect understanding of what another intended to convey through their action. It is, however, on such tenuous bases that actors proceed to interact, and to demur from or assent to one another's proposals. In fact, we noted in the Epilogue to Chapters 4 and 5 how propriety seems able to emerge alongside moral knowledge that is tacitly held and very rarely – if ever – openly discussed.

(iv)   Moral narrative crystallizing in espoused narrative

Dr. McGregor and his colleagues had still to determine the guidance that would be issued to Remembrance Hospitals' staff. Discussing and agreeing these guidelines, consulting upon them and seeking approval, all involved a wider circle of associates in ethical sense-making. A moral narrative assumes a more settled form as its essence is disclosed in draft guidance, stated in discussions, referenced in disagreement, recorded in the minutes of meetings, transformed into black humour, chewed over by staff and patient representatives, discussed with family. Increasingly, a particular moral narrative is reported (or resisted) in others' statements and expressed (or resisted) through others' action.

As the moral narrative becomes a shared understanding of 'how we should do things' it is less a process of sense-making and more a process of engaging others in enacting a particular vision of the good. Eventually Remembrance Hospitals published its guidance. It would have signified a vision of the good that may never have been expressed in response to the influenza outbreak in 2009. But publication is itself enactment of a moral narrative. By authorizing some actions and de-legitimizing others, the publication of guidelines alters the moral landscape. It does so by redefining, to employ a phrase I used earlier, who may do what to whom, when and with what consequences.

As we consider all of the preceding activity, we should recognize that Dr. McGregor and his associates are not just *deciding* what to do. They are engaging as ethical actors. They are meeting, articulating, imagining, prompting, proposing, empathizing, comparing, objecting, projecting and re-inhabiting the roles of doctor, nurse, spouse, partner, carer, parent, neighbour and friend. They are learning, influencing, planning, negotiating, adapting, managing and coordinating. They are creating an ethical environment now, in the present, by preparing for ethical challenge in the future.

(v) Moral narrative manifesting in interaction

Had a serious pandemic materialized, the moral narrative would have been observed in its most complete incarnation. At an individual level, Dr. McGregor stated his conviction that in the event of a pandemic, it would be for clinicians like him to 'lead from the front'. When the time came, his actions would either express his moral narrative or belie his stated beliefs. Not infrequently, differences become apparent between what individuals and organizations say they believe (their espoused values) and what we infer are their 'true' beliefs on the basis of their behaviour (their enacted values).

In moral discourse, the gap between espoused and enacted values is apt to be condemned as an expression of individual or organizational hypocrisy, a failure of conviction, commitment or moral courage. In other fields, however, it is viewed rather more kindly. In studies of organizational culture, for example, the difference between espoused and enacted values is more likely to be ascribed to lack of insight, lack of skill, or an uncongenial environment for learning, than to character weakness or decadence [52]. How far Dr. McGregor's colleagues implement the hospitals' policies may depend on their character, and on their commitment to the moral narrative those policies express. It will also rest on their skill, on what others do, and on whether the policies are workable.

So far we have worked outwards and looked towards the future, tracing the path of moral narrative from Dr. McGregor's sense of himself, in the current time, as an instigator of ethical enactment. We should now step back to consider what preceded his action.

(vi) Moral narrative circulating the social arena

Matthew McGregor did not draw his moral quandary inchoate from the maelstrom of everyday experience. The prospect of pandemic influenza had already been constructed as an object of concern through the combined efforts of many others. In fact, as we shall see in a moment, it had been made an object of specifically ethical concern. But is being constituted as an object of ethical concern the same thing as coming into being as a moral narrative? I suggest not. The two processes are, however, related.

The UK Chief Medical Officer first drew attention to the threat of pandemic influenza in 2002 [53]. By 2005 he could report that 'major planning activity has taken place in this and many ... other countries', including the inception of Committee on the Ethical Aspects of Pandemic Influenza at the Department of Health. Advice was needed to consider such issues as:

> Who, for example, should have priority for drugs or vaccines if they are in short supply? On what basis should 'critical care' beds be allocated? Should NHS staff be expected to come to work to help others, even if this impacts on their caring for their own families? What are the implications of not sending someone to hospital if beds are at full capacity? [54]

The CMO's Committee shortly issued a document introducing a set of guiding ethical principles [55–57]. Further meetings, a round of public consultation, and publication of a more definitive version of their initial blueprint followed [58]. The framework the Committee produced, however, operated at a high level of abstraction. It explained broad principles for the benefit of policy-makers and planners, but contained little tangible guidance for clinicians or managers. The work that would be needed to transform ethical abstractions into moral narrative – collective understandings and actions that produce fair, effective and humane treatment of patients and staff in organizations under pressure – remained the responsibility of others.

Consider, for example, the potentially conflicting duties to care for patients and to care for sick family members. When Dr. McGregor argued that during a crisis healthcare professionals would owe their first duty to their patients, over and above a commitment to their families, he was drawing upon a central tenet of professional ethics: patients' welfare should come first. It was a first principle that stood unchallenged by the disasters he had witnessed before. A significant difference between pandemic illness and major incidents such as a terrorist attack or other 'big bang' disaster is the likelihood that the professional's family or other intimates may themselves require care or demand isolation from the source of infection. Should the healthcare professional's obligation extend to putting the welfare of patient-strangers before the welfare of their patient-family? If it did, should employers enforce that obligation? If so, how? Would punitive action be justified in the event of a breach? The ethical principles proposed by the Committee afforded little assistance in settling such questions and the Committee made no claim that they could. Their document is not, of itself, a moral narrative in the sense in which I have described narrative.[7] Rather, it adumbrates principles that may contribute towards, assist in developing and become a part of moral narrative.

We may conclude that Remembrance Hospitals' emergent moral narrative owes its existence to, is not yet present within, but may become a part of, the social arena in which pandemic influenza has been constituted as an object of ethical concern.

We need finally to consider how moral narrative comes into existence around the periphery of its purposeful core. We have thus far concentrated on how the moral narrative comes into being amongst those it most immediately concerns, that is, the staff and patients

---

[7] The framework document refers to discussion of a number of scenarios that were used by the committee to test the lucidity of the ethical principles. In so far as they contributed to a developing vision of how the good or the right could be achieved in specific circumstances, those scenarios and those discussions come closer to constituting a moral narrative than does the framework document itself.

of Remembrance Hospitals and the other healthcare providers that surround it. But the moral narrative will not be limited to a small coterie of people intimately involved or immediately affected. Just as the moral narratives that emerged from the outbreak of SARS have done [27,28,35–40], moral narratives continue to structure ethical sense-making in other quarters.

(vii) Moral narrative in the awareness of peripheral players

The moral narrative emerging through Remembrance Hospitals' preparation for pandemic influenza has extended beyond the confines of McGregor's workplace. It involves family. It will have moved outwards to include friends, medical students, perhaps conference attendees, or readers of journal articles, and so on.

The moral narrative that was about how to prepare for pandemic will by now have been modified by the course of events. Perhaps it has become part of a narrative about preparing for mild pandemics as well as serious ones. Or the experience of the 2009 pandemic in Remembrance Hospitals may have begun to help answer some of the enduring questions of duty, such as whether family or patients should come first and how organizations should respond to professionals who put their family first. It may in time be merged into wider moral narratives; or it may be wholly subsumed by them.

The distinctiveness of moral narrative: an example of financial retrenchment

I have argued throughout the book that moral leadership concerns itself with orchestrating an organizational moral narrative. But if 'we dream in narrative, day-dream in narrative, remember, anticipate, hope, despair, believe, doubt, plan, revise, criticize, construct, gossip, learn, hate and love by narrative' then what makes a narrative a *moral* narrative [22]? I have made clear that I see no sharp distinction between the moral and the non-moral, the ethical and the practical, so it might seem odd to claim that moral narratives can be distinguished from any other narrative [59].[8] I think that we can do so, and moral narratives appear to express the following elements of moral enactment:

(i)   Referencing narrative and normative expectations within a moral community.

(ii) Identifying morally relevant events, causes and consequences.

(iii) Attributing moral status to acts and to actors.

(iv) Acting, reacting, and making moral judgements.

(v)   Reckoning the moral context, such as justifications and excuses [9].[9]

---

[8] Different schools of linguistic analysis recognize a variety of different genres against which it is possible to map this account of moral narrative. Pursuit of such theoretical coherence would take us too far from the chief aim of the current discussion. See, however, reference 59.

[9] This structure includes many of the components of Labov and Waletzky's highly specified structural model of narrative form which consists of (i) an abstract, summarizing the subject matter; (ii) orientation, which provides information about the time, place, situation and participants; (iii) complicating action which recounts what happened and what happened next; (iv) evaluation, summarizing what the events mean to the narrator; (v) the resolution, recounting how it ended; and (vi) a coda which returns the perspective to the present. See reference 9.

I argued in Chapter 1 that moral leadership consists of three major phases. First, moral leaders recognize the need for moral action as they begin to make sense of their experience; second, moral leaders involve others around them in making deeper moral sense of the situation; third, moral leaders seek the commitment of others to acting out a shared vision that includes appropriate solutions. The task across all three phases is to assemble an organizational moral narrative that contains the five elements listed above. Sense-making thus begins the task by assembling the basic elements of the moral narrative; the elements are refined with further, deeper sense-making; and enacting the shared vision embeds each element of moral narrative in the life of the group.

Moral narrative will, then, generally start with moral intentions; interaction renders elements of the moral narrative visible to others; and many moral narratives will settle, eventually, as lasting outcomes [60].[10] Such outcomes include the harm prevented, the justice done, the good secured; individual memories or the collective memory of the group and organization; and lasting differences in those who were involved, differences in their emotional composure, their character, their social skills, their knowledge, their wisdom.

In this section we see how the five elements of narrative are composed within an everyday moral narrative of resource management at Brickvale Hospital NHS Trust. Brickvale Hospital serves an old industrial and commercial district, one that has long provided a home for immigrants to Britain from all over Europe and the former British Empire. The hospital, like the area, has been through troubled times. Structural reorganization within the NHS did not favour it, and, unpopular with junior doctors, it was seriously weakened when it lost several training posts. But in the past decade both Brickvale Hospital and its surrounding area have started to pull themselves up by their bootstraps. The hospital used PFI[11] funding to regenerate its estate, and has pressed forward with imaginative ways to meet the health needs of its various African, Caribbean and Asian communities. But there are historical inequities in NHS provision, with those poorer parts of the country that were ill served by medicine when the NHS was created remaining significantly under-resourced. And the health inequality associated with poverty means that the people Brickvale serves need more resources than their wealthier neighbours, not less. Brickvale has never received, and is unlikely in future to receive, the funding it requires if it is to serve its stakeholders as well as it might.

At the time of my meeting with its medical director, Dr. Edward Evans, Brickvale Hospital was 'in turnaround'. 'In turnaround' was the management-speak of the moment, and it meant taking drastic steps to slash an often long-standing financial deficit. Like other hospitals in my study, Brickvale was also grappling with the government's policy of shifting care for chronic conditions into community settings [61]. This required Primary Care Trusts to commission and fund General Practitioners to provide a range of treatments hitherto the preserve of hospital specialists, and hitherto a source of revenue for the hospital.

In the sample of narrative that I analyse here, the Trust's medical director explained how his clinical role sustained his capacity to offer moral leadership in these difficult circumstances. Dr. Evans, in common with most medical directors, had chosen to retain some clinical responsibilities. This was partly because he enjoyed clinical work, partly because he wanted to preserve his professional identity, and partly to retain the collegial bonds that

---

[10] 'Spontaneous ethical coping', however, is non-deliberative so it may arrive without any conscious intent. See reference 60.

[11] The Government's Private Finance Initiative was a means of funding new public buildings, such as hospitals and schools, without the debt appearing in the public sector borrowing requirement.

went with being a member of the clinician community. He told me that when doctors tried to claim the moral high ground in their arguments with 'management', he could challenge them as a fellow professional standing on the same ground. He then gave me the example that appears below.

The interview extract is reproduced almost verbatim, with very minor cuts. In the discussion that follows the extract, I analyse the structure and content of the moral narrative, according to the summary headings appearing alongside the transcript.

In the middle of [turnaround] we've been doing stuff around commissioning intentions. The difficulty here is that there's the PCT on one arm saying 'We want less of this', there's a specialist on another arm saying 'You can't do this', there's GPs saying 'Well look, we can do some of it but clearly can't do all of it' and it's really where the higher moral ground is.

Identifying morally relevant events

That's the bit of where I have to try and provide a bit of balance . . . [Hospital consultants are] saying, 'These commissioning intentions are potentially dangerous to patients and we're not going to play ball and we will go to the press' and everything else.

Referencing narrative and norms of the moral community

My general response to that is 'Well there is some truth in what you say and I'll engage with the PCT's Medical Director about the bits that we think are the truth, or we'll try and get to the bottom of the truth and use some other people to look at it. At the same time you can go to anyone you like, you're free, we have a whistle-blowing policy . . . . But if you want to look after your patients and your service what's the best thing to do? The best thing is to try and do all this in a comfortable manner behind closed doors rather than create anxiety, unfair anxiety for your patients and your population.'. . . It's worked partially because they've managed to not talk to every journalist. But we do have journalists on our back and we had the MP in here on Friday . . . .

Acting, reacting, and judging

What you need in systems, you do need a bit of dissent . . . . Listen to the people who are dissenting. Sometimes [they are claiming the] high moral ground, but where it comes from is personal interest . . . . Sometimes there is real proper, it's not personal interest, it's actual proper dissent, 'This is wrong, be careful'. . . . It's very easy to lose all the dissent because everyone feels frightened or threatened, jobs and everything else but I sense that doctors will always dissent . . . and they know how to dissent in the highest possible places . . . .

Attributing moral status

It's about listening to it. In this case there was some truth in what they were claiming about the higher moral ground. There's obviously some stuff in it that's very personal . . . but recognizing that, it would be wrong of me not to acknowledge and deal with it if they raise a problem about patients. (Dr. Evans, Brickvale Hospital NHS Trust)

Reckoning the moral context

(i) Referencing existing narrative and norms within a moral community

The origins of moral narrative lie within existing normative expectations of a community. Fitting moral narratives cohere with precedent moral narratives that already anchor the value commitments of a group, and incorporate the explicit and tacit norms that guide group behaviour.

In Dr. Evans' narrative, the 'higher moral ground' that doctors are asserting is, of course, their explicit duty to safeguard the interests of patients, and, perhaps, tacit expectations about the proper approach to patient advocacy.

> [Hospital consultants are] saying, 'These commissioning intentions are potentially dangerous to patients and we're not going to play ball and we will go to the press' and everything else.

The jealously guarded prerogative of clinical judgement, and the ethical imperative commanding doctors to place patients' interests before all other concerns, make this higher moral ground a fertile source of ethical conflict. Medical leaders are frequently obliged to negotiate the path of change in face of the truth in the assertion that any alteration in the present way of doing things could jeopardize patient safety. The present way may be imperfect, but generally its risks are known. The future may promise improvements, but it also brings with it unanticipated risks and unforeseen consequences. Couched in terms of patient benefit or safety, arguments that may be generated by professional rivalry, 'specialty arrogance', self-interest or simple resistance to change can all be made by dissenters to seem morally compelling.

(ii) Identifying morally relevant events, causes and consequences

To be fitting, moral narratives rest on accurate moral sense-making. Moral significance has to be assigned to events, their moral meaning explicated and the responsibilities they invoke identified. Narrative identifies the morally relevant events, and adumbrates causes and consequences. In many of the examples we have considered, medical leaders have had to undertake sensitive and demanding inquiries before they could claim to have reliable knowledge of events and their causes. Here, Evans and his interlocutors were drawing on their common knowledge of key events. They knew about the policy background, about the commissioning proposals, about the reasons for disagreement between the PCT, the GPs, the hospital and individual consultants.

> In the middle of [turnaround] we've been doing stuff around commissioning intentions. The difficulty here is that there's the PCT on one arm saying 'We want less of this', there's a specialist on another arm saying 'You can't do this', there's GPs saying 'Well look, we can do some of it but clearly can't do all of it .... That's the bit of where I have to try and provide a bit of balance.

Morally relevant causes and consequences remained, however, a source of contention. Which of these interlocutors is right about the consequences for various groups of patients of new approaches to providing care? The continuing dissent was founded in continuing predictive uncertainty. It may well be that it was also founded in self-interest, anxiety and 'initiative fatigue'. But what sustained it was insoluble, legitimate uncertainty about the future, giving rise to two opposing 'sub-narratives'.

One 'sub-narrative' asserted that chronically ill patients' interests will be best met by care outside hospital in primary care settings, that doctors should strive to meet their interests in this way, and that doctors reluctant to do so should be called to account on behalf of those patients. The other asserted that patients' interests are best served by specialist care in safe settings, that it is doctors' fiduciary duty to protect their patients from the vagaries of ill-thought-through health policies, and that it would be morally blameworthy not to protest against them on patients' behalf. Each sub-narrative thus sought to vindicate the normative expectations that it represented.

(iii) Attributing moral status to acts and actors

To be fitting, moral narratives must assign a moral status to acts and actors that is consistent with reasonable normative expectations. The causes of events, and the intentions of actors, play a critical role in moral narrative.

At the beginning of Chapter 5 I referred to a decision by the editors of the British Medical Journal to discourage use of the word 'accident' in articles discussing medical and other harms. This is a small but revealing example of the role that narrative plays in moral sense-making. First, a single concept can point to an extensive moral hinterland. In the case of 'accident' the concept imports assumptions of causation (the event was unpredictable and therefore could not be prevented) and an understanding of the mechanism of blame (no harm was intended; unless someone failed through carelessness or neglect to prevent it there is no one to blame). Second, narrative definitions are important. How we understand a situation determines what we will do about it. The BMJ editors believed that continuing to view preventable injuries as accidents implied that they were unavoidable, and this in turn led to a continuing failure to prevent them.

The perpetrator's intentions determine whether a death that follows administration of morphine is murder, manslaughter, mercy killing, gross negligence, negligence, medical mistake or a side effect of palliative care; hence they also define the moral status of the healthcare professional who administered the drug. But this process also works the other way around. The high moral status of an actor, for example a doctor, may promote a (sometimes mistakenly) benign assessment of intentions and hence a (sometimes mistakenly) benign assessment of the act [62,63].

The moral status Dr. Evans accords to both 'dissent' and 'dissenters' is a less dramatic instance:

> Listen to the people who are dissenting. Sometimes [they are claiming the] high moral ground, but where it comes from is personal interest .... Sometimes it's actual proper dissent, [they're saying] 'This is wrong, be careful'.

The dissent that flows from a genuine commitment to patient interest acquires a different moral status from the dissent that arises from self-interest. And dissenting doctors who make themselves unpopular to defend the interests of their patients are granted a different moral status from dissenting doctors who stake a claim to the moral high ground apparently for personal advantage. Again, the relationship between the moral status of the act and the actor may be an observably circular one. When the respected 'real dissenter' speaks, it may sound more like 'real dissent' than when the awkward colleague holds forth to espouse the exact same view.

In the moral narratives we have examined throughout the book, patients most frequently appear as trusting and innocent ciphers. (When we noted one exception, Dr. Seddon's encounter with families of patients who had suffered harm, it was a dramatic one.) Medical directors' assessments of the moral character of their colleagues, on the other hand, ran the gamut from moral hero to moral leper. That patients were for the most part (there were exceptions) granted the benefit of unsullied moral status is consistent with the ethical aspirations of the medical profession. However, the very consistency with which patients' blamelessness was invoked might, perhaps, provoke a degree of skepticism.

(iv) Acting, reacting and making moral judgements

Moral narratives come into being as people act and react around their ethical intuitions and convictions. Every action provokes a reaction, and every action and reaction is liable to moral judgement. Out of the several action-reaction-judgement sequences in Edward Evans's narrative, one will suffice to make the point.

Dr. Evans believed that dissent was vital to 'systems', but also that dissent should not adversely impact on patients. He thereby challenged his consultants to demonstrate their good faith by refraining from disruptive public protestation.

> But if you want to look after your patients and your service, what's the best thing to do? The best thing is to try and do all this in a comfortable manner behind closed doors rather than create anxiety, unfair anxiety for your patients and your population.

If Dr. Evans's colleagues were credibly to claim the moral high ground, they would be obliged to respond to this challenge with constraint. When it was clear that they had done so, it had the effect both of expressing a shared moral narrative and of reinforcing their moral status as trustworthy professionals.

Of course, a far less charitable interpretation of this sequence of action and reaction could be offered. Patients' interests, Dr. Evans argued, would be better served by keeping quiet than by making trouble. Did he make judicious use of exactly the same moral high ground as his consultants, in order to suppress damaging public debate? We cannot know. But we can observe that if we came to this conclusion we would be attributing moral status to him and his actions through a sequence of actions and reactions leading to moral judgement. The alternative interpretation is simply the reverse of the narrative of vice and virtue, action and reaction, and final judgement that Dr. Evans composed.

(v) A reckoning of the moral context, such as justifications and excuses

The moral reckoning expresses one or more perspectives on the norms, expectations, events, moral statuses, actions, reactions and judgements woven through the moral narrative. The moral reckoning expresses the end point of the narrative in hand. Moral leadership in medicine is about bringing into focus, pursuing and instating the moral reckoning that best addresses the normative expectations of all those with a stake in healthcare organizations.

Dr. Evans concluded with a balancing statement that expressed the way in which normative expectations could best be realized. His statement acknowledged two sets of expectations: the normative expectations of patients, that their health interests would be promoted and protected; and the normative expectations of doctors, that their advocacy on behalf of patients would be properly heard. It was Dr. Evans's responsibility to manage, and to respect, these expectations. It would be wrong, he asserted, to allow inter-professional rivalry, organizational interests or personal dislike to override them.

The narrative turn in social research and ethics

The quotation from Sartre with which I opened this chapter appeared in an influential article on narrative accounts of human action, published in 1987 by psychologist Jerome Bruner; Jane Elliott quotes the same words again nearly twenty years later in a comprehensive survey of narrative analysis in social research [7,64]. Narrative analysis has spread across an increasing number of fields in the social sciences and medical humanities, so my purpose in this part of the chapter is to locate my study in relation to that diversity in narrative research.

Narrative social research

Narrative research is both a method (researchers seek to elicit narrative) and a phenomenon of study (researchers analyse narrative, whether elicited in interview or occurring naturally). Narrative social research has tended to focus on one or more of the three categories first proposed by Mishler [65]: on the content of narrative, on its structure, or on its performance. Elliot adopts this typology to review the ways in which narrative analysis has been used in social research, and it makes a convenient place to start the comparison with my approach [66].[12]

The first category, which draws on the representational capacity of narrative, has perhaps been the dominant form in narrative social research. Narrative data are collected, and narrative accounts of social life are published, because narrative is capable of conveying information with great economy. The objective has been to achieve a deep understanding of individual experience, using this as the foundation for modest generalization. This approach to narrative has a long history in social research. A reputable method in the repertoire of 'Chicago school' sociologists [67][13] the 'quantitative turn' in sociology dismissed it from the sociological mainstream on grounds that it was non-scientific and non-generalizable.

Over the past thirty or so years social research turned back to narrative, in part as a result of the growing acceptance of qualitative social research and in part the result of increased interest in narrative across many disciplines [3,68,69]. The complex content densely encoded in individual life histories makes narrative inquiry ideally suited to understanding personal and group identity. Clandinin and Connelly, two leading proponents of life narrative research in education, outline the status of narrative as follows:

> [L]ife – as we come to it and as it comes to others – is filled with narrative fragments, enacted in storied moments of time and space, and reflected upon and understood in terms of narrative unities and discontinuities . . . . Experience is what we study, and we study it narratively because narrative is a key form of experience and a key way of writing and thinking about it . . . . Narrative is both the phenomenon and the method of the social sciences. [68(p17–18)]

Although detailed analysis of a very small sample of life narratives has come to epitomize narrative social research, it is not restricted to it. Introducing narrative research Riessman, for example, discusses Ginsburg's study of thirty-five abortion activists, while Elliot cites Franzosi's study of 1,000 narrative presentations of labour disputes [70,71].

A second approach to narrative social research introduced consideration of the structure of narrative, that is, the ways in which different narrative forms shape the content and message the narrative conveys. This strand in research emphasizes the extent to which different narrative forms are part of a cultural 'tool kit' that individuals draw upon both to

---

[12] For a different typology and a useful overview of a decade of research on illness narratives see reference 66.

[13] Reference 67 is generally cited as the green shoot of narrative research, subsequently trampled under the iron boot of positivist-quantitative sociological orthodoxy.

make sense of experience and to communicate with one another. As an exemplar of this approach Elliot cites Williamson's study of the iconography of HIV/AIDS: Williamson argued that the illness was represented as a gothic-horror story, assimilating the startling new disease to familiar cultural conventions [72]. This type of research is primarily concerned with the contribution of narrative to sense-making and shared understanding.

A third approach, again concerned with the form of narrative as much as its representational content, has been to investigate the emergence of narrative in its social context. The emphasis in this research has been to identify how narratives are constructed and achieved in the flow of everyday activity. Drawing on the analytic tools of socio-linguistics, conversation analysis and discourse analysis this approach to narrative has been strongly oriented towards an investigation of story-telling in everyday settings [73].[14] In all of these fields, the narrative or stories are treated as being constitutive of social life: socio-linguistic genre theory, for example, 'invites us to see culture as a system of [narrative] genres ... through which we *enact* community' (emphasis added) [59(p1637)].

The preponderance of narrative research has taken as its focus the composition of individual life narratives and the authoring of identity, although socio-linguistics in particular has been interested in the production of narrative within groups. It is probably research into organizational learning that has been most influential in promoting the view that group activity is directed, developed, synchronized and harmonized according to narrative [74–79].[15] Perhaps because of the difficulty of researching managerial elites, much of the research in this idiom has observed lower-status employees and community workers. Moreover, organizational narrative research has tended to treat 'narrative' as synonymous with 'storytelling'. As David Boje summarized, employees 'tell stories to predict, empower, and even fashion change .... They tell stories about the past, present and future to make sense of and manage their environment' [80–82]. When compared with the muscular language dominant in business management, the notion of story-telling may seem 'somehow weak effete and soft' [68(p27,29)]; but in their study of hospital management Currie and Brown argue that 'narrating' within organizations is an important way of constituting legitimacy and, ultimately, power.

> In a sense, organizations literally are the narratives that people author in networks of conversations ... an accumulation of continuous and (sufficiently) consistent story lines that in turn maintain and objectify 'reality' ... [I]ndividuals and groups author sensemaking/constructing narratives which permit people to organize their experiences ... in ways that facilitate prediction, comprehension, and control in organizations. [83–88]

This study had its starting point in grounded theory, but came to have greater affinity with all three narrative research orientations above. First, it became a study of narratives of experience, and in common with the first approach has an interest in the content of narrative. Second, it became a study of narrative form, the distinctive genre of moral narrative. Third, while it is not a study of the production of narrative in its social context – I worked with reported narratives – I share with socio-linguistics the view that culture is 'a system of [narrative] genres ... through which we enact community' [59(p1637)].

---

[14] A good representative selection of essays, including a discussion of narratives of illness, appears in reference 73.

[15] Key texts in this field are identified in references 74–77. See also references 78 and 79.

Narrative in ethics

There are several slightly different projects through which narrative has become part of ethics in general, and medical ethics in particular. Alasdair MacIntyre's work played an influential role, introducing a narrative version of *phronesis* (practical wisdom) to virtue ethics. What is humanly good, MacIntyre argued, may be ascertained by reference to the narrative unity of human lives, and to the ethical goals of the social practices in which we participate. According to MacIntyre, narrative is important because it gives us reasons for acting. In a much-quoted passage, he argues:

> I can only answer the question 'What am I to do' if I can answer the prior question 'Of what story or stories do I find myself a part?'. . . To be the subject of a narrative that runs from one's birth to one's death is . . . to be accountable for the actions and experiences which compose a narratable life. It is, that is, to be open to being asked to give a certain kind of account of what one did or what happened to one. [21(p216–17)]

Being able to give 'a certain kind of account' supplies a teleological aspect to our lives, lives that would otherwise be ungrounded in meaning. MacIntyre's assertion of the centrality of narrative is one that this study has echoed. But it would seem that by and large MacIntyre envisaged virtuous actors deciding and justifying decisions through narrative, rather than enacting morality or orchestrating group moral action.

Beyond the confines of virtue ethics, a variety of narrative approaches have in various ways challenged the pre-eminence of what Walker called the theoretical-juridical model. Viewing human life as an essentially meaning-making activity, narrative theorists concur that 'the meanings we look for and seek to construct in our lives are not collections of propositions' [89]. For narrative ethicists, 'doing ethics', whether as a theorist or as an ordinary moral agent, draws on skills in sense-making and story-telling. In the sphere of medicine, this has resulted in four slightly different visions of narrative ethics: edification by narrative; a patient-narrative ethic: moral narratives as a supplement to rule-based methods; and integrated narrative-based ethics.

Edification by narrative

Well-established in the medical humanities, this version of narrative ethics does least to upset traditional rule-based applied moral theorizing. Study of morally edifying literatures and patient or professional 'narratives of witness' is believed to contribute to moral development and moral perception [90,91]. The use of patient narratives of witness, that is, patient narratives of illness and of medical treatment, has obvious affinity with the genre of a patient-narrative ethic to which we turn next.

A patient-narrative ethic

The patient-narrative ethic challenges both scientific biomedicine and traditional professional ethics. Greenhalgh and Hurwitz describe this narrative ethic when they argue that medicine, as a practice, is founded in narrative. Narratives 'are the phenomenal form in which patients experience ill health' [15(p7)][111]. It follows, then, that:

> understanding the narrative context of illness provides a framework for approaching a patient's problems holistically, as well as revealing potential diagnostic and therapeutic options which we ignore at the patient's peril. Furthermore, illness narratives provide a medium for education of the patient and professional, and expand and enrich the research agenda. [15(p7)]

To overlook the narrative structure of patient experience is thus to fail to fulfil the aims and potential of the practice of medicine. Not only does ethical medical practice rest upon respect for patient narratives; but doctors' reasoning is also narrative in nature, a process of narrative reconstruction of patient narrative [16,92,93] The primary interest is in patients' biographies, and how these might influence decision-making, inform doctors' understanding of illness and contribute to the canon of professional knowledge.

A narrative approach to bioethics focuses on the patients themselves: these are the moral agents who enact choices. Theirs are the lives ruptured by the *peripeteia*, or the transformative event, that the cases highlight. The descriptions, analyses, and interpretations of their journeys through the moral realms of illness become our tradition, our storied past, the collectively held touchstones that enable us to know what to do next. Known to us in rich, earthy, singular complexity, these stories of individual patients form our professional canon, both in ethics and in clinical medicine. [18(p.xi)]

The defining feature of this particular narrative approach to bioethics is a focus on the patient as a moral agent, someone making decisions on their own behalf, or someone whose wishes ought to be respected by surrogate decision-makers. Decisions or courses of action are best justified by how well they serve the life narrative of the patient, a life narrative that is situated within other narratives that should also, as far as possible, be heard.

In ideal form, narrative ethics recognizes the primacy of the patient's story, but encourages multiple voices to be heard and multiple stories to be brought forth by all those whose lives will be involved in the resolution of a case. Patient, physician, family, nurse, friend, and social worker, for example, may all share their stories in a dialogical chorus that can offer the best chance of respecting all the persons involved in a case. [94]

The chief focus of the patient-narrative ethic is doctors' relationships with patients; one of its central tenets, that 'doing ethics' entails attending to narrative in clinical practice [16, p159)]. The patient-narrative ethic thus comprehensively decentres the project of principle-driven bioethics, without necessarily demolishing it.

Moral narratives as a supplement to rule-based ethics

Perhaps the most common approach to incorporating narrative into medical ethics is to treat narratives as a supplement to propositional moral reasoning. The larger claim is that narratives serve 'a central epistemic function in the discovery of, justification, or application of ethical knowledge – a role that fills the gaps inherent in any analytical, rule-based method' [95,96]. This approach seeks to augment theoretical-juridical reasoning by providing an additional sense-making element [97]. The conviction remains that medical ethics is centrally concerned with doctor-patient relationships and life-changing decisions. These individual decisions can be better made, so the argument goes, if we use the human propensity for narrative as a resource for understanding.

This approach differs from the patient-narrative ethic in contemplating a much broader range of potentially relevant narratives. Doctors' and other professionals' narratives, and broader moral narratives, are just as useful as a means of 'filling the gaps' in analytical method.

Although narrative ethics of this sort has gained ground and credibility, rigorous empirical study of how ethical or moral narrative is produced in medical settings remains elusive [98].[16] (There is of course a substantial body of empirical ethics scholarship of the non-narrative variety.) Jordens and Little's study of narrative genre in clinical ethical reasoning supplies, however, a compelling example of the purchase to be gained by a socio-linguistic analysis of narrative reasoning about ethical challenges. They identify a 'policy genre' within their interview data, a mode of narrative that, they argue, 'is the unfolding of practical wisdom in speech ... [it] is evidently the appropriate choice of genre in a situation where a display of ethical identity is called for ... [and it] encodes norms about order and disruption' [59(p1643)].

Integrated narrative-based ethics

Ethicist Howard Brody is one of few theorists who have proposed a comprehensive framework for integrating narrative data into ethical reasoning. He argues for a mode of 'narrative equilibrium' where agents search for coherence between 'top'-level abstract ethical principles, 'middle'-level concepts and categories contained in cultural narratives, and 'bottom'-level particulars expressed in life narratives and illness narratives [13(p230ff)].

Brody's central concern remains moral reasoning and moral justification in professional medical ethics. This initially seems far removed from the concerns in this study. Interestingly, though, in a discussion of not whether, but how, to tell the truth about a grim prognosis, he depicts the enactment of medical ethics as a narrative interaction between doctor and patient. The manner in which bad news is broken is an exhibition of ethical expertise, he argues, and this expertise rests on a narrative relationship between the two parties.

> To do a *morally decent job* ... of disclosing a grim diagnosis, the physician must attend to many particular details that cannot be encompassed by a principled analysis. Most of these details lie within the unfolding narrative of the patient's life and of the patient's relationship with the physician. [13(p230ff)] (emphasis in original)

Brody's conviction that ethical expertise entails enacting values, and that enactment depends on narrative, finds a counterpart in my argument about moral leadership at organizational level. There is much in the present study that has echoed Brody's description of 'doing a morally decent job' by attending to demands of enactment and the challenges of relational narratives.

Moral narrative: a final word

In the next chapter I move on to examine the implications of my study, both for conceptualizing the field of organizational ethics and for fostering the development of moral leadership.

But before I do so, I want again to offer the final words in a chapter to the medical leaders who participated in the research. What follows is one medical leader's narrative of action, a vivid example of how propriety is expressed in the narrative structure that I discussed above.

---

[16] Reference 98 is flawed but thought-provoking; the authors seem unaware of the meaning of narrative beyond 'story', and of research into how narrative is constructed in daily life. What becomes apparent is the paucity of empirical research in narrative medical ethics, and the conventions of scholarship in bioethics which permit unapologetic anecdotage.

This is a moral narrative about taking responsibility for processes culminating in the dismissal of a hospital chief executive. Those were circumstances that, as far as this leader was concerned, clearly called for the exercise of moral judgement. Very much more is conveyed in this short extract of transcript than I explain in my accompanying comments, including the character and attitudes of the speaker. Yet my fairly terse explanatory comments are already half as long again as the extract itself, without even making much reference to those issues of character and attitude. I have selected this narrative as a final sample of evidence from the interviews because it demonstrates so clearly what a rich medium of communication narrative is.

§1. There were tales of inappropriate behaviour towards other execs and towards the non-execs. The Chief Exec had a very combative approach to relatively junior managers. Then it became obvious that coteries of people would, for no apparent reason, be held in particular regard. Then they were just dropped and new ones picked up. There were difficulties around finance. A number of things were railroaded through the Board.

The opening makes reference to the normative expectations of the management community, which are apparent in implied abuses of bureaucratic propriety: favouritism, unpredictability, lack of restraint, and financial irregularity. This opening identifies morally relevant 'trigger' events, attributes moral status to actions, and hints at an attribution of degraded moral status to the CEO that is confirmed later in the narrative.

§2. So a number of the execs came to see me with concerns. They said 'You've got to do something about this'. I said 'Well forgive me – but why me?' And they said 'Because you're a certain type of personality; and the rest of us are professional managers so if this all goes belly up, we've lost our jobs completely'.

The consequences of the CEO's actions – managerial revolt – are spelled out. Then the narrative shifts perspective and new morally relevant events, causes and consequences are introduced. These are the actions of colleagues, and the medical leader's response. A fresh theme of collegial obligations and collegial propriety emerges to supply a new strand in the moral narrative, the justifiability of the actions the medical leader will take. The leader assigns himself a positive moral status, a person who takes robust action but does not seek power.

§3. I had to satisfy myself that what they were asking me to do was right, and that there was no other way forward.

We learn about the medical leader's actions, reactions, and moral judgement. These reflect the sense-making stage of narrative development and contain a suggestion of inquisitorial propriety. The medical leader took steps to find out whether what was being alleged was true, and whether it would be right to proceed to take further action.

§4. Then I coordinated a response and we made it apparent to the Chairman that we didn't feel the situation could continue. Eventually the Chief Exec resigned, and virtually the entire Board went too.

The medical leader acts to orchestrate a response, which comes to a head in presentation of a shared moral narrative to the chairman. This presentation activated the hierarchical structure of bureaucratic propriety, including the accountability of the CEO to the chairman and the accountability of the Board of directors for management at the senior level of the organization. The action references further normative expectations, that the chairman would be responsive to such a narrative and that other members of the Board felt it right to resign in the circumstances.

§5. This was certainly, for me, a case of moral and ethical judgement. It wasn't just to do with organizational efficiency. If the Chief Exec had said 'Look, this is the reasoning, there may be one or two shortcuts through good employment practice because the organization is in a fix', and I'd believed that, I might have accepted that the end justified the means. I'd have had disquiet about it.

The reckoning of the moral context starts at this point, with elaborated justification of the leader's actions. The first justification refers to bureaucratic propriety, and the tension between maintaining the viability of the organization and maintaining procedural rectitude. At this stage in the narrative, the leader argues that in some situations corporate viability would be the first priority, an expression of bureaucratic propriety.

§6. But all I could see was normal working practices being overridden for no good reason, a very centralist way of dealing with things, use of senior managers in a way which was manipulative, and so on.

Concluding that the CEO was not acting as he did to serve the needs of the organization, a negative attribution of moral status is made on grounds of bureaucratic impropriety.

§7. It was an open and shut case. Not only was this person doing things very badly and very wrongly, but the consequences of it being unchecked were potentially horrendous for patients.

The narrative culminates with the most powerful and morally compelling justification, the one that truly makes this 'an open and shut case': fiduciary propriety. Even if the medical leader was not justified in acting as they did as a matter of bureaucratic propriety, they believe they were justified by reference to the interests of patients. This concluding comment on fiduciary propriety reflects why the medical leader perceived this to be 'a case of moral and ethical judgement'.

Further reading

Brody H. *Stories of Sickness*. 2nd edn. New York: Oxford University Press; 2003.

Johnson M. *Moral Imagination: Implications of Cognitive Science for Ethics*. Chicago: University of Chicago Press; 1993.

Code L. Narratives of responsibility and agency: reading Margaret Walker's Moral Understandings. *Hypatia*. 2002;**17**(1): 156–73.

Card C. Responsibility ethics, shared understandings, and moral communities. *Hypatia*. 2002;**17**(1):141–55.

Walker MU. Morality in practice: a response to Claudia Card and Lorraine Code. *Hypatia*. 2002;**17**(1):174–82.

Gabriel Y. *Storytelling in Organizations: Facts, Fictions, and Fantasies*. Oxford: Oxford University Press; 2000.

Lam V. *Bloodletting & Miraculous Cures*. London: Fourth Estate; 2005.

References

1. Sartre J-P. *Nausea*. New York: New Directions Publishing; 1964, p. 56.

2. Johnson M. *Moral Imagination: Implications of Cognitive Science for Ethics*. Chicago: University of Chicago Press; 1993.

3. Riessman CK. *Narrative Analysis*. London: Sage; 1993.

4. Labov W. The transformation of experience in narrative syntax. In: Labov W, ed. *Language in the Inner City: Studies in the Black English Vernacular*. Philadelphia: University of Pennsylvania Press; 1972, pp. 354–96.

5. Polkinghorne DE. *Narrative knowing and the human sciences*. Albany: State University of New York Press; 1985.

6. Bruner J. The narrative construction of reality. *Critical Inquiry.* 1991;**18**:1–21.

7. Bruner J. Life as narrative. *Social Research.* 1987;**54**(1):11–32.

8. Bruner J. *Actual Minds, Possible Worlds.* Cambridge, MA: Harvard University Press; 1986.

9. Labov W, Waletzky J. Narrative analysis: oral versions of personal experience. *Journal of Narrative and Life History.* 1997 [reprint: original 1967];**7**(1–4):3–38.

10. Kleinman A. *The Illness Narratives: Suffering, Healing, and the Human Condition.* New York: Basic Books; 1988.

11. Frank AW. *The Wounded Storyteller: Body, Illness, and Ethics.* Chicago: University of Chicago Press; 1995.

12. Mattingly C, Garro LC, eds. *Narrative and the Cultural Construction of Illness and Healing.* Berkeley: University of California Press; 2000.

13. Brody H. *Stories of Sickness.* 2nd edn. New York: Oxford University Press; 2003.

14. Clark JA, Mishler EG. Attending to patients' stories: reframing the clinical task. *Sociology of Health and Illness.* 1992; **14**(3):344–72.

15. Greenhalgh T, Hurwitz B, eds. *Narrative Based Medicine.* London: BMJ Books; 1998.

16. Hunter KM. *How Doctors Think: Clinical Judgment and the Practice of Medicine.* New York: Oxford University Press; 2006.

17. Lindemann Nelson H, ed. *Stories and their Limits: Narrative Approaches to Bioethics.* New York: Routledge; 1997.

18. Charon R, Montello M, eds. *Stories Matter: The Role of Narrative in Medical Ethics.* New York: Routledge; 2002.

19. Chambers T. *The Fiction of Bioethics: Cases as Literary Texts.* New York: Routledge; 1999.

20. Barthes R. Introduction to the structural analysis of narratives. In: Heath S, ed. *Image – Music – Text.* Glasgow: Collins; 1966/1977.

21. MacIntyre A. *After Virtue.* 3rd edn. London: Duckworth; 2007.

22. Hardy B. Towards a poetics of fiction: an approach through narrative. *Novel.* 1968; **2**:5–14.

23. Maines DR. Narrative's moment and sociology's phenomena: toward a narrative sociology. *Sociological Quarterly.* 1993; **34**(1):17–38.

24. Slote M. *The Ethics of Care and Empathy.* New York: Routledge; 2007.

25. Walker MU. *Moral Understandings: A Feminist Study in Ethics.* 2nd edn. New York: Oxford University Press; 2007.

26. Jonsen AR. *The Birth of Bioethics.* Oxford: Oxford University Press; 1998.

27. Ruderman C, Tracy CS, Bensimon CM, Bernstein M, Hawryluck L, Zlotnick Shaul R, et al. On pandemics and the duty to care: whose duty? who cares? *BMC Medical Ethics.* 2006;**7**(5).

28. Thompson AK, Faith K, Gibson J, Upshur R. Pandemic influenza preparedness: an ethical framework to guide decision-making *BMC Medical Ethics.* 2006;**7**(12).

29. Barr HL, Macfarlane JT, Macgregor O, Foxwell R, Buswell V, Lim WS. Ethical planning for an influenza pandemic. *Clinical Medicine, Journal of the Royal College of Physicians.* 2008;**8**(1):49–52.

30. Letts J. Ethical challenges in planning for an influenza pandemic. *New South Wales Public Health Bulletin.* 2006;**17**(10):131–4.

31. Garrett JE, Vawter DE, Prehn AW, DeBruin DA, Gervais KG. Ethical considerations in pandemic influenza planning. *Minnesota Medicine.* 2008 Apr;**91**(4):37–9.

32. Upshur REG, Faith K, Gibson JL, Thompson AK, Tracy CS, Wilson K, et al. Ethics in an epidemic: ethical considerations in preparedness planning for pandemic influenza. *Health Law Review.* 2007;**16**(1):33–9.

33. Payne K. Ethical issues related to pandemic flu planning and response. *AACN Advanced Critical Care.* 2007; **18**(4):356–60. 10.1097/01. AACN.0000298627.07535.76.

34. Kotalik J. Preparing for an influenza pandemic: ethical issues. *Bioethics.* 2005;19(4):422–31.

35. Singer PA, Benatar SR, Bernstein M, Daar AS, Dickens BM, MacRae SK, *et al.* Ethics and SARS: lessons from Toronto. *BMJ.* 2003;327(7427):1342–4.

36. Bernstein M. SARS and ethics. *Hospital Quarterly.* 2003;7(1):38–40.

37. Gostin LO, Bayer R, Fairchild AL. Ethical and legal challenges posed by severe acute respiratory syndrome: implications for the control of severe infectious disease threats. *JAMA.* 2003 Dec 24;290(24):3229–37.

38. Hsin DH-C, Macer DRJ. Heroes of SARS: professional roles and ethics of health care workers. *Journal of Infection.* 2004; 49(3):210–5.

39. Reid L. Diminishing returns? Risk and the duty to care in the SARS epidemic. *Bioethics.* 2005;19(4):348–61.

40. Dwyer J, Tsai DF-C. Developing the duty to treat: HIV, SARS, and the next epidemic. *Journal of Medical Ethics.* 2008;34(1):7–10.

41. Pandemic (H1N1) 2009 briefing note 21 2010: Available from: http://www.who.int/csr/disease/swineflu/notes/briefing_20100610/en/index.html.

42. Ball J. SPI-M-O committee: lessons learned 2010. Available from: http://www.dh.gov.uk/prod_consum_dh/groups/dh_digitalassets/@dh/@ab/documents/digitalasset/dh_118907.pdf.

43. Scientific Pandemic Influenza Advisory Committee (SPI): subgroup on modelling: modelling summary 2010. Available from: http://www.dh.gov.uk/prod_consum_dh/groups/dh_digitalassets/@dh/@ab/documents/digitalasset/dh_122957.pdf.

44. Rothstein MA. Currents in contemporary ethics. *The Journal of Law, Medicine & Ethics.* 2010;38(2):412–9.

45. Pahlman I, Tohmo H, Gylling H. Pandemic influenza: human rights, ethics and duty to treat. *Acta Anaesthesiologica Scandinavica.* 2010;54(1):9–15.

46. Simonds AK, Sokol DK. Lives on the line? Ethics and practicalities of duty of care in pandemics and disasters. *European Respiratory Journal.* 2009 August 1, 2009; 34(2):303–9.

47. Ng ES, Tambyah PA. The ethics of responding to a novel pandemic. *Annals Academy of Medicine.* 2011;40(1):30–5.

48. Godlee F. Conflicts of interest and pandemic flu. *BMJ.* 2010;340(c2947).

49. Harris RF. Jab fears. *Current biology.* 2009;19(24):R1096–7.

50. Atkinson P. *Medical Talk and Medical Work: The Liturgy of the Clinic.* Thousand Oaks, CA: Sage; 1995.

51. Strauss A, Fagerhaugh S, Suczek B, Wiener C. *Social Organization of Medical Work.* Chicago: University of Chicago Press; 1985.

52. Argyris C, Schön DA. *Organizational Learning: A Theory in Action Perspective.* Reading, MA: Addison-Wesley; 1978.

53. *Getting Ahead of the Curve: a strategy for combating infectious diseases (including other aspects of health protection).* Department of Health; 2002.

54. *On the State of the Public Health: Annual Report of the Chief Medical Officer,* 2005, p. 49.

55. Sharpe VA. Taking responsibility for medical mistakes. In: Rubin SB, Zoloth L, eds. *Margin of Error: The Ethics of Mistakes in the Practice of Medicine.* Hagerstown, MD: University Publishing Group; 2000, pp. 183–94.

56. Committee on Ethical Aspects of Pandemic Influenza (CEAPI) 2009. Available from: http://webarchive.nationalarchives.gov.uk/+/www.dh.gov.uk/en/Publichealth/Flu/PandemicFlu/DH_065163.

57. CEAPI's Approach to the Ethical Issues. Available from: http://www.dh.gov.uk/prod_consum_dh/groups/dh_digitalassets/@dh/@en/documents/digitalasset/dh_080762.pdf.

58. Responding to pandemic influenza:the ethical framework for policy and planning 2007. Available from: http://www.dh.gov.uk/prod_consum_dh/groups/dh_digitalassets/@dh/@en/documents/digitalasset/dh_080729.pdf.

59. Jordens CFC, Little M. In this scenario, I do this, for these reasons: narrative, genre and ethical reasoning in the clinic. *Social Science & Medicine.* 2004;**58**(9):1635–45.

60. Dreyfus HL, Dreyfus SE. What is moral maturity? A phenomenological account of the development of ethical expertise. In: Rasmussen D, ed. *Universalism v Communitarianism: Contemporary Debates in Ethics.* Cambridge: MIT Press; 1990, pp. 237–63.

61. White Paper: Our Health, Our Care, Our Say: New Direction for Community Services: Department of Health; 2006.

62. Shipman Inquiry. Safeguarding patients: lessons from the past – proposals for the future: *Cm* 6394; 2004.

63. R v Adams Unreported 1957.

64. Elliott J. *Using Narrative in Social Research.* London: Sage; 2005.

65. Mishler EG. Models of narrative analysis: a typology. *Journal of Narrative and Life History.* 1995;**5**(2):87–123.

66. Hydén L-C. Illness and narrative. *Sociology of Health & Illness.* 1997;**19**:48–69.

67. Thomas WI, Znaniecki F. *The Polish Peasant in Europe and America.* New York: Dover; 1918.

68. Clandinin DJ, Connelly FM. *Narrative Inquiry: Experience and Story in Qualitative Research.* San Francisco: Jossey Bass; 2000.

69. Maines DR. *The Faultline of Consciousness.* New York: Aldine de Gruyter; 2001.

70. Ginsburg FD. *Contested Lives: The Abortion Debate in an American Community.* Berkeley: University of California Press; 1989.

71. Franzosi R. *From Words to Numbers; A Journey in Science.* Cambridge: Cambridge University Press; 2003.

72. Williamson J. Every virus tells a story. In: Carter E, Watney S, eds. *Taking Liberties.* London: Serpent's Tail; 1989, pp. 69–80.

73. Thornborrow J, Coates J. *The Sociolinguistics of Narrative.* Amsterdam: J. Benjamins; 2005.

74. Brown JS, Duguid P. Organizational learning and communities-of-practice: toward a unified view of working. *Learning, and Innovation Organization Science: Special Issue: Organizational Learning* 1991;**2**(1):40–57.

75. Orr JE. Sharing knowledge, celebrating identity: war stories and community memory in a service culture. In: Middleton DS, Edwards D, eds. *Collective Remembering: Memory in Society.* Beverley Hills, CA: Sage Publications; 1990.

76. Zuboff S. *In the Age of the Smart Machine: The Future of Work and Power.* New York: BasicBooks; 1988.

77. Jordan B. Cosmopolitical obstetrics: some insights from the training of traditional midwives. *Social Science and Medicine.* 1989;**28**(9):925–44.

78. Gabriel Y. *Storytelling in Organizations: Facts, Fictions, and Fantasies.* Oxford: Oxford University Press; 2000.

79. Calman KC. *A Study of Storytelling, Humour and Learning in Medicine.* London: The Stationery Office; 2000.

80. Boje DM. The storytelling organization: a study of story performance in an office-supply firm. *Administrative Science Quarterly.* 1991;**36**:106–26.

81. Boje DM. *Storytelling Organizations.* London: Sage; 2008.

82. Bowles N. Storytelling: a search for meaning within nursing practice. *Nurse Education Today.* 1995;**15**(5): 365–9.

83. Currie G, Brown AD. A narratological approach to understanding processes of organizing in a UK Hospital. *Human Relations.* 2003;**56**(5):563–86.

84. Brown AD. A narrative approach to collective identities. *Journal of Management Studies.* 2006;**43**(4):731–53.

85. Brown AD, Stacey P, Nandhakumar J. Making sense of sensemaking narratives. *Human Relations.* 2008;**61**(8):1035–62.

86. Brown AD, Gabriel Y, Gherardi S. Storytelling and change: an unfolding story. *Organization.* 2009;**16**(3):323–33.

87. Storey J, Holti R. Sense-making by clinical and non-clinical executive directors within new governance arrangements. *Journal of*

Health Organization and Management. 2009;23(2):149–69.

88. Hibbert P, McInnes P, Huxham C, Beech N. Characters in stories of collaboration. *International Journal of Sociology and Social Policy.* 2008;28(1/2):59–69.

89. Murray TH. What do we mean by 'narrative ethics?'. In: Lindemann Nelson H, ed. *Stories and their Limits: Narrative Approaches to Bioethics.* New York: Routledge; 1997, pp. 3–17.

90. Nussbaum M. *Love's Knowledge: Essays on Philosophy and Literature.* New York: Oxford University Press; 1990.

91. Hunter K. Narrative, literature, and the clinical exercise of practical reason. *Medicine & Philosophy.* 1996;21(3): 303–20.

92. Hunter KM. *Doctors' Stories: The Narrative Structure of Medical Knowledge.* Princeton: Princeton University Press; 1991.

93. Greenhalgh T. Narrative based medicine in an evidence based world. In: Greenhalgh T, Hurwitz B, eds. *Narrative Based Medicine.* London: BMJ Books; 1998.

94. Hudson Jones A. narrative in medical ethics. In: Greenhalgh T, Hurwitz B, eds. *Narrative Based Medicine.* London: BMJ Books; 1998.

95. Childress JF. Narratives versus norms: a misplaced debate in bioethics. In: Lindemann Nelson H, ed. *Stories and Their Limits: Narrative Approaches to Bioethics.* New York: Routledge; 1997, pp. 252–72.

96. Tomlinson T. Perplexed about narrative ethics. In: Lindemann Nelson H, ed. *Stories and their Limits: Narrative Approaches to Bioethics.* New York: Routledge; 1997, pp. 123–33.

97. Charon R. Narrative contributions to medical ethics; recognition, formulation, interpretation and validation in the practice of the ethicist. In: DuBose ER, Hamel RP, O'Connell LJ, eds. *A Matter of principles? Ferment in US Bioethics.* Valley Forge: Trinity Press International; 1994, pp. 260–83.

98. Churchill LR, Schenk D. One cheer for bioethics: engaging the moral experiences of patients and practitioners beyond the big decisions. *Cambridge Quarterly of Healthcare Ethics.* 2005;14: 389–403.

Moral leadership for ethical organizations

This book is subtitled 'Building Ethical Healthcare Organizations', and in this chapter I consider the implications of my study for doing just that. The discussion falls into three parts. First I temporarily set aside our concern with moral leadership and look at the emergence of healthcare organizational ethics as a bioethical 'sub-specialty'. I consider the reasons for its rise, and review its current form and content. Next I consider current approaches to healthcare organizational ethics, questioning whether applied normative analysis is the best way to proceed. Readers of earlier chapters will not be surprised to discover that I find applied normative analysis to have yielded limited benefits, or that I suggest that a focus on expressive moral behaviours could enhance our understanding of how to build ethical organizations. I then ask what healthcare organizational ethics ought to be about. In the third and final part of the chapter I return to my analysis of moral leadership as an expressive moral behaviour. I ask how ethical expertise is learned, and how we might set about developing the moral leadership that secures ethical behaviour in organizational settings.

Building ethical organizations: learning from healthcare organizational ethics

My own starting point for thinking about healthcare organizational ethics is the question 'what do patients, and those who care about them, normatively expect of healthcare organizations?' A part of the answer is that they normatively expect their confidence and trust in healthcare organizations to be justified, and the components of confidence and trust were discussed in Chapter 5.

This analytical focus is warranted by findings from empirical inquiry into patients' perceptions of care. For example, when patients in the USA were asked what factors affected their assessment of care providers, it was confidence and trust in the provider alongside treatment with respect and dignity that ranked highest. These appeared to be more important to the majority of respondents than were autonomy and shared decision-making [1–4].[1] As the authors of that study remark, these findings at least invite consideration whether bioethics has accorded sufficient prominence to confidence, trust and respect, alongside its central concern for autonomy, in ethical models of healthcare.

Whether or not respect for autonomy should be dislodged from its position as the reigning first principle of US bioethics, we have good reason to question whether it is the most useful starting point for an ethics of healthcare organization. We have already seen,

---

[1] See references 1–3. From a different perspective, and perhaps suggesting why it is that patients do not focus on issues of choice, see reference 4.

for example, that an ethics of healthcare organization must concern itself with decisions made on behalf of those who are not participants in decisions because they are not yet patients, with decisions where patients may no longer be alive, with decisions where the autonomous desires of some must be over-ridden in the interests of others, and so on. Expressing impassioned advocacy, demonstrating respect for others' moral agency, deciding in accordance with equity, acting with transparency, and exhibiting neutrality, have all assumed greater importance in my discussion than have respecting patients' own autonomy or facilitating patients' participation in decisions. This emphasis has derived, of course, from clinical leaders' views of healthcare organizations and their demands. I return later in this discussion to the question whether the findings from my study suggest the right focus for healthcare organizational ethics.

The emergence of healthcare organizational ethics

A different starting point for healthcare organizational ethics is supplied by having recourse to the existing literature. At the time that I started this research, scholars still viewed healthcare organizational ethics as a new field of inquiry [5(p25),6].[2] Its boundaries remain somewhat indistinct, and the task of identifying what has been published in the field rather depends upon how we define it. A search using the MeSH term 'institutional ethics' in PubMed retrieves articles published from the mid 1970s onwards, and at the date of writing over 2,700 journal pieces are cited in that part of the database [7–11].[3] So whereas scholarly interest in organizational ethics is a fairly recent phenomenon, it would seem that a piecemeal practitioner literature had been accumulating almost unnoticed during the four decades that dramatic beginning-of-life and end-of-life decisions attracted most academic and press attention. Those 2,700 items do not, though, constitute anything like a comprehensive catalogue of organizational ethics. If we were to add to the 'institutional ethics' literature all the publications that discuss just apologizing for medical error, the citation count would pass the 3,000 mark; adding all of the relevant material on medical harm and the material on healthcare regulation would render it a vast field.

The majority of the 2,700 publications have appeared in practitioner journals; many are descriptive or exhortatory; and only a fraction are based on empirical research. But after some thirty years of growth on the margins of bioethics, organizational ethics (particularly organizational ethics in managed care) began to assume greater prominence in the 1990s. Two notable journal special issues, an American Medical Association report and four book-length treatments were published between 1999 and 2001. These were followed by a fifth text derived from a field study of organizational ethics in 2003 [5,12–20]. This literature, which builds on some of the earlier scholarship, has sought to bring a degree of coherence to the concept of organizational ethics. Taken as a whole, the early 'institutional ethics' literature reflects American and (to a lesser extent) Canadian preoccupations; but interest in organizational ethics is burgeoning worldwide [21,22].[4]

---

[2] 'Organizational ethics is a new frontier for health-care ethics': reference 5, p. 25. See also reference 6.
[3] Interestingly, the very earliest are publications in law journals, and include discussion of abortion rights and prisoners' access to medical treatment. Some examples of early concerns are listed in references 7–11.
[4] The interest is often joined to interest in how healthcare leaders approach organizational ethical difficulties, apparent in the literature reviewed by Žydžiūnaite and colleagues: see reference 21. See also reference 22.

What accounts for this convergence of international scholarly and practitioner concern on healthcare organizational ethics? While part of the explanation is undoubtedly bioethicists' eager pursuit of novel moral problems, increased interest in the field reflects a number of factors: complex changes in the global environment in which healthcare organizations operate; the growth of managed care in the USA, and attendant US health reform controversies; US hospital accreditation requirements; the maturation of clinical ethics as a field; a greater appreciation of organizations as distinct systems; and cultural shifts in attitude towards the responsibilities of organizations in general. I take each of these in turn.

First, as we noted in Chapter 1, all developed healthcare systems have experienced three related changes in healthcare culture: increasing 'industrialization' in patterns of care provision, greater 'institutionalization' in the form of standardized, protocol-driven practice, and 'diffusion of the health agenda' so that health is the responsibility of a broader range of agencies including social care, education and policing [23–25]. These three trends are as apparent in Europe as they are in North America, and they affect universal health coverage systems such as Canada and the UK as much as they do mixed health coverage systems such as in the USA [26–28].[5] They shape the nature of the challenges facing healthcare organizations in all three jurisdictions, and influence healthcare organizational ethics on both sides of the Atlantic.

Second, the rapid rise of managed care in the United States and recent healthcare reforms have generated enormous conflict and moral controversy over the nature and powers of provider organizations. The US controversies are mirrored in healthcare reforms in other countries. The global changes mentioned above and these local changes are not unrelated. Managed care and other healthcare reforms are in part a response to these worldwide shifts because of the pressure on health systems – including cost pressure – that the changing global systems generate. Managed care and other reforms become, in turn, drivers for yet further local change. When citizens observe or experience unwelcome change in healthcare provision at a national or local level, it is reform that appears to be the problem. Reform becomes the symbol of organizational dilemmas that are a consequence of deeper underlying changes.

Third, an immediate stimulus to the development of healthcare organizational ethics as a field was supplied by new requirements imposed on American hospitals by the Joint Commission for the Accreditation of Healthcare Organizations (hereafter JCAHO). This influential and powerful body accredits the vast majority of US hospitals, rendering them eligible to claim reimbursement for care they provide to uninsured citizens through government Medicaid and Medicare programmes [29(p60),30].[6] The JCAHO lent its weight to the development of organizational ethics when in 1995 it inaugurated a new standard – 'organization ethics' – for regulatory review [31]. Once a voluntary activity among the well-intentioned, organizational ethics moved into the mainstream of healthcare regulation in the USA.

Fourth, as clinical ethics has matured as a field there has been far greater appreciation of how organizations and their practices shape clinical ethics. This is in part because the decisions that clinical ethics confronts are a consequence of social and organizational cultures and practices. For example, where terminally ill patients are encouraged to agree

---

[5] Approx. 60% of US healthcare expenditure is by government. However, it is difficult to locate accurate figures. See reference 26. The same source for the statistic has been cited as recently as 2010–2011; see references 27 and 28.

[6] Around 80% of US acute hospitals are JCAHO accredited. See references 29 and 30.

an end-of-life care plan recognized by provider organizations, there are likely to be fewer difficult decisions when and if they lose capacity; the converse of course applies [32–34]. It is also in part because 'the interpenetration of organizational and clinical ethical decisions is becoming increasingly obvious'; there is evidence that when clinical ethics committees resolve individual problems they are increasingly likely to follow up with recommendations for organizational changes to prevent the problem recurring [18(p31)]. In addition, the maturation of the field has brought with it some criticism of the individualistic focus of professional ethics. There is a cogent argument that if clinical ethics problems are shaped by the organizational context, it is (at least at times) unjust to hold professionals individually responsible when they arise [35].

Fifth, the increased recognition of the part that organizations play in shaping ethical problems is matched by increased recognition of the part that organizations play in producing medical harm, as well as in shaping professionals' responses to medical harm. In Leape's seminal paper published in 1994, he argued that error sprang from both individual acts and systemic forces, and management of error must therefore address both sources. A focus on systems error was further entrenched in Kohn *et al.*'s landmark publication on safer health systems, and 'systems thinking' has become part of patient safety discourse and practice around the world [36].

Finally, as organizations have assumed a size and power larger than many nation states there has been greater determination to hold them accountable for harm they do. It has long been possible, through legal doctrines such as vicarious liability, to hold organizations responsible for the acts of employees. Additionally, a fiction of corporate personality permits moral agency, and moral responsibility, to be imputed to them. Several jurisdictions are now prepared to hold organizations responsible for criminal offences where culpability has hitherto rested upon proof of individual intent [37–48].[7] As corporate personality has become a more compelling fiction, so corporate responsibility has become a more compelling social and moral fact [49].[8]

Organizational ethics is assuming greater prominence, so the question of how its nature and scope are to be conceptualized has become more pressing. Given that bioethics as a whole has found no one moral theory satisfactory [50(Ch10)], that moral life in the 'back regions' of medicine has been patchily described, that healthcare organizations are extraordinarily diverse and complex, and that healthcare systems operate at many different levels, determining its proper content presents formidable problems. Two approaches to the subject matter can be discerned in the literature: one 'aetiological' and one 'topographical'. These approaches converge on a common set of concerns, but each diverges in its emphasis and in its implications for scholarship and practice.

'Aetiological' and 'topographical' approaches to organizational ethics

The 'aetiological' approach proceeds by considering the source of normative dilemmas in the changes affecting healthcare organizations worldwide, and also by considering the source of normative dilemmas in the nature of organizational systems themselves. Agich

---

[7] E.g. The Corporate Manslaughter and Corporate Homicide Act 2007 in the UK. See references 37–48 for discussion of corporate killing in the USA, Canada and Europe.

[8] On corporate personality see, for example, reference 49.

epitomizes this approach in his analysis of deep but ill-understood changes in conceptions of healthcare and medical management; as do Boyle *et al.* in their organization-as-system analysis [16,51]. The 'topographical' approach proceeds by mapping the already visible features of the ethical landscape within healthcare organizations. Spencer and co-authors [18] exemplify a 'topographical' analysis when they argue for an organizational ethics that integrates clinical ethics, business ethics and professional ethics, and examine in detail the relationship between the three.

The development of the 'aetiological' approach can be traced back to an influential article by Thompson, who was among the first to articulate the need for a systematic 'mid-level' treatment of bioethical issues [52,53]. Ethical analysis, he argued, had tended to oscillate between micro-level (doctor-patient) concerns such as consent, and macro-level (society-patient) concerns such as regulating reproductive technologies. What bioethics was overlooking was the nature of intermediate institutions such as the hospital, and how they shaped the moral experience of healthcare. By spelling out critical changes in contemporary health systems and the pressures these create in organizations, scholars such as Khushf, Cribb, Morreim, Rodwin, Wong and Annas have facilitated the emergence of an 'aetiological' approach to organizational ethics even if some of these have not consciously promoted it [23–25,54–57].

The hallmark of the 'aetiological' approach is an attempt to understand how healthcare management and healthcare organizations function. Where others have left conceptions of 'management' unexamined, Agich considered how different management functions (clinical management, resource management, administrative management) impose different normative demands. Equally, where others have left 'the organization' largely unexamined, for Boyle *et al.* different understandings of organizational dynamics are what bring ethical issues into visible relief. Boyle *et al.* consider whether organizations are best treated as 'rational' systems, 'natural' systems or 'open' systems. Each approach, they contend, highlights different moral features in the life of the organization.

The rational systems approach draws attention to issues such as the development of rules, the dissemination of policy, procedural infractions and the penalties for rule breaking. The key areas in which such an approach locates ethical trouble are poor implementation or violation of protocols and procedures. The natural systems approach directs attention to the way in which workers' informal discretion is used to the benefit or detriment of an organization and its stakeholders. For example, overworked clinicians may be tempted to neglect bureaucratic tasks in order to fulfil normative expectations of 'hands-on' care. Natural systems analysis is a mainstay in sociological accounts of welfare bureaucracies, and it brings to the surface how ethical choices confront all 'street-level bureaucrats' (including doctors) who deliver services in situations of limited resource [58,59]. Finally, open systems analysis draws attention to how the internal moral world of the organization develops in response to the challenges of an external environment. For instance, hospitals' ethical climates are shaped in part by the demands imposed by health insurers and regulators. This is not a simple relationship, in so far as healthcare providers may choose their response to external forces, including regulation. They may approach regulation in the spirit of being 'trustees' for patients' interests and surpass regulatory requirements; they might be satisfied with mere 'technical compliance'; they could even elect a strategy of 'efficient breach' of legal obligations [60].

Boyle *et al.*'s approach has the advantage of generating cross-cutting principles as well as interesting examples of organizational ethical tribulation. They find potential ethical trouble in the temptation to trade compliance for integrity, in multiple conflicts of interest, and in the need to balance professional discretion (such as clinical autonomy) with bureaucratic control (such as treatment protocols). But the curious feature of their analysis is a seeming reluctance to rank ethical difficulties in terms of their significance. An administrator's disquiet about keeping redundancy plans secret is presented in such a way that it appears equivalent to participating in a conspiracy to conceal dangerous medical malpractice [16(p170ff,185ff)]. Granted, it is a foundational principle of organizational ethics that ostensibly minor moral lapses can have grave impacts on patient care. But medical professional standards are so central to the intrinsic goods and hazards of health-care, that they seem to me to warrant a central place in any account of a healthcare organization's key responsibilities.

Turning to the topographical approach, the most influential and conceptually ambitious has been Spencer et al. [61].[9] Their aim is to rationalize and integrate a disjointed array of healthcare ethical codes and commitments into a single comprehensive programme of healthcare organizational ethics. The purpose of such a programme is 'to produce a positive ethical climate where the organizational policies, activities, and self-evaluation mechanisms integrate patient, business and professional perspectives in consistent and positive value-creating activities that articulate, apply and reinforce its vision' [18(p6)].

The mechanism they adopt to conceptualize organizational ethics is an analysis of the moral agency of the corporation, followed by consideration of the content in, and relation-ships between, clinical ethics, business ethics and professional ethics. They do, it is true, sketch the changing patterns of American medicine; but they do so only to supply a descriptive backcloth to their argument for an integrated organizational ethics programme. The value in their approach lies in their discussion of the ethical implications of each of the three domains. Its limitation is precisely that these three domains remain distinct in their analysis, despite their attempt to blend them into an all-encompassing 'systems' approach [62].[10]

They join other commentators in drawing upon stakeholder theory to map the account-abilities of the healthcare organization [15]. But this stakeholder analysis is vulnerable to the criticism that stakeholder theory provides limited insight to organizations confronting a central organizational dilemma: conflict between the demands of different groups where each believes that their needs should take priority [63].[11] So for example, in ordinary circumstances it is clear that patients, as primary stakeholders, take priority over employee interests. But does that apply in situations of pandemic infection to the extent that employees should be expected to put themselves at risk? Or, using Peppin's example, how can stakeholder theory help to rank the interests of anti-abortion campaigners against the interests of physicians who are pro-choice [64(p545)]?

The limited purchase of stakeholder theory becomes most apparent when Spencer et al. turn to professional ethics. Their map of accountabilities shows that the primary concern for eight out of their ten stakeholder groups is professional competence. The logical conclusion would be that securing patient safety, managing error and regulating profes-sional competence would be activities at the heart of an organizational ethics programme. And yet these issues hardly feature in their analysis. The closest they come to it is in their

---

[9] E.g. Spencer et al.'s approach is adopted by reference 61.
[10] But cf. reference 62.
[11] For similar criticism see reference 63.

discussion of reciprocal responsibilities between healthcare organizations and the professionals who deliver care, where they modestly propose that an organizational ethics programme 'should be the site for professional ethics issues to be discussed and resolved should the professional standards not be met' [18].

It may be that Spencer and colleagues do not conceive of organizational ethics as being essentially concerned with issues of professional competence and medical harm because of the nature of the relationship between US hospitals and their physicians. Some organizations (an increasing proportion, as a result of managed care and other reforms) have been built on a 'staff model' in which physicians are hospital employees. More usually, however, a patient's 'attending physician' has not been a hospital employee but, as Hall put it, one of a hospital's most highly valued 'customers' [17(p24)]. It is attending physicians who bring in the paying patients on which clinical facilities rely; the upshot seems to be a degree of administrative deference to internal professional regulation that is absent in the UK.[12] Spencer et al.'s approach to issues relating to professional standards is unimpeachably pragmatic, and it is redolent of the *realpolitik* that inevitably surrounds organizational ethics. But their topographical approach to organizational ethics is more than a little constrained by stakeholder theory and the existing geography of moral responsibilities.

In a 'field study' of the organizational ethical problems facing managed care organizations, Pearson, Sabin and Emanuel have combined elements of the aetiological and the topographical approach [5]. They carried out their study from a 'pragmatic ethics' orientation, the lineage of which can be traced to the work of John Dewey [65].[13] Its central claim is that 'efficacy in practical application provides a standard for the determination of truth in the case of statements, rightness in the case of actions, and value in the case of appraisals' [20,66]. Pearson and his colleagues used this as a lens through which to evaluate the organizational-level ethical work these organizations were doing. The real value of their study is that it identified, more systematically than other studies, the organizational ethical issues that were of central concern to leaders in American healthcare organizations, and then went on to ascertain what might be exemplary ethical strategies for addressing them [5].[14] The study's approach to understanding the processes of organizational ethics, and their method for judging what might constitute an exemplary ethical strategy, stand out as especially valuable.

The first two dimensions of Pearson et al.'s definition are unexceptional. One is 'articulation of a moral compass for the organization' [5(p26)]. The other, which they term the deliberative aspect, unsurprisingly entails addressing 'the inevitable conflicts among basic values – "good versus good" – in a systematic manner' [5(p26)]. This deliberative aspect is central to virtually all accounts of ethics. It is their third dimension that is of real interest:

> A robust organizational ethics must include management processes that lead to doing the right thing. Vision statements and moral deliberation that do not result in more worthy performance are at best a waste of time and resources and at worst, a duplicitous effort to

---

[12] The JCAHO, however, requires a 'zero-tolerance' approach to employee bullying.

[13] A good introduction is identified in reference 65.

[14] Their summary of these problems appears on pp. 18–19. They group them into seven ethical domains: confidentiality, community benefits, vulnerable populations, medical necessity and coverage decisions, end-of-life care, organizational ethics programme issues, and consumer empowerment.

clothe organizational wolves in the clothing of ethical sheep. This practical, quality improvement phase completes the organizational ethics cycle. [5(p26)]

If the language in which they describe the third dimension does not stir the soul, the point is one well made. It reveals that being able to deliberate, to choose between values and elect one good over another, is perhaps not the defining difficulty of organizational ethics. Working out what might best be done in the face of ethical challenge, conducting and/or coordinating the organizational activities that seem to be mandated and judging the effect of the organization's actions on all those involved would seem to be the better part of it. It was this conviction that motivated their study, a search for exemplary ethical strategies more than a search for exemplary ethical deliberation.

How did they judge what would be an exemplary ethical strategy? They summarized their criteria as follows:

- a coherent formulation of an organizational problem or challenge that reflects an awareness of conflicting values
- a plan of considered action to manage the ethical tension . . .. This plan must embody a way of specifying and balancing key ethical values
- a set of consistently applied procedures that . . . constitute a plausible means . . . for managing the conflict of ethical values
- a mechanism to evaluate the effectiveness of the implementation. [5(p22-3)]

These interesting criteria are not the criteria for evaluating a one-off ethical choice. They are criteria for evaluating a complex course of ethical conduct. According to these criteria, the ethical skills upon which the organization relies are to some degree deliberative (criterion one). But they are to a far greater degree strategic, procedural and managerial (criteria two, three and four). There is clearly some convergence between my own account of moral leadership and the approach that Pearson and co-authors adopt towards organizational ethics, but their work lacks a compelling foundation in ethical theory.

Exceeding Churchill and Schenk's 'one cheer' for bioethics, we might therefore charitably offer 'two cheers' for organizational ethics as it stands at present [67]. Questions about how we should do organizational ethics, both in theory and in practice, connect with far broader controversies about the nature of bioethics and the nature of ethical expertise. In the next section I dip a toe into that debate by considering the approach that bioethics more broadly has taken to its subject matter. This discussion may be of greater interest to theorists than to those looking for an account of ethical expertise, but it underpins my later claims about what ethical expertise looks like.

Building ethical organizations: what does it mean to do organizational ethics?

Whatever the differences between aetiological and topographical approaches to organizational ethics, a great deal of the scholarship shares a common starting point: the view that morality and ethics is about making and justifying moral decisions, and evaluating choices. Boyle et al. describe morality as the lived experience of making choices, and ethics as systematic reflection on lived experience [16(p13)]. Spencer et al. explicitly categorize organizational ethics as a branch of applied ethics, that is, the use of general moral norms to make and evaluate moral decisions about concrete situations [18(p17)].

What is problematic about this orientation to the field of healthcare organizational ethics? Quite simply, it suggests a radically incomplete view of ethics as a practice. According to this approach to organizational ethics, what people are 'doing' when they are 'being ethical' is *reasoning*: they are choosing between available options and courses of conduct. But it is evident from Boyle and Spencer's own texts that this is not, in fact, a particularly apt account of what is involved in 'doing' organizational ethics. Pearson *et al.*, as we have seen, make this even more starkly apparent.

For a start, organizational ethics clearly means developing and implementing organizational policies and ethics programmes. This in turn entails more than merely choosing between available policy options. It must involve all of the following and more: scanning the environment for actual or potential organizational trouble; making sense of possible moral troubles that appear on the horizon; deciding whom to tell, and how, and 'performing the telling' appropriately; gathering further 'organizational intelligence'; investigating the causes of trouble; imagining a range of ways to address it, weighing the benefits and disadvantages of different approaches; exploring the implications of policy with colleagues; judging the validity of objections and proposed amendments; engaging in complex moral negotiation with frequently uncooperative organizational factions; drawing patients, carers and the public into discussion as moral interlocutors; determining when inquiries and apologies are appropriate; and performing gestures of restitution. Lived experience of making choices, systematic reflection on lived experience or the use of general moral norms to make and evaluate moral decisions about concrete situations hardly begins to scratch the surface of all of this activity.

How are we to account for such a glaring discrepancy between what organizational ethics is said to be about, and what organizational ethics seems to entail? And does it matter? The incongruity seems to arise out of the continuing influence of versions of applied ethics that dominated the field during the development of bioethics. And the incongruity matters because it prevents us from creating a useful general account of what healthcare leaders ought to be doing to create ethical organizations. In the next section I discuss why applied ethics may not supply the most productive source of guidance for healthcare organizational ethics.

The problem with treating bioethics as applied ethics

Here I must tread carefully. It is very difficult to generalize about the intellectual currents that have shaped the field of bioethics, without being vulnerable to well-placed criticism that such generalizations fail to take bioethics' diversity into account. André observes that the term bioethics suggests 'a specific, technical sort of work, the activity of concluding that some choices are, and others are not, ethically right'; but that even a cursory survey reveals 'every kind of examination of the moral dimensions of healthcare, health policy, the biological sciences, and cultural stances toward health and sickness' [68(p.xi)]. André's point is indisputable. But bioethics has been, and remains, centrally concerned with articulating and applying moral norms relevant to fateful decisions in medical treatment and research. Moreover, the field as a whole has paid far more attention to ethical deliberation than it has to ethical enactment.

As Crigger explains in her intellectual ethnography of bioethics, the core literature in bioethics explores the moral character of 'those moments of intersection between medicine and biomedical science and the human life cycle that are among the most highly charged philosophically, theologically, emotionally, and politically' [69]. Organizational ethics is in some respects a deliberate counter to this perspective, but it is not immune to its effects. It remains caught within a particular conception of the ethical.

That conception of the ethical is the theoretical-juridical model that we encountered in previous chapters. The theoretical-juridical model (TJM) represents, in Margaret Walker's view, the prevailing consensus on what moral philosophy, and thus ethical theorizing, is. But the TJM, she proposes, is simply one – somewhat misleading – model of moral life. It is a model centred on three core propositions: that the task of moral philosophy is to discover and validate moral knowledge; that moral knowledge consists in a completely general theory, which explains and justifies all true moral judgements; and that an adequate moral theory will be analogous to a 'scientific' theory [70(p44)].

The TJM contains five significant assumptions about the nature of moral life. The codifiability assumption is the view that all essential moral knowledge will be propositional in form, capable of being stated and taught. The nomological assumption is that such propositional knowledge will consist in law-like generalizations that correspond with the actual moral judgements about what to do in particular situations. The logical priority assumption is that these law-like generalizations are where essential moral knowledge resides, rather than in the concrete processes of living a moral life. The assumption of systematic unity creates the expectation that all relevant moral knowledge will be reducible to a very few, non-contradictory and internally consistent general rules. And the assumption of impersonality proposes that the one moral code holds true for everyone irrespective of their needs or relationships (e.g. lover, spouse) with other moral actors. These assumptions, Walker concluded:

> define code-like theory building, testing, and fine tuning, with standard appeal to 'intuitions' and vulnerability to intuition-based counter-examples, as the premier genre of, and perhaps simply what to do, in ethics.

Walker's detailed examination of the TJM arose out of feminist scepticism regarding its universalist claims. The TJM is a model born, some have argued, of male philosophical reflection on the social facts of male lives. But feminist critics have not been alone in rejecting the implications and applications of the TJM, including in the field of bioethics. Articles critical of the 'applied TJM' approach to bioethics appear in the literature from the early 1980s [71–74], as members of the 'white male establishment' who tried to do 'applied TJM' in the field of clinical ethics found it unsatisfactory.

Of many critical articles, two early papers by Hoffmaster are among the most widely cited [75,76]. In them he summarized what has become the orthodox account of the shortcomings in bioethicists' use of applied ethics. But Hoffmaster was not the first critic; Caplan, for example, had early on criticized the 'engineering model' of applied ethical reasoning [77].

Decisions in bioethics are not and cannot be made by reference to law-like norms

Challenging the nomological assumption, Hoffmaster argued that bioethicists themselves had already shown the principles underpinning applied medical ethics to be both essentially contested and vague. 'Essentially contested' principles are those that invoke insoluble disagreement before they are even applied. So, for example, the notion of autonomy had already, by the time of Hoffmaster's article in 1994, come to be defined in at least four mutually exclusive ways. Turning to vagueness, if the test of applied ethics was how well it generated solutions to difficult problems, it was of concern that a single principle frequently generated multiple interpretations. Those who disagreed, for instance, about physician-assisted dying, disagreed whether respect for autonomy would be best served by permitting the practice or by prohibiting it.

Hoffmaster's article indicated that the nomological assumption is further undermined by the experience of doing bioethics. When bioethicists engage in effective moral action, it looks rather unlike the kind of activity anticipated in applying a principle. Caplan's account of attaining the status of moral guru within his hospital's emergency department is both entertaining and instructive in this respect. He recounted how each summer, patients with respiratory disease converged upon the hospital for oxygen therapy. With only two oxygen units available, staff sought his help developing a set of criteria by which to allocate this scarce resource:

> My first response ... was to see what various philosophers and theologians had to say about issues of micro-allocation and ethics . ... Some defended a criterion of merit, some a criterion of need, some a criterion of social utility, and some a random lottery . ... But ... it occurred to me that it might be possible to solve the allocation problem by ameliorating the source of the scarcity. I asked some of the emergency room staff if Medicaid/Medicare covered the provision of air conditioners in the homes of persons suffering from respiratory ailments. It turned out, much to everyone's surprise, that the machines could be prescribed and the cost reimbursed. [77]

This efficacious moral action was hardly dependent, Caplan observed, on analytical rigour or moral sophistication.

The logical priority assumption is based in reliance on deductive reasoning to generate correct solutions to moral problems. The postulate is that when a valid norm is logically applied it will generate a morally right solution. But as Hoffmaster pointed out and as Caplan's example confirms, important moral work deciding how to define the situation may be accomplished independently of applying any moral norm. When Caplan defined the problem as one of resource procurement rather than resource allocation, he determined the outcome in such a way that philosophically fine-tuned principles of fairness were rendered secondary.

The assumption of systematic unity has proved problematic for bioethics from the beginning, as deontological and consequentialist norms came into stark conflict. Parents' and doctors' wish to transplant the organs of anencephalic infants was an early example of the incommensurable moral conclusions that might be derived from faithful application of either the Kantian imperative or a utilitarian felicific calculation [78]. And as Jonsen has observed, attempts to generate a general theory for bioethics have foundered on the same problem. Whether they gave primacy to deontological principles, consequentialist leanings or ontological analysis of the values essential to practice, each approach was judged to be equally unsatisfactory [50(p331)].

In sum, a singular and striking effect of 'applied TJM' has been to distort the relationship between the bioethical imagination, the formulation of ethical foci and actual ethical practice. TJM aspires to differentiate morality from other domains, such as prudence, etiquette and law, and to detach it from practice so that it may be represented in an abstract and consistent theoretical system. 'Unfortunately' concluded Hoffmaster, 'the philosophical project of generating moral knowledge ultimately displaces morality from the experience in which it is founded' [75(p1424)]. I now want to consider the effects of that displacement on bioethics as a discipline.

Bioethics in the distorting mirror of the theoretical-juridical model

Not so long ago, Agich asked:

> What kind of *doing* is ethics consultation? This rather odd way of phrasing the question is intended to call attention to the fact that our question is itself unusual and is, remarkably, not a central theme in the literature. [79(p7)]

The nomological assumption has made normative dilemmas and normative conflicts the core concern of bioethics, and pushed broader questions about the actual practices of ethical endeavour out to the periphery. It is the nomological assumption (common to all approaches to medical ethics that involve applying general principles to particular cases [79(p7)])[15] that seems responsible for the paucity of analysis around what kind of 'doing' ethics actually is.

Agich observed that the belief that clinical ethics expertise is grounded in 'possession of *ethical* knowledge' is so widespread that little attention has been paid to 'the type of *practical* knowledge involved' [79(p14)]. Is ethical knowledge then not practical knowledge? Agich's distinction between the ethical and the practical is itself, I think, a Freudian slip, a symptom of the problem he is striving to address. He seems to have meant to contrast theoretical ethical knowledge with practical ethical knowledge, what he calls the 'canon' and the 'discipline' of ethics consultation. We get close to a sense of what 'doing ethics' is about when he describes the 'discipline' of ethical consultation as 'practical actions, behaviours, cognitions, communications, deliberations, judgements and perceptions' through which the substantive and procedural 'rules' of ethics consultation come to be practically enacted [80(p36)].

The nomological assumption has made pervasive a belief that ethics, and by implication ethical life, is all about making choices. This has helped instate 'fateful decisions' as bioethics' leading concern [81]. It could be argued that it is not just the nomological assumption that is operational here, but also a Western narrative convention that tends to focus attention on a moment of *peripeteia*, a point where stories and lives take a decisive turn [82].[16] This combination of nomological and narrative assumptions produces the question that appears at the end of the following paragraph;

> What do you do if you find out that a medical colleague is guilty of malpractice? Is it worth it to become a whistle-blower? How do you explain to a weakened patient that the allotted time for a hospital stay is up? Is it worth it to make a special application for extra days? An already disabled child may be the victim of abuse by the mother's boyfriend. Should you inquire further? An operation must be done on a homosexual who has not been tested for HIV. Should you request the test?
>
> Is such a level of problem solving worthy of being called bioethics? [83]

That final question is, surely, only intelligible when healthcare is viewed through the prism of bioethics' fascination with fateful decisions.

At this point it might be objected that it is only deontological and consequentialist theories that are vulnerable to this critique of applied ethics. Do other orientations towards

---

[15] Agich differentiates applied ethics, casuistry and principlism, but the TJM underpins them all.
[16] On narrative structure see Chapter 6. Reference 82 is a very interesting discussion of the influence of a dominant narrative of rescue on American medicine.

bioethics – such as virtue ethics and narrative ethics, which have both made some headway in the field – exhibit similar faults [84–86]?[17] The short answer is that while they do not share all of the shortcomings of 'applied TJM', nor do they yet offer a wholly satisfactory alternative. Neither suffers from the constraints of theoretical-juridical reasoning, but equally neither offers a compelling account of moral action.

Virtue ethics eschews the rule-based reasoning that characterizes the TJM, and locates moral capability in the character of the moral agent. As Annas has noted, virtue requires doing the right thing for the right reasons, and may be likened to 'a skill exercised on the materials of your life' [87(p522)]. The concept of *phronesis* or practical wisdom that is central to virtue ethics suggests that ratiocination must at least lead into expressive behaviour. Philosophical analysis remains firmly centred, however, on how to reason according to virtue, rather than on the repertoire of actual social practices in which virtue finds tangible expression.

Jackson, for example, bases her account of virtue ethics in Foot's 'root notion' of moral virtue as 'goodness of the will'. This goodness means that a moral agent

> must act well, in a sense that is given primarily at least by *his recognition of the force of particular considerations as reasons for acting*: that and the influence that this has on what he does. [88,89] (emphasis added)

In their account of *phronesis* Beauchamp and Childress press further into the territory of 'doing', and hint that practical wisdom may have as much to do with designing courses of conduct as it does with choosing between them.

> A person of practical wisdom knows which ends to choose, knows *how* to realize them in particular circumstances, and carefully selects from among the range of possible actions, while keeping emotions within proper bounds. [90] (emphasis added)

What is the 'knowing how' that Beauchamp and Childress have in mind? They do not go on to clarify it, but the extract above implies that 'knowing how' is the intellectual capacity to develop a plan of action, rather than the expressive behaviours that bring it to fruition. Their conception of *phronesis* thus challenges the 'engineering model' of applied ethics ('practical wisdom' is an apt description of Caplan's reasoning in response to the oxygen unit shortage describe earlier) but does not go beyond cognition into expressive action.

MacIntyre's work constitutes a bridge between virtue ethics and narrative ethics, because he envisaged a narrative version of *phronesis*: we use narrative to figure out what is humanly good, asking ourselves how we can bring narrative unity to our lives and the social practices in which we participate. Whilst MacIntyre's assertion of the centrality of narrative is one that this account echoes, it is clear that, in common with other virtue theorists, MacIntyre's interest lay primarily in what virtuous actors decided and how they justified their decisions.

Decisions and justifications generally remain the focal concern for other, non-virtue approaches to narrative ethics. Questioning the norm-driven codification of theoretical-juridical ethics, narrative ethicists contend 'the meanings we look for and seek to construct

---

[17] I do not discuss casuistry because I see it as less a departure from applied ethics than is claimed. Advocates differentiate it by emphasizing its inductive nature, but it nevertheless approaches ethics as a matter of utilizing maxims, principles and rules to resolve unusually challenging cases. See references 84–86.

in our lives are not collections of propositions' [91]. In narrative ethics, 'doing ethics' certainly entails using sense-making and story-telling tools in order to make moral decisions; but does 'doing ethics' also go beyond making decisions into implementing decisions? For some, notably Howard Brody, 'doing ethics' is as much about 'doing a morally decent job' of executing decisions as it is of making decisions. But the body of scholarship in narrative ethics has in common with that of virtue ethics rather limited discussion of expressive behaviour.

I have not discussed care ethics here, although there is much that is promising in that approach for thinking about the components of moral action. Readers of previous chapters will already know that I am attracted by Walker's expressive-collaborative model as an account of moral understanding and moral performance, and I shall discuss it again shortly. Before I do so, I consider how social theorists of morality might help us to understand what healthcare organizational ethics should look like.

Sociological perspectives on ethics at work

After more than thirty years of talk, theory, and clinical practice, we bioethicists still know far too little about what patients, subjects, and healthcare professionals are up to, morally. [67]

The bioethics literature is liberally interlaced with articles in which opponents claim that either that philosophical analysis or sociological research is barking up the wrong tree when it comes to understanding bioethical concerns [92,93]. The problem is that each has a different view on what it is important to say about what people are doing when they are doing 'something ethical' in medical settings.

At the risk of considerable oversimplification, it is possible to identify three overarching themes in social theory. The first theme, characterized by Charles Bosk's landmark study of American surgeons in training *Forgive and Remember*, is an 'occupational moralities' theme. In 'occupational moralities' studies the chief interest lies in how a distinctive set of moral values is expressed in the activities of specific professional groups. The second theme, exemplified by Renée Anspach's elegant study of decision-making in a neonatal intensive care unit published as *Deciding Who Lives*, is a 'decisional realities' theme. 'Decisional realities' research exposes the difference between bioethical prescription and the decision processes observed in everyday medical settings. The third theme is socio-logical examination of bioethics as a social movement, an approach represented in Renée Fox and Judith Swazey's *Observing Bioethics*. I include it for purposes of completeness, but it is not of concern to us here.

Whether a study is one of 'occupational moralities' or 'decisional realities', each offers a sociological perspective. That is of course obvious, but the implications are easy to overlook. We should note first that the sociological gaze is directed towards the activity of individuals as it takes place within a particular social context. Sociological studies therefore take as their object of interest precisely those features that bioethics has tended in the past to overlook: the role that collectivities play in both structuring and labelling whatever behaviour passes for ethical activity. Because the best studies of decision processes in medical settings take care to investigate how healthcare organizations give shape to the ethical actions of professionals, patients and carers, there is much in them that is instructive for organizational ethics [94].[18]

---

[18] An exemplary and very rich study is reference 94.

But while a sociological perspective usefully directs attention to the social context that shapes decisions, it less usefully relegates in importance individual psychological explanations. Moral philosophers commonly criticize sociology for over-emphasizing the role of social structures, and for downplaying the importance of individual moral reasoning. These moves, philosophers argue, obscure the moral responsibility of individuals. This criticism is not, however, my main concern. The more pressing one is whether a description of 'doing ethics' that makes no reference to individual intentions or moral reasons can capture what needs to be caught about ethical action.

The difficulty is most readily apparent when we consider actions conventionally understood to be either ethical or unethical by virtue of the intent that underlies them. A nurse administers morphine in a dose sufficient to depress respiration: how we describe this action depends upon whether it is intended to relieve pain and has the unfortunate side effect of depressing respiration, or whether it is intended to depress respiration and hasten death [95–97].[19] We cannot identify this behaviour as 'being ethical' unless we identify the intent that defines the act, and also the moral reasons that define it as an act whose rightness rests upon intent. This is a rather obvious example of how intent defines an action and determines our moral assessment of it, but there were others less so in this study. Consider, for example, Dr. Iliffe (Graveldene NHS Trust): a committed Christian opposed to abortion, she nevertheless participated in appointing a gynaecologist to lead the abortion service. She reasoned that she was right to do so. Was her participation in the appointment panel an expression of ethical expertise or lack of moral conviction? That depends upon her reasons for doing it, as well as, to some degree, our own judgement of the circumstances.

Occupational moralities: 'doing ethics' in day-to-day work

The lineage of the first sociological theme may be traced back to Durkheim's treatment of morality as a collectively constituted social fact, and his insight that every occupational group works to establish and sustain a distinctive set of moral norms and values [98].[20] Durkheim viewed 'moral elements – whether the collective conscience, collective sentiments, collective representations or moral rules – as powerful forces controlling the socialized individual' [99(p424)]. Works in this vein such as Freidson's landmark studies of professionalism, Bosk's study of surgeons in training and Chambliss's studies in nursing ethics [100–103] have delineated the moral understandings that underpin professional activities and considered, to a greater or lesser degree, how these values are sustained by organizational arrangements.

A penchant for C. Everett Hughes's sociological dictum to 'humble the proud, and elevate the humble' has permeated such research [104,105]. This tradition, with its tendency towards self-righteous admonishment of healthcare professionals, has not endeared it to the

---

[19] It should be noted that where morphine is used in appropriate dosages, the patient's pain acts as an antagonist and inhibits the side effects of the drug. It has therefore been argued that the old ethical chestnut of the doctrine of double effect may now be dispensed with. The claim that morphine does not have unwanted side effects rests, however, upon the drug being delivered in just the right dosage; so it seems to me that the doctrine of double effect retains some utility as a means of understanding the overall circumstances. A very cogent recent article is reference 97. See also references 95 and 96.

[20] Durkheim treated ethics as rules enforced by sanctions but later recognized that morality included an element of idealism.

medical or bioethical mainstream. There is a rich seam of sociological inquiry to be mined here, however. A summary invariably does it a disservice, but using Bosk and Chambliss as examples we can extrapolate three elements that are particularly suggestive: the routinization of ethical work; the relationship between occupational and organizational moralities; and the relationship between individual and organizational power.

In this literature 'being ethical' is an aspect of occupational identity, and it is embedded in occupational activity. It thus has no apparent independent existence; ethical enactment is just what you do at work. In Bosk's study of surgical training, therefore, the practice of the ethical is subsumed into surgeons' practices of clinical responsibility and surgical training. Bosk concluded his study with the claim 'that postgraduate training is above all things an ethical training ... the moral and ethical dimensions of training are not bracketed from all other concerns but are instead built into everyday clinical life' [102(p190)]. In Chambliss's study of nursing ethics, the ethical is subsumed into nurses' role and position in the hospital hierarchy: nursing ethics 'is the ethics of powerless people; the ethics of witnesses, not decision makers; the ethics of implementers, not choosers; the ethics of those whose work goes unnoticed' [103(p87)].

Each of these accounts is a valuable corrective to the assumption that 'morality' is a special compartment of behaviour, somewhat separate from the mundane drudgery of daily work routine. Chambliss calls attention to how a great deal of moral work becomes invisible to those who are doing it, habituated as they are to the hospital environment and to conventional ways of managing ethical activity. He recalls, for example, the head nurse in a paediatric research unit who, when interviewed, could not think of any 'ethical problems' associated with her work. As his study demonstrates, such statements are not necessarily made because informants lack moral imagination, nor because their conduct is morally deficient. It may be because the ethical problems so stark to outsiders are adequately managed as a matter of organizational and occupational routine. Similarly, Bosk argues, rightly in my view, that managing error is one of the most important moral tasks undertaken in a self-regulating profession, even if it is not recognized as such by insiders. His study calls attention to how inculcating the values, processes and practices of this moral task is an integral part of the training routine.

Durkheim's attentiveness to occupational morality preceded the pre-eminence of the organization. Studies of occupational morality indicate that transcending occupational tribalism is a task central to healthcare organizational ethics, and that medical leaders will have to nimbly traverse occupational cultures if they are to orchestrate an organization-wide morality. An organizational-level ethics contends that healthcare organizations are (sociologically speaking) and must be (morally speaking) more than simply a loose collection of occupational moralities making their own way within a 'vast system of organized irresponsibility' [106(p95)].[21]

Finally, Chambliss's and Bosk's inquiries into occupational morality make readily apparent how 'doing ethics' is action done from positions of relative power and relative powerlessness: patient/caregiver, nurse/doctor, junior doctor/consultant, manager/doctor, middle manager/executive. Virtually all moral negotiation will be done at an 'uneven table' [107]. All across healthcare organizations subordinates and superordinates are bound together in layers of mutual dependence, a dependence that can stifle moral action.

---

[21] Phrase attributed to C. Wright Mills; see reference 106, p. 95.

Decisional realities: 'doing ethics' as making fateful decisions

After his excursus into surgical training Bosk went back into the field to study life-and-death decisions (this time in genetic counselling) and was frankly disappointed to discover that as 'an ethnographer seeking medical action I was Ishmael on the wrong boat' [108]. Anspach subtitled her study of withdrawing and withholding treatment of severely disabled and dying neonates *Fateful Choices in the Intensive Care Nursery*. And Zussman introduced his account of ethics in intensive care by making crystal clear that the key contribution sociology could make to medical ethics was increased understanding of how momentous decisions are made [109].

> If sociology cannot tell us how matters of medical ethics should be resolved, it can tell us how, in fact, they are resolved. It can tell us when medical treatments are likely to be terminated or continued, under what conditions, and for what reasons. It can tell us who does receive dialysis or a heart transplant, under what circumstances, by what decision making process. Perhaps most important, sociology can tell us what values underlie those decisions, how those values articulate with other values, how they emerge from the interests and influences of different groups or organization. [110]

Commenting more recently from a European perspective, Borry *et al.* reviewed empirical studies of, inter alia, decision-making for newborns, decision-making in organ transplantation, decision-making in end-of-life care, decision-making for those in persistent vegetative state and decision-making around genetic testing; Hedgecoe described decision-making in pharmacogenetics; Scully *et al.* investigated how lay people decide about sex selection [111–113]. All of these studies have posed important questions about the ways decision-making processes are commonly represented in the bioethical literature, and have thus raised doubts about some of its moral prescriptions. At the same time, however, they indicate that much empirical bioethics shares with philosophical bioethics an assumption that decisions are where the moral action is [114,115].[22]

There is a very clear example of this in Anspach's discussion of activity in the neo-natal ICU. After twelve pages detailing the ebb and flow of sad events that led up to one fateful decision, Anspach reports:

> The parents reluctantly agreed to the decision to withdraw life support, and Matthew died that afternoon.[116(p160)][23]

But we are told almost nothing about what happened after the parents assented to the decision. Who told what to whom about it? How were they told? Did they concur with the moral basis for the decision? Was baby Matthew medicated into an easeful death, or did he choke out his life in uncomprehending, primal panic? Why? Who cared for his parents, how, and with what intentions? Was anything learned from the events leading up to Matthew's death? When Matthew's parents brought an action for malpractice, how did the hospital respond? Did parents of children in the ICU experience a loss of confidence and

---

[22] Pearlman *et al.* (reference 114) noted 'the majority of empirical research in ethics concentrates on life and death decisions for terminally ill patients'. The range has widened but decisions still dominate, paralleling the focus on the consultation in medical sociology.

[23] She briefly recounted how afterwards 'staff struggled to make sense of their complicated and conflictual relationship' with the child's parents, who sued for malpractice.

trust? In Anspach's otherwise illuminating study we learn very much less than we might about the 'ethics of performing' as distinct from the 'ethics of deciding'. The scope of empirical studies has rarely extended to that stage in the ethical process that in Holm's study of healthcare professionals was identifiable as implementation (and perhaps subsequent modification) through the organization [117–119].[24]

Notwithstanding, there are worthwhile lessons to be learned from decisional realities research. Situating decision-making activity within the complex organizational division of labour that characterizes modern medicine, such research shows how the organizational setting comprises multiple groups of actors: patients, doctors, nurses, social workers, lab technicians, managers, sometimes an ethicist. Decision realities research recognizes the occupational tribalism identified in occupational realities research, but goes further by paying attention to all the players – patients and lay caregivers included – who participate in negotiating care. It proceeds by paying attention to what needs to be done to get decisions made by differently situated actors with different goals, perspectives, knowledge, languages and needs. No single participant possesses an objective, all-embracing view of the actuality; all must negotiate their understandings of reality as well as their decisions. And 'decisional realities' research recognizes that organizational decisions are not bounded in time. Decisions do not emerge in a smoothly engineered sequence from information to decision. Information is itself a consequence of earlier decisions about what data to gather, for example, or how to interpret it.

Anspach's study amply demonstrates the consequences of these organizational realities. When uncertainty surrounds differently situated actors, their access to the resources available for resolving uncertainty has an important effect on outcomes. Predicting and prognosticating about a baby's uncertain future are integral features of decision-making in the NICU [116(p57)]. Anspach observed that NICU physicians and nurses relied on diagnostic technology, direct perception and social interaction in order to assess an infant's condition. But because physicians and nurses accessed those resources in different ways, they came to develop different perspectives. The two groups tended to compose different prognostic stories and project different endings, with different versions of reality and different values culminating in ethical disagreement.

Anspach also noted the expressive strategies that professionals employed in the decision-making process. These included, for example, referring to expert authority and presenting a united professional front. Among the repertoire of persuasive techniques that Anspach observed was 'an almost canonical script' [116(p97)] deployed in decision-making conferences with parents. Starting with a recitation of test results it moved through a summary of the infant's medical history to a statement of the moral consequences of continuing treatment. Designed to present parents with the ineluctable conclusion that terminating life support was the 'only medically sound and morally correct alternative' this script appears to be the NICU equivalent of the organizational moral narratives I have reviewed in this study [116(p97)].

So although the 'ethics of performing' has received less attention than it should even in social theory, sociological studies of the 'ethics of deciding' help to point the way towards understanding how ethics beyond decision-making is done.

---

[24] Hurst et al. (reference 118) found no earlier reports on what was done in the face of ethical problems regarding resources, but see reference 119.

What can we learn from business ethics?

In an interesting contrast with bioethics, which has not been overly concerned with modelling decision-making, business ethics teems with conceptual frameworks. Many elaborate Rest's parsimonious four-stage model of the ethical decision process, which makes a useful starting point here because it has supported the conventional view of what doing ethics is about: it focuses on individuals and it focuses more on cognition than interaction [120,121].[25] For Rest, an individual moral agent (a) recognizes a moral issue; moves to (b) making a moral judgement; proceeds with (c) establishing a moral intent; and finally (d) perseveres with his or her intended action in the face of obstacles. Much subsequent research has been concerned with the pattern of moral reasoning that leads to moral judgement, and has paid particular attention to the discontinuity between moral judgement and moral action.[26]

Jones elaborated Rest's basic model to incorporate the insight that an individual's ethical behaviour is shaped by the characteristics of the issue that has stimulated a response. His much cited 'issue contingent model' has given rise to a great deal of research activity endeavouring to predict when subjects will respond to ethical challenge, based for example on how 'intense' the ethical challenge appears to be [122]. I do not review this research enterprise in detail here because it takes us too far from the main path of our argument, and, in any event, has not had the purchase that was hoped for it [123,124].[27] Two features are worth noting, however.

One is that research in business ethics has until fairly recently been overwhelmingly focussed on the ethics of deciding, rather than the ethics of performing. It has therefore made extensive use of vignettes and scenarios in empirical research, with modest returns. A recent review of empirical research concluded that 'a more meaningful study of the ethical decision making process [than survey research conducted using unengaged undergraduate participants] might be to conduct in-depth interviews with individuals who have engaged in the ethical decision making process' [125]. This realization that pen and paper surveys of business undergraduates fail to capture the realities of moral behaviour in organizations had already been reached by some of those educating for moral leadership in organizations, notably Mary Gentile and colleagues [126]. I return to Gentile's work on educating for ethical expertise at the end of this chapter.

In addition, although Rest's model and those that elaborate upon it remain largely focussed on explaining individual responses to moral challenge, empirical research indicates that 'significant others' are a major influence on ethical behaviour in organizations. As the term 'significant *others*' implies, however, business ethics is still overwhelmingly concerned with understanding individual moral capability. Well-regarded works, such as Jackall's study of how organizational life shapes *un*ethical behaviour, have apparently failed to prompt consideration of how collective life in organizations might equally be the well-spring of ethical behaviour [106]. There has been little discussion of the moral resilience of groups or networks, and the notion of moral leadership for 'collective moral wisdom' that is suggested by the present study seems not to have assumed any prominence.

---

[25] Bioethicists have occasionally drawn on Rest's model, for example reference 120.

[26] So-called 'akratic failure'.

[27] They possess limited predictive power (reference 123) but cf. reference 124.

Grounding healthcare organizational ethics in an expressive-collaborative model of morality

In a preceding section, I concluded that the theoretical-juridical model in moral philosophy had distorted the relationship between the bioethical imagination and actual ethical practice. While it has challenged the terrain of bioethics, organizational ethics remains caught within a conception of moral life that is inconsistent with its own practice. I then argued that although sociological inquiry has also been captivated by fateful choices and dilemmatic decisions, studies of occupational morality and decisional reality are of real value to healthcare organizational ethics. They have afforded insight into how everyday ethical issues are managed as a matter of routine, and, for good or ill, may never intrude into moral awareness; and they have shown how intra-group and inter-group interactions shape moral decision-making in organizations. Then I noted that business ethics has offered ways of understanding individual moral decisions, but is only just beginning to consider the ethics of collaborative implementation. What is needed is a model of moral action capable of capturing such insights.

In previous chapters I have presented a model of moral leadership in medicine that correlates with Margaret Walker's expressive-collaborative model of morality. This model foregrounds the challenge of performative moral action, and situates moral leadership squarely in a context of collaborative and collective ethical activity. It will come as no surprise that I argue that the same model supplies a worthwhile approach to healthcare organizational ethics. In this part of my discussion, I reprise the key features of Walker's expressive-collaborative model for readers who may not have read, or have forgotten what I wrote in, earlier chapters.

According to Walker's model the central practice of morality is the continuing mutual negotiation of responsibility within moral community.

> An expressive-collaborative model looks at moral life as a continuing negotiation among
> people, a practice of mutually allotting, assuming, or deflecting responsibilities of important
> kinds, and understanding the implications of doing so. As a philosophical model, this
> representation of morality functions both descriptively and normatively. Descriptively, it
> aims to reveal what morality 'is' – what kinds of interactions go on that can be recognized as
> moral ones. Normatively, it aims to suggest some important things morality is 'for' – what
> in human lives depends on there being such practices, and how these practices can go better
> or worse. [70(p67)]

Moral community creates the conditions for mutual understanding; and continued attempts at mutual moral understanding are what create the conditions for moral community. To live morally means to be continually negotiating our responsibilities and the responsibilities owed by others, through concrete practical action. Engaging in moral practice in this way, we are made responsible to ourselves, and we are responsible to others, for the moral sense we make with our lives. What emerges from this unceasing social negotiation is moral equilibrium in Walker's sense: knowledge of what to expect morally of others, and knowledge of what others expect morally of us.

Narrative is a critical mode of moral engagement, the form in which moral problems are represented and moral responsibilities negotiated. Walker proposed that three kinds of narrative are central to moral negotiations: narratives of relationship that are based primarily in trust and integrity; narratives of moral identity that record the values that a person has exhibited through their actual actions; and narratives of value that connect narratives of relationship and of identity by expressing shared understandings of what is morally important to a group or moral community. In Chapter 6 I suggested we should add to these three kinds of narrative a fourth kind, moral narratives that recount how concrete moral challenges arise and are resolved.

Walker's expressive-collaborative model maps morality around practices of responsibility. The fundamentally important point is this: being held responsible, being exempted from responsibility and being excluded from responsibility are the basic relations of morality. An ethics of responsibility serves to 'put people and responsibilities in the right places with respect to each other' [70(p84)]. These understandings of mutual responsibility and accountability subsist as normative expectations and when breached elicit those feelings that Strawson identified as 'reactive attitudes', responses such as resentment, guilt or remorse that are the literal embodiment of our social expectations [127,128]. Moral responsibilities cannot be demarcated in any 'sharp, principled, or noncircular' way [70 (p103)]. Responsibilities tend to appear more 'moral' when the stakes are high, when failing to meet a responsibility seems to reflect upon the character of a person, or when there are important responsibilities to be enforced but formal mechanisms, such as the law, decline to enforce them.

The focus of the expressive-collaborative model is morality in action and it is in practices of responsibility that Walker locates moral life.

> Practices of responsibility include attributing some states of affairs to human agency; taking ourselves and others to be (variously) answerable for these; setting terms of praise- and (more elaborately) blameworthiness, excusability, and exculpation for what is or is not done and for some of what ensues as a result; and visiting, (in judgment, action, speech, or feeling) forms of commendation, or of criticism, reproof, or blame, on those judged in those terms . . .. But practices of responsibility are not only ones of assignment. They also include ones of accepting or refusing, deflecting or negotiating, specific assignments of responsibility. They are given ways of contesting, defending or excusing oneself; inviting or limiting one's exposure to expectations or damages; showing regret, contrition, or remorse (or contempt, indignation or derision) over one's (alleged) responsibility: offering apologies, reparations, compensations, restitutions. A more or less rich repertoire of feelings, experienced and expressed, accompany these realizations and interactions. [70(p100)]

Walker goes on to categorize the practices of responsibility in functional terms, suggesting that they might be grouped as follows: assigning blame and approval (a 'manipulative' function); informing us of our responsibilities (a 'regulative' function); eliciting emotional responses such as guilt, satisfaction or anger (an 'expressive' function); and promoting conceptions of agency (a 'definitional' function).

Medical leaders' own accounts of moral leadership suggested that it could be best understood as a course of collaborative conduct through which shared moral narratives were expressed in action. I grouped their practices of responsibility together in a rather different way than Walker: I clustered distinctive practices of responsibility together and identified them as behavioural proprieties, patterns of behaviour that express the normative expectations associated with particular healthcare organizational challenges. Narrow though my range of participants and data sources was, the version of moral leadership independently derived from data turned out to be consistent with and informative of Walker's moral philosophy.

This study did not set out to investigate the plausibility of Walker's expressive-collaborative model of morality, and neither was it designed as a study of narrative. It has nevertheless discerned that expressed, collaborative narratives are central to moral leadership in healthcare organizations. It may therefore be seen as a contribution to the 'empirically saturated reflective analysis of what is going on in actual moral orders' without which 'ethics has nothing to reflect on but moral philosophers' own assumptions and experiences' [70(p11)].

Whether we are doing organizational ethics in practice or in theory, my argument is that we should be doing it according to an expressive-collaborative model of morality. What we must now add to Walker's abstract model are the concrete issues with which organizational ethics ought to be concerned.

Building ethical organizations: what should we focus on?

The concept of organizational ethics has yet to be widely espoused in the UK. However, work by scholars from the USA and Canada has started to define the field: healthcare organizational ethics concerns the theories and practices that enable moral challenges arising at the mid-level of healthcare systems to be identified and managed. It is apparent from the existing literature of institutional ethics and organizational ethics that such moral challenges are more varied than the 'fateful decisions' that have tended to attract attention in bioethics; and they touch every aspect of healthcare organization, not only the direct provision of medical services.

With what issues, specifically, should organizational ethics be concerned? There are three avenues towards an answer to this question: asking what organizational moral challenges preoccupy those in healthcare organizations; asking what organizational moral challenges scholars have identified; and then asking what moral challenges ought to have been identified but seem for whatever reason to have been overlooked.

What organizational ethical issues actually preoccupy professionals?

This first avenue has received some attention from contributors around the world [5,6,15,21,129–131].[28] Central to the organizational ethics that emerges from empirical inquiry are, perhaps unsurprisingly, dilemmas arising from unlimited medical need and limited resource [5(p156)].[29] These issues are significantly shaped, in the case of the USA, by the design of medical insurance plans, limits on benefit coverage and the huge number of uninsured citizens. There is an affinity between the other resource-related concerns that arise in Canada, the UK and Scandinavian countries: anxiety about resource allocation decisions being influenced by remote political directives, and sometimes out of alignment with local health needs; concerns about reduced staffing levels and other cost-saving measures; difficulties around funding expensive drugs, particularly those with regulatory approval but not included in local drug formularies; and the influence of resource scarcity on clinical decisions, for example admission to the intensive care unit [130,132,133].

---

[28] Internationally, see reference 21. For an intriguing insight into how national cultures affect perception of organizational ethical issues see reference 129. From the USA see references 5 and 15. From Canada see references 6, 130 and 131.

[29] There is a useful synopsis of topics listed in reference 5, p. 156.

In addition to the dominant concern with issues of resource, confidentiality is discussed by Saeed, and also by Pearson *et al.*, who treat it as a representative example of 'systems that foster exemplary ethical principles and tenets of medicine, e.g. autonomy, beneficence, nonmaleficence and confidentiality' [5(p156),129]. Canadian clinical ethicists and Scandinavian decision-makers have identified a wider range of issues, including anxieties about the moral climate of the organization and its effect on staff (somewhat akin to NHS medical leaders' concern for collegiality); conflicts of duty (somewhat akin to NHS medical leaders' concern for fiduciary obligations); and disclosure of medical error (somewhat akin to NHS medical leaders' concern for clinical performance and medical harm).[30]

In stark comparison to the importance NHS medical leaders placed on concerns around managing medical harm, however, this issue is hardly touched on in Pearson's study; is only hinted at in Ozar's; appears to be something of a minority interest among clinical ethicists in Silva's; and receives scant attention in other studies. My study affords a view of organizational ethics from the particular, and therefore partial, perspective of medical directors. Medical directors' responsibilities for performance management, clinical quality and addressing patient complaints about care draw attention to the moral troubles associated with these domains; moreover, performance managing consultant colleagues and morally managing iatrogenic injury carry burdens of enduring uncertainty and genuine sorrow. It is unsurprising, therefore, that medical directors chose to foreground these concerns.

Empirical inquiry into organizational ethics has drawn on the views of varied professional populations, and consistent with 'decisional realities' research the study findings clearly reflect the different perspectives of differently situated actors. They equally clearly suggest that a comprehensive picture of healthcare organizational ethics will only emerge from research that spans all of the healthcare professions, including the managerial professions.

What do scholars propose organizational ethics should be about?

Loewy captures the general tenor of feeling among many scholars when she cites Avishai Margalit's view:

> A civilized society is one whose members do not humiliate one another, while a decent society is one in which the institutions do not humiliate people. [134]

The 'institutional humiliation' that I think Loewy had in mind was the humiliation of being without, and of being denied, in a society of plenty. Her comments reflect how managed care controversies and insurance coverage issues have been at the forefront of organizational ethical concern in North America. But access to the care that people need is not the only issue to have concerned organizational ethicists, as we have noted.

Boyle *et al.* discuss twenty representative scenarios. (It is not clear whether they were cases Boyle and colleagues had encountered in practice, or were fictions based on practical experience.) About half of these concern the financial bottom line, in one way or another: for example, the ethical status of the organization's investment policy, whether health insurance benefits should extend to same-sex partners, financial probity, aggressive marketing, commercial gifts, the management of charitable fundraising and the popularity of unproven complementary therapies. Some raise issues of organizational reputation and

---

[30] See references 130,132 and 133.

integrity, including spiritual integrity in faith-based hospitals and the conflict between secular and religious moral norms [135].[31] Others concern the reciprocal obligations of organizations and their staff; and one considers an egregious example of medical harm. This is a reasonably fair representation of the concerns of the field as a whole, at least as they have emerged in the primarily North American literature. The UK-based clinician reviewing that list might experience a degree of relief: whatever the vexations of working in the NHS, its structure and funding, and the reach of UK equality law into public institutions, means that many of those issues simply do not arise for consideration.

What else ought to concern moral medical leaders?

Most empirical research in healthcare ethics identifies ethical affronts that participants seem not to notice, or do not perceive to be morally problematic, or that they do not report to investigators, or towards which they acquiesce. Studies of organizational ethics are no exception to this general rule. I cannot comment on what went unnoticed by study respondents elsewhere, but there were striking omissions from the concerns reported to me. During the period that my interviews took place, an independent inquiry was discovering that the general health problems of people with learning disabilities were systematically neglected; an employee network was establishing that black and minority ethnic staff faced widespread discrimination; and an influential General Practitioner body reported that patient well-being was seriously compromised by poor hospital discharge procedures [136–138]. In the period since then major failures in care for the elderly have been revealed in two hospitals, and the Parliamentary and Health Service Ombudsman has reported further cases which suggest systemic ageism is not restricted to a few isolated organizations [139–141]. I have selected these examples out of the cornucopia of concerns that never arose for discussion, because they point to fundamental problems concerning ethical perception and ethical enactment, and therefore major problems for moral leadership.

Disregarding the healthcare needs of people with learning difficulties, treating minority ethnic staff less favourably and neglecting elderly people in hospital are all manifestations of institutionalized discrimination [132].[32] This is discrimination that is embedded in the ways that institutions work: in policies and practices that, because they are just 'the way things are', permit harmful decisions and behaviours to pass unnoticed or to be tolerated. Institutional discrimination is reminiscent of the un-remarked cruelty of hospital life that was apparent to Chambliss but utterly taken for granted by hospital staff and totally invisible to them [103]. This type of discrimination obviously poses a real challenge to ethical perception. Institutional discrimination also poses a challenge to ethical enactment, because to address institutional discrimination leaders must identify and change attitudes and behaviours that have hitherto passed unnoticed, remained unremarked or been viewed as unexceptionable. Changing such attitudes and behaviours entails contending with what people take to be common sense.

At the beginning of this chapter, I argued that the starting point for healthcare organizational ethics should be the policies and practices that secure patient confidence and trust in

---

[31] There is an informative collection of essays on institutional integrity edited by Iltis; see reference 135.

[32] On institutional discrimination in care of the elderly, see also reference 132.

healthcare organizations. I suggest that the five proprieties I have discussed – fiduciary, bureaucratic, collegial, inquisitorial and restorative – each in their way make a vital contribution to building, maintaining and repairing confidence and trust. Healthcare organizational ethics in North America has been founded in moral challenges that are, on my account, primarily fiduciary, bureaucratic and collegial concerns. A healthcare organizational ethics that correlated with the moral anxieties of NHS medical leaders would make central the moral challenges inherent in preventing, investigating and repairing medical harm, and thus the demands of inquisitorial and restorative propriety.

I did not of course interview patients for my study: is it a 'doctor-centred' theory that places concerns about professional competence, unintended medical harm and discriminatory neglect right at the heart of organizational ethics? Quite the contrary: this, I suggest, would be a truly patient-centred organizational ethics. People seeking care repose their trust and confidence in both individual clinicians and the institutions of care. If institutional agents fail to take the steps required to secure all patients' wellbeing, or if they fail to attend compassionately to harm when it has been done, then these institutions have failed in their most fundamental moral responsibilities – whatever other worthwhile ends they may have achieved.

MacIntyre has argued that practices like those that make up medicine, and the internal goods such as health that they pursue, are reliant upon institutions like hospitals, and the external goods such as money that they supply. The danger as he sees it is that practices are vulnerable to institutions' corrupting power [142]. Here I argue the opposite may be true too. In keeping their implied promise to patients to protect them from harm, healthcare institutions may indeed protect medical practice from its own tendency towards corruption. How well mid-level healthcare organizations discharge their specific responsibilities for assuring the quality of medical work is a measure of the organization's integrity.

Building ethical organizations: learning expressive moral leadership

The task of building ethical healthcare organizations entails developing and sustaining expressive ethical behaviour among professionals, and developing and sustaining able moral leadership. What has to be learned and taught in order to realize these goals? This study indicates that two courses of action lie before us. The first centres on the organizational setting in which people work: we must learn how to build organizations that do not confront professionals with invidious choices, or require them to compromise basic values in order to properly care for patients [143–151].[33] The second centres on the people who work in organizations: we must learn how to promote ethical artistry and moral leadership. It is this second course of action, educating people to become ethical artists and moral leaders, which I discuss in this final part of the book.

I should acknowledge a basic difficulty at the outset. I intend to claim that basic medical education, and then postgraduate training and development, should aim to develop at least some of the moral expertise recounted by the medical leaders in my study. This of course assumes that the medical leaders I interviewed did recount genuine moral expertise, as well as that I have properly understood what they were telling me. This difficulty is an instance of the 'credentials' problem that has been known to moral philosophers for over

---

[33] Discussion in the literature considers the issue both in relation to ethical challenges for junior doctors and also as a more general leadership concern; see references 143–151.

two millennia: how is one supposed to know who a moral expert is, particularly if one is a novice? It is a philosophical problem that remains substantially unresolved [152–155]. The difficulty is that of circularity: in order to identify the experts, we need to understand the practice of morality; but in order to understand the practice of morality, we need to consider the activity of those we know to be experts. I am proceeding therefore on the basis that the medical leadership I have described in the book is at least indicative of the form moral leadership takes, but I make no claim that my account is exhaustive.

There are three points to recall before I turn to considering how people might learn to be moral leaders in medicine.

First, I have argued that everyone is potentially a moral leader. All moral leadership entails some foundational moral understanding. So, this discussion of learning moral leadership is as much about learning ethics in basic medical education as it is about training for leadership. I have focussed on the education of doctors because that is what I know about, but the discussion has relevance to other healthcare professions too.

Second, expressive moral behaviour is the action of a specific individual (or group) responding to a specific context. Individual (or group) capability and organizational context each impose their own demands on the practitioner. To break bad news well will call on different skills in a stressed junior doctor meeting a patient for the first time in an under-funded emergency department, than those skills mobilized by an experienced oncologist conversing with patients she knows in the comfort of her own consulting rooms. These two situations are utterly different. To simply categorize them both as 'breaking bad news' obscures the challenges supplied by the need to learn new skills (in the first case) or to resist habituation (in the second); the demands of the situations in which individuals and groups find themselves, and the extent to which they may control or compensate for environmental factors; and the moral responsibilities of the organization to avoid placing patients and professionals in circumstances where compassionate care is unachievable [156].[34]

Third, moral expertise is significantly the cultural property of a functioning group or network. Moral expertise comes to reside in the narratives of identity, relationship, value and moral history that bind groups and networks together and that direct group energies towards tasks such as protecting patient dignity. The moral expertise of the group lies in its assumptions about how it is right to behave, in its normative expectations of group members' behaviour, and in its willingness to hold group members to account: conscious or unconscious understandings that 'this is the way we do things round here'. What this implies for those of us learning to be morally capable individuals is that we must learn how to be morally capable as members of a group: how to lead, follow, collaborate, influence, give moral support, promote accountability and generally comport ourselves to build collective moral capacities.

Helping healthcare professionals to learn expressive ethical expertise

What does moral leadership call upon people to know and to be able to do? If, as I believe, it means working with others to create, realize and perform the best possible moral narrative in the circumstances it encompasses all of the capacities that appear below, and probably more:

---

[34] Cf. reference 156.

(i)   apprehending moral trouble in the context of practice;

(ii)   recognizing and managing reactive attitudes to breaches of normative expectation;

(iii)   making preliminary moral sense of a situation in light of narratives of identity, relationship, value and fact;

(iv)   considering the claims of practice standards, normative expectations and proprieties;

(v)   investigating and inquiring into past events and current feelings;

(vi)   formulating and trying out narratives of facts, meanings and moral reasons;

(vii)   comprehending and taking into account others' narratives of fact, meaning, and moral reason;

(viii) imagining, mentally rehearsing and modifying narratives of action;

(ix)   managing one's own and others' responses to conflicting narratives, mediating between them and negotiating fitting outcomes;

(x)   experiencing morally appropriate responses: e.g. compassion, regret, remorse;

(xi)   expressing ethically significant behaviours appropriate in the circumstances: e.g. demonstrating neutrality; exhibiting empathy; speaking as an advocate; speaking as a witness; eliciting and repeating testimony; listening to narratives of distress; performing an apology;

(xii)   comporting the self: e.g. accepting responsibility; withholding judgement; making balanced judgements on the facts; evaluating one's actions; persisting in the face of doubt, hostility and setbacks; managing anger, fear, partiality, boredom, vindictiveness, envy, threats, imprecations and all the everyday impediments to ethical enactment.

This, clearly, anticipates a long journey of development accompanying different stages in professional life. It could be that in the early years the greatest challenge is to recognize basic patient normative expectations, master basic medical proprieties, develop a reflective response to normative challenge, and learn essential ways of comporting the self. Early in a professional career, one must know how to narrate and what to listen for from a junior position. Later, senior professionals will develop a wider appreciation of the moral dimensions of their work, expand their mastery of propriety and realize that they may play a significant role prompting, mediating and negotiating organizational narratives. At this stage, one must know how to narrate and what to listen for from a position of seniority.

How well do we currently prepare clinicians for this kind of practice? Theoretical-juridical understandings of morality have presented educators with the task of preparing moral agents to make sound choices, and justify them according to moral reasons. Virtue-based theories invited educators to consider how moral agents could develop the practical reason that enabled them 'to do the right thing for the right reason, in the appropriate way – honestly, courageously and so on' [87(p516),157–159]. During its first twenty-five or so years, medical ethics education thus concentrated on developing normative expertise and/or individual moral character; and it by and large assumed that appropriate moral action would follow from sound justifications and decisions [160,161].[35]

---

[35] It should be noted that there have been two rather divergent strands in ethics education. One is a focus on cognitive skills and propositional moral knowledge; the other is a focus on development of virtuous moral character.

While the development of normative expertise and the development of character have both been perceived to be desirable, it has been the development of normative expertise that has tended to dominate curricula [162].[36] In the UK, a consensus-based 'Core Curriculum' has set out the substantive content that the medical ethics community recommends be taught [163,164]. The Association of American Medical Colleges has required students to be taught 'knowledge of the theories and principles that govern ethical decision making, and of the major ethical dilemmas in medicine' [165]. Surveys of curricula in the USA and Canada reveal that a tiny fraction of course hours is spent on ethics education (a mere one percent) generally in the pre-clinical years; and that although there is some bedside teaching much time is spent in lectures or small groups discussing cases, empirical studies, moral philosophy and literary narratives [166–168].

Consistent with the focus on developing moral judgement, controversy has tended to arise over the subjects addressed in ethics education or over the role of moral theory. For example, Christakis and Feudtner called for greater concentration on the day-to-day ethical concerns that preoccupy junior doctors, a call echoed by many [169–171]; André and others have pressed for more attention to be paid to facilitating moral perception [120,172–174]; and Cowley advanced the interesting proposition that teaching moral theory merely gets in the way of moral development [175].

There is no doubt, however, that winds of change are blowing through ethics instruction in both basic medical education and post-qualification training. Significantly driven by greater understanding not only of the nature of the moral challenges that junior doctors face, but also of the difficulties they experience in realizing their moral aspirations, the focus is shifting towards developing expressive ethical skills. Teachers are focussing on developing empathic response, 'ethical mindfulness', ability to negotiate from a position of disadvantage, development through mentorship, how to communicate about error, and so on [107,146,148,176–184].[37] But such initiatives have been inhibited, I think, by lack of an adequate underlying theory and description of moral action in healthcare organizations.

It is very difficult to design effective ways of learning expressive ethical expertise if there is insufficient understanding of what expressive ethical performance looks like. Observing the limitations of ethics education in Canadian medical schools for example, Singer noted that moral reasoning is

> only one piece of the puzzle ... [T]he doctor must recognize situations as an ethical dilemma; possess the relevant knowledge of norms, laws and policies; analyze how this knowledge applies to the situation at hand; and demonstrate the skills needed to communicate and negotiate this situation in practice. [185]

While Singer rightly differentiated between three distinct facets of moral reasoning – perception, knowledge and analysis – the complexity of expressive moral action was reduced to broad notions of communication and negotiation. Some other attempts to define 'clinical ethical competency' have been similarly reductive, amounting to little more than 'applying ethical concepts and principles to real-life cases, real-life people' [186].[38]

---

[36] In Bloom's taxonomy of educational objectives; the cognitive domain.
[37] In relation to nursing see also reference 107.
[38] See also reference 182.

This incomplete understanding of expressive ethical expertise has been matched by limited understanding of moral medical leadership. The NHS Medical Leadership Competencies Framework, for example, is intended to underpin medical leadership development. It includes as one item out of twenty-four 'acting with integrity' and further guidance tells us only that this means 'take appropriate action if ethics and values are compromised'. Given that – as we have seen throughout this book – medical managers are essentially suspended between moral contradictions, this is a singularly unhelpful suggestion. What tests medical leaders' integrity and moral ingenuity is determining and implementing the least worst compromise, not avoiding compromise altogether. American medical leaders have been offered an equally thin description of moral competency [187,188].[39] In fairness, these unhelpful descriptors may be as much a manifestation of the inanity of competency frameworks as they are a manifestation of the paucity of our understanding of moral leadership. Or maybe not?

My view, it hardly needs to be stated, is that we should approach the development of moral expertise across medical education and training as the development of narrative, expressive, collaborative capabilities. Encouragingly, ethics education being the vast industry that it is, there are others who are already working on developing ethical artistry as an expressive ability.

Among the most interesting developments is the work that has been led by business ethicist Mary Gentile [126]. She argues that individuals need to believe that they can voice their values without alienating others; to believe that when they do so it can really make a difference; and to have confidence that they are able to communicate their convictions. She has developed a programme that enables individuals to learn how to voice their values in difficult situations by formulating and rehearsing an effective 'script' before they encounter real moral hazard. Gentile presents a persuasive argument that – parsed into the vocabulary I have used in this book – aspects of expressive collaborative moral action can be learned by trying out practices of responsibility in a safe environment.

This 'pre-scripting' approach only enables people to learn a few aspects of expressive collaborative morality, though. Gentile's programme is subtitled 'how to speak your mind when you know what's right', and thus while it is an exciting project it is one that is seriously incomplete. In terms of the list of expressive collaborative capacities I set out above, it deals only with some of those that become relevant after sense-making has started: formulating and trying out narratives of facts, meanings and moral reasons; comprehending and taking into account others' narratives of fact, meaning and moral reason; imagining, mentally rehearsing and modifying narratives of action; and managing one's own and others' responses to conflicting narratives. It does not address issues of moral awareness or

---

[39] The NHS Medical Leadership Competency Framework describes acting with integrity as: 'Uphold personal and professional ethics and values, taking into account the values of the organisation and the culture, beliefs and abilities of individuals; communicate effectively with individuals, appreciating their social, cultural, religious and ethnic backgrounds and their age, gender and abilities; value, respect and promote equality and diversity; take appropriate action if ethics and values are compromised.' See reference 187. See also reference 188: 'Assure that health service activities reflect ethical standards, comply with all pertinent legal and regulatory requirements ... and incorporate risk management principles and practices. E.g. identification and analysis of an ethical issue in a health care setting (e.g., access to bone marrow transplant) and effective communication of a recommended resolution.'

perception; or sense-making; or broader behaviours such as attentiveness to others. The notion of 'pre-scripting' also raises questions about how individuals learn what an 'effective' script is in particular organizational or professional cultures. Again, parsed into the vocabulary of my own account, how do people come to know what scripts are mandated by the demands of propriety?

Finally, even in Gentile's innovative programme, it is individual moral capability that remains the firm focus of developmental activity. How much difference might it make to our healthcare organizations if we were to set out to develop the moral capacities of groups, assisting them to build a morally resilient group culture and develop practices that sustain the group and its new members over time?

Programmes such as Gentile's demonstrate, however, that there are promising new avenues to explore. I hope that readers of this book will seize the opportunity to rethink the development of clinical ethical artistry and moral leadership; and I would be delighted to hear from those who are already, like Gentile, experimenting with how to teach expressive collaborative moral action.

We have in the past invited our future healthcare leaders to learn how to justify their decisions by reference to prevailing moral norms. This is no mean task, and it is not an unimportant one. Knowing how to analyse morally sensitive situations and knowing how to evaluate possible responses to them are very significant aspects of narrative practice. But where normative analysis is too dominant in our teaching of ethics or moral leadership, we misrepresent and disparage the demanding tasks of real moral artistry. We thereby unintentionally mislead the professionals we aspire to enlighten, and inadvertently fail the patients and carers whose interests we hope to promote.

We all of us have to make ourselves ready for the times that we are granted the privilege of moral responsibility and the prospect of moral accomplishment. To do so we need to nurture our capacity to express moral narratives in action. Then, to recall the words of Denise Levertov's poem, we will hear our whole selves saying and singing what we know: *we can* [189].

Further reading

André J. *Bioethics as Practice*. Chapel Hill: University of North Carolina Press; 2002.

Lindemann H, Verkerk M, Walker MU, eds. *Naturalized Bioethics: Toward Responsible Knowing and Practice*. Cambridge: Cambridge University Press; 2009.

Rasmussen LM, ed. *Ethics Expertise: History, Contemporary Perspectives, and Applications*. Dordrecht: Springer; 2005.

Gentile MC. *Giving Voice to Values: How to Speak Your Mind When You Know What's Right*. New Haven: Yale University Press; 2010.

Kritek PB. *Negotiating at an Uneven Table: Developing Moral Courage in Resolving Our Conflicts*. 2nd edn. San Francisco: Jossey Bass; 2002.

References

1. Joffe S, Manocchia M, Weeks JC, Cleary PD. What do patients value in their hospital care? An empirical perspective on autonomy centred bioethics. *Journal of Medical Ethics*. 2003;29(2):103–8.

2. Narenda DP. What do patients value in their hospital care? A response to Joffe et al. *Journal of Medical Ethics*. 2004;30(6): 610–2.

3. Joffe S, Manocchia M, Weeks JC, Cleary PD. Author's reply. *J Med Ethics* [serial on the Internet]. 2003. Available from: http://jme.bmj.com/content/29/2/103.abstract/reply.

4. Agledahl KM, Førde R, Wifstad Å. Choice is not the issue. The misrepresentation of healthcare in bioethical discourse. *Journal of Medical Ethics*.

5. Pearson S, Sabin J, Emanuel EJ. *No Margin, No Mission: Health-care, Organizations, and the Quest for Ethical Excellence.* New York: Oxford University Press; 2003.

6. McDonald F, Simpson C, O'Brien F. Including organizational ethics in policy review processes in healthcare institutions: a view from Canada. *HEC Forum.* 2008; **20**(2):137–53.

7. Rozovsky LE. Abolish medical staff on hospital boards. *Hospital Trustee.* 1977; Nov-Dec **1**(3):5–6.

8. Cunningham Jr R. Of snake oil and science: hospital marketing must never ignore the professional ethic that grows out of patient trust. *Hospitals.* 1978;**52**(8): 79–82.

9. Umbeck P. The church related hospital in a secular society. *Bulletin American Protestant Hospital Association.* 1977; **41**(5):14–5, 28–9.

10. Doughty E. Purchasing ethics and the supplier. *Hospital Equipment Supplies.* 1975;**21**(4):6ff.

11. Are ethics of industry appropriate to medical care? *Hospital Trustee* 1979;**3**:5ff.

12. Bishop LJ, Cherry MN, Darragh M. Organizational ethics and health care: expanding bioethics to the institutional arena. *Kennedy Institute of Ethics Journal.* 1999;**9**(2):189–208.

13. Kushner T, Heilig S, Häyry M, Takala T, eds. Special section. *Issues in Organization Ethics and Healthcare* 2000.

14. Khushf G, ed. Special issue. *The Case for Managed Care* 1999.

15. Ozar D, Berg J, Werhane PH, Emanuel LL. *Organizational Ethics in Healthcare: Toward a Model for Ethical Decision-making by Provider Organizations.* AMA Institute for Ethics National Working Group Report: American Medical Association 2000.

16. Boyle PJ, DuBose ER, Ellingson SJ, Guinn DE, McCurdy DB. *Organizational Ethics in Health Care: Principles, Cases, and Practical Solutions.* San Francisco, CA: Jossey-Bass and AHA Press; 2000.

17. Hall RT. *An Introduction to Healthcare Organizational Ethics.* New York: Oxford University Press; 2000.

18. Spencer EM, Mills AE, Rorty MV, Werhane PH. *Organization Ethics in Health Care.* New York: Oxford University Press; 2000.

19. Weber LJ. *Business Ethics in Healthcare.* Smith DH, Veatch RM, eds. Bloomington: Indiana University Press; 2001.

20. Anderlik MR. *The Ethics of Managed Care: A Pragmatic Approach.* Bloomington: University of Indiana Press; 2001.

21. Žydžiūnaite V, Suominen T, Åstedt-Kurki P, Lepait D. Ethical dilemmas concerning decision-making within health care leadership: a systematic literature review. *Medicina (Kaunas).* 2010;**46**(9):595–603.

22. Shale S. Managing the conflict between individual needs and group interests – ethical leadership in health care organizations. *The Keio Journal of Medicine.* 2008;**57**(1):37–44.

23. Khushf G. The case for managed care: reappraising medical and socio-political ideals. *Journal of Medicine and Philosophy.* 1999;**24**:415–33.

24. Khushf G. The value of comparative analysis in framing the problems of organizational ethics. *HEC Forum.* 2001; **13**(2):125–31.

25. Cribb A. Reconfiguring professional ethics: the rise of managerialism and public health in the U.K. National Health Service. *HEC Forum.* 2001;**13**(2):111–24.

26. Bitton A, Kahn JG. Share of healthcare expenditures. *Journal of the American Medical Association.* 2003;**289**:1165.

27. Kemble SB. A better idea for United States healthcare: the balanced choice proposal. *The Hawai Medical Journal, a Journal of Asia Pacific Medicine.* 2010;**69**(12): 294–7.

28. Caronna CA. Clash of logics, crisis of trust: entering the era of public for-profit health care? In: Pescosolido BA, Martin JK, McLeod JD, Rogers A, eds. *Handbook of the Sociology of Health, Illness, and Healing.* New York: Springer; 2011, pp. 255–70.

29. Wiener C. *The Elusive Quest: Accountability in Hospitals*. New York: Aldine de Gruyter; 2000.

30. Walshe K. *Regulating Healthcare: A Prescription for Improvement?* Maidenhead: Open University Press; 2003.

31. Schyve PM. The evolution of external quality evaluation: observations from the Joint Commission on Accreditation of Healthcare Organizations. *International Journal For Quality in Health Care*. 2000;**12**:255–8.

32. Chan R, Webster J. End-of-life care pathways for improving outcomes in caring for the dying. *Cochrane Database of Systematic Reviews*. 2010(1).

33. Gomes B, Higginson I. Factors influencing death at home in terminally ill patients with cancer: a systematic review. *BMJ*. 2006;**332**:515–21.

34. LaMantia MA, Scheuneman LP, Viera AJ, Busby-Whitehead J Hanson LC. Interventions to improve transitional care between nursing homes and hospitals: a systematic review. *Journal of the American Geriatric Society*. 2010;**58**(4).

35. Brecher B. The politics of professional ethics. *Journal of Evaluation in Clinical Practice*. 2010;**16**:351–5.

36. Kohn LT, *et al.*, ed. *To Err is Human: Building a Safer Health System*. Washington DC: Institute of Medicine: National Academy Press; 2000.

37. Meister Jr DJ. Comment: criminal liability for corporations that kill. *Tulane Law Review*. 1990;64.

38. Wells C. Corporate manslaughter: A cultural and legal form. *Criminal Law Forum*. 1995;**6**(1):45–72.

39. Wells C. The reform of corporate criminal liability. In: De Lacy J, ed. *The Reform of United Kingdom Company Law*. London: Cavendish; 2002, pp. 301–6.

40. Wells C. Corporate criminal responsibility. In: Tully S, ed. *Research Handbook on Corporate Legal Responsibility*. Cheltenham: Edward Elgar; 2007.

41. Ridley A, Dunford L. Corporate killing – legislating for unlawful death? *Industrial Law Journal*. 1997;**26**(2):99–113.

42. Samanta A, Samanta J. Charges of corporate manslaughter in the NHS may be brought if patients die after clinical negligence. *BMJ*. 2006;**332**(7555):1404–5.

43. Gobert J. The Corporate Manslaughter and Corporate Homicide Act 2007 – Thirteen years in the making but was it worth the wait? *The Modern Law Review*. 2008;**71**(3):413–33.

44. Gray DP. Proposed new law on manslaughter: implications for the NHS and doctors. *British Journal of General Practice*. 2001;**51**:156–7.

45. Childs M. Medical manslaughter and corporate liability. *Legal Studies*. 1999; **19**(3):316–38.

46. Belcher A. Corporate killing as a corporate governance issue. *Corporate Governance: An International Review*. 2002;**10**(1):47–54.

47. Clarkson C. Kicking corporate bodies and damning their souls. *Modern Law Review*. 1996;**59**:557.

48. Langsford H, Clark B. A rebirth of corporate killing: lessons from America in a new law for scotland. *International Company and Commercial Law Review*. 2005;**16**(1):28–37.

49. Werhane PH. *Persons, Rights, and Corporations*. Englewood Cliffs, NJ: Prentice Hall; 1985.

50. Jonsen AR. *The Birth of Bioethics*. Oxford: Oxford University Press; 1998.

51. Agich GJ. The importance of management for understanding managed care. *Journal of Medicine and Philosophy*. 1999;**24**:518–34.

52. Thompson DF. Hospital ethics. *Cambridge Quarterly of Healthcare Ethics*. 1992;**3**: 203–10.

53. Wolpe PR. From bedside to boardroom: sociological shifts and bioethics. *HEC Forum*. 2000;**12**(3):191–201.

54. Rodwin MA. *Medicine, Money and Morals*. New York: Oxford University Press; 1993.

55. Morreim H. *Balancing Act; The New Medical Ethics of Medicine's New*

Economics. Washington DC: Georgetown University Press; 1995.

56. Wong K. *Medicine and the Market Place: The Moral Dimensions of Managed Care.* Notre Dame, IN: University of Notre Dame Press; 1998.

57. Annas GJ. *Some Choice: Law, Medicine, and the Market.* New York: Oxford University Press; 1998.

58. Blau PM. *The Dynamics of Bureaucracy.* Chicago: University of Chicago Press; 1955.

59. Lipsky M. *Street-Level Bureaucracy: Dilemmas of the Individual in Public Services.* New York: Russell Sage Foundation; 1980.

60. Spielman B. Organizational ethics programs and the law. *Cambridge Quarterly of Healthcare Ethics.* 2000;**9**: 218–29.

61. Kurlander JE, Danis M. Organizational ethics in health care. In: Ashcroft R, Draper H, Dawson A, McMillan J, eds. *Principles of Health Care Ethics.* New York: John Wiley; 2007, pp. 593–600.

62. Rorty MV, Werhane PH, Mills AE. The *Rashomon* effect: organization ethics in health care. *HEC Forum.* 2004;**16**(2):75–94.

63. Loewy RS. The 'ethics' of organizational/ institutional ethics in a pluralistic setting: conflicts of interests, values, and goals. *McGeorge Law Review.* 2008;**39**:703–18.

64. Peppin JF. Business ethics and health care: the re-emerging institution-patient relationship. *Journal of Medicine and Philosophy.* 1999;**24**:535–50.

65. Fesmire S. *John Dewey and Moral Imagination: Pragmatism in Ethics.* Bloomington, IN: Indiana University Press; 2003.

66. Fins JJ, Miller FG, Bacchetta MD. Clinical pragmatism: bridging theory and practice. *Kennedy Institute of Ethics Journal.* 1998; **8**(1):37–42.

67. Churchill LR, Schenk D. One cheer for bioethics: engaging the moral experiences of patients and practitioners beyond the big decisions. *Cambridge Quarterly of Healthcare Ethics.* 2005;**14**: 389–403.

68. André J. *Bioethics as Practice.* Chapel Hill: University of North Carolina Press; 2002.

69. Crigger B-J. As time goes by: an intellectual ethnography of bioethics. In: de Vries R, Subedi J, eds. *Bioethics and Society: Constructing the Ethical Enterprise.* Upper Saddle River, NJ: Prentice-Hall; 1998, p. 196.

70. Walker MU. *Moral Understandings: A Feminist Study in Ethics.* 2nd edn. New York: Oxford University Press; 2007.

71. Fox R, Swazey JP. Medical morality is not bioethics: medical ethics in China and the United States. *Perspectives in Biology and Medicine.* 1984;**27**:336–60.

72. McCullough LB. Methodological concerns in bioethics. *Journal of Medicine and Philosophy.* 1986;**11**:17–37.

73. Light DW, McGee G. On the social embeddedness of bioethics. In: De Vries R, Subedi J, eds. *Bioethics and Society: Constructing the Ethical Enterprise.* Upper Saddle River, NJ: Prentice Hall; 1998.

74. Wolpe PR. The triumph of autonomy in American bioethics: a sociological view. In: de Vries R, Subedi J, eds. *Bioethics and Society: Constructing the Ethical Enterprise.* Upper Saddle River, NJ: Prentice Hall; 1998.

75. Hoffmaster B. Can ethnography save the life of medical ethics? *Social Science & Medicine.* 1992;**35**(12):1421–31.

76. Hoffmaster B. The forms and limits of medical ethics. *Social Science & Medicine.* 1994;**39**(9):1155.

77. Caplan A. Can applied ethics be effective in health care and should it strive to be? *Ethics.* 1983;**93**(2):311–9.

78. Harrison MR, Meilander G. The anencephalic newborn as organ donor. *Hastings Center Report.* 1986;**16**(2):21–3.

79. Agich GJ. What kind of doing is clinical ethics? *Theoretical Medicine.* 2005;**26**:7–24.

80. Agich GJ. The question of method in ethics consultation. *The American Journal of Bioethics.* 2001;**1**(4):31–41.

81. Kass L. Practising ethics: where's the action? *The Hastings Center Report.* 1990;**20**(1):5–12.

82. Chapple H. *No Place for Dying: Hospitals and the Ideology of Rescue.* Walnut Creek, CA: Left Coast Press; 2010.

83. Guillemin J. Bioethics and the coming of the corporation to medicine. In: de Vries R, Subedi J, eds. *Bioethics and Society: Constructing the Ethical Enterprise.* Upper Saddle River, NJ: Prentice Hall; 1998. p. 73.

84. Jonsen AR, Toulmin S. *The Abuse of Casuistry: A History of Moral Reasoning.* Berkeley: University of California Press; 1988.

85. Arras J. The revival of casuistry in bioethics. *Journal of Medicine and Philosophy.* 1991;**16**:9–51.

86. Kopelman L. Case method and casuistry: the problem of bias. *Theoretical Medicine.* 1994;**15**:21–37.

87. Annas J. Virtue ethics. In: Copp D, ed. *The Oxford Handbook of Ethical Theory.* Oxford: Oxford University Press; 2005, pp. 515–36.

88. Foot P. *Natural Goodness.* Oxford: Clarendon Press; 2001, p. 14.

89. Jackson J. *Ethics in Medicine.* Cambridge: Polity Press; 2006, p. 11.

90. Beauchamp TL, Childress JF. *Principles of Biomedical Ethics.* 5th edn. Oxford: Oxford University Press; 2001, p. 34.

91. Murray TH. What do we mean by 'narrative ethics?'. In: Lindemann Nelson H, ed. *Stories and their Limits: Narrative Approaches to Bioethics.* New York: Routledge; 1997, pp. 3–17.

92. Fox RC, Swazey JP. *Observing Bioethics.* New York: Oxford University Press; 2008.

93. Hoeyer K. 'Ethics wars': reflections on the antagonism between bioethicists and social science observers of biomedicine. *Human Studies.* 2006;**29**:203–27.

94. Heimer CA, Staffen LR. *For the Sake of the Children: The Social Organization of Responsibility in the Hospital and the Home.* Chicago: University of Chicago Press; 1998.

95. Quill TE, Dresser R, Brock DW. The rule of double effect – a critique of its role in end-of-life decision making. *New England Journal of Medicine.* 1997;**337**(24):1768–71.

96. Fohr SA. The double effect of pain medication: separating myth from reality. *Journal of Palliative Medicine.* 1998; **1**(4):315–28.

97. Foster C, Herring J, Melham K, Hope T. The double effect effect. *Cambridge Quarterly of Healthcare Ethics.* 2011; **20**(1):56–72.

98. Hall RT. *Emile Durkheim: Ethics and the Sociology of Morals.* New York: Greenwood Press.

99. Pope W, Cohen J, Hazelrigg L. On the divergence of Weber and Durkheim: a critique of Parson's convergence thesis. *American Sociological Review.* 1975;**40**: 417–27.

100. Freidson E. *Profession of Medicine: A Study in the Sociology of Applied Knowledge.* Chicago: University of Chicago Press; 1970.

101. Freidson E. Process of control in a company of equals. In: Freidson E, Lorber J, eds. *Medical Men and their Work: A Sociological Reader.* Chicago: Aldine-Atherton; 1972, pp. 185–201.

102. Bosk CL. *Forgive and Remember: Managing Medical Failure.* 2nd edn. Chicago: University of Chicago Press; 2003.

103. Chambliss DF. *Beyond Caring: Hospitals, Nurses, and the Social Organization of Ethics.* Chicago: Chicago University Press; 1996.

104. Anspach R, Mizrachi N. The field worker's fields: ethics, ethnography and medical sociology. In: de Vries R, Turner L, Orfali K, Bosk C, eds. *The View From Here: Bioethics and the Social Sciences.* Oxford: Blackwell; 2007, pp. 48–66.

105. Bosk C. Irony, ethnography, and informed consent. In: Hoffmaster B, ed. *Bioethics in a Social Context.* Philadelphia: Temple University Press; 2000, pp. 199–220.

106. Jackall R. *Moral Mazes.* New York: Oxford University Press; 1988.

107. Kritek PB. *Negotiating at an Uneven Table: Developing Moral Courage in Resolving Our Conflicts.* 2nd edn. San Francisco: Jossey Bass; 2002.

108. Bosk CL. *All God's Mistakes: Genetic Counseling in a Pediatric Hospital.* Chicago: University of Chicago Press; 1992. p. xvii.

109. Zussman R. Sociological perspectives on medical ethics and decision-making. *Annual Review of Sociology.* 1997;**23**: 171–89.

110. Zussman R. *Intensive Care: Medical Ethics and the Medical Profession.* Chicago: University of Chicago Press; 1992. p. 3.

111. Borry P, Schotsman P, Dierickx K. What is the role of empirical research in bioethical reflection and decision-making? An ethical analysis. *Medicine, Health Care and Philosophy.* 2004;**7**:41–53.

112. Hedgecoe A. It's money that matters: the financial context of ethical decision-making in modern biomedicine. In: de Vries R, Turner L, Orfali K, Bosk C, eds. *The View From Here: Bioethics and the Social Sciences.* Oxford: Blackwell; 2007.

113. Scully J, Shakespeare T, Banks S. Gift not commodity? Lay people deliberating social sex selection. In: de Vries R, Turner L, Orfali K, Bosk C, eds. *The View From Here: Bioethics and the Social Sciences.* Oxford: Blackwell; 2007.

114. Pearlman RA, Miles SH, Arnold RM. Empirical research in medical ethics. *Theoretical Medicine.* 1993;**14**:197–208.

115. Atkinson P. *Medical Talk and Medical Work: The Liturgy of the Clinic.* Thousand Oaks, CA: Sage; 1995.

116. Anspach RR. *Deciding Who Lives: Fateful Choices in the Intensive Care Nursery.* Berkeley: University of California Press; 1993.

117. Holm S. *Ethical Problems in Clinical Practice: The Ethical Reasoning of Healthcare Professionals.* Manchester: Manchester University Press; 1997, p. 145.

118. Hurst SA, Hull SC, DuVal G, Danis M. Physicians' responses to resource constraints. *Archives of Internal Medicine.* 2005;**165**:639–44.

119. Strech D, Synofzik M, Marckmann G. How physicians allocate scarce resources at the bedside; a systematic review of qualitative studies. *Journal of Medicine and Philosophy.* 2008;**33**:80–99.

120. Maxwell B, Racine E. Should empathic development be a priority in biomedical ethics teaching? A critical perspective. *Cambridge Quarterly of Healthcare Ethics.* 2010;**19**(4):433–45.

121. Rest J. *Moral Development; Advances in Research and Theory.* New York: Praeger; 1986.

122. Jones TM. Ethical decision making by individuals in organizations; an issue contingent model. *Academy of Management Review.* 1991;**16**(2): 366–95.

123. Loe TW, Ferrell L, Mansfield P. A review of empirical studies assessing ethical decision making in business. *Journal of Business Ethics.* 2000;**25**:185–204.

124. Ajzen I. Attitude, structure and behavior. In: Breckler SJ, Greenwald AG, eds. *Attitude Structure and Function.* Hillsdale, NJ: Lawrence Erlbaum; 1989, pp. 241–74.

125. McMahon JM, Harvey RJ. The effect of moral intensity on ethical judgment. *Journal of Business Ethics.* 2007;**72**:335–57.

126. Gentile MC. *Giving Voice to Values: How to Speak Your Mind When You Know What's Right.* New Haven: Yale University Press; 2010.

127. Walker MU. *Moral Repair: Reconstructing Moral Relations after Wrongdoing.* Cambridge: Cambridge University Press; 2006, p. 24.

128. Strawson PF. Freedom and resentment. In: Strawson PF, ed. *Studies in the Philosophy of Thought and Action.* New York: Oxford University Press; 1968.

129. Saeed KS. How physician executives and clinicians perceive ethical issues in Saudi Arabian hospitals. *Journal of Medical Ethics.* 1999;**25**:51–6.

130. Silva DS, Gibson J, Sibbald R, Connolly E, Singer PA. Clinical ethicists' perspectives on organizational ethics in healthcare organizations. *Journal of Medical Ethics.* 2007;**34**:320–3.

131. Wall S. Organizational ethics, change and stakeholder involvement; a survey

of physicians. *HEC Forum*. 2007; **19**(3):227–43.

132. Mamhidir A-G, Kihlgren M, Sørlie V. Ethical challenges related to elder care. High level decision-makers' experiences. *BMC Medical Ethics*. 2007;**8**:3.

133. Kälvemark S, Höglund A, Hansson M, Westerholm P, Arnetz B. Living with conflicts-ethical dilemmas and moral distress in the health care system. *Social Science & Medicine*. 2004;**58**(6):1075–84.

134. Margalit A. *The Decent Society*. Translated by Naomi Goldblum. Harvard: Harvard University Press; 1996.

135. Smith Iltis A, ed. *Institutional Integrity in Health Care*. Dordrecht: Kluwer Academic; 2003.

136. Michael SJ. *Healthcare for All: report of the independent inquiry into access to healthcare for people with learning disabilities*: Department of Health; 2008.

137. Santry C. Minority staff get worse deal on jobs, pay and grievances. *Health Service Journal*. 7 August 2008;3–5.

138. A Very Present Danger: restricted circulation report 2007. Available from: http://www.nhsalliance.org/documents/ survey-reports/, http://www.nhsalliance. org/press-releases/article/date/2007/03/ institutionalised-contempt-puts-patients-at-risk/.

139. *Investigation into outbreaks of Clostridium difficile at Maidstone and Tunbridge Wells NHS Trust*. Healthcare Commission; 2007.

140. Francis R. *The Mid Staffordshire NHS Foundation Trust Inquiry*. Department of Health; 2010.

141. Abraham A. *Care and Compassion: Report of the Health Service Ombudsman on ten investigations into NHS care of older people*. Parliamentary and Health Service Ombudsman; 2011.

142. MacIntyre A. *After Virtue*. 3rd edn. London: Duckworth; 2007, pp. 194ff.

143. Dailey J. Modeling manipulation in medical education. *Advances in Health Sciences Education. Theory and Practice*. 2010;**15**(2):291–5.

144. Lopez L, Katz J. Perspective: creating an ethical workplace: reverberations of resident work hours reform. *Academic Medicine*. 2009;**84**(3):315–9.

145. Higginson J. Perspective: limiting resident work hours is a moral concern. *Academic Medicine*. 2009;**84**(3):310–4.

146. McDougall R. Combating junior doctors' '4am logic': a challenge for medical ethics education. *Medical Ethics*. 2009;**35**(3): 203–6.

147. Martinez W, Lo B. Medical students' experiences with medical errors: an analysis of medical student essays. *Medical Education*. 2008;**42**(7):733–41.

148. Cordingley L, Hyde C, Peters S, Vernon B, Bundy C. Undergraduate medical students' exposure to clinical ethics: a challenge to the development of professional behaviours? *Medical Education*. 2007; **41**(12):1202–9.

149. Aroskar M. Healthcare organizations as moral communities. *Journal of Clinical Ethics*. 2006;**17**(3):255–6.

150. Austin W. The ethics of everyday practice: healthcare environments as moral communities. *Advances in Nursing Science*. 2007;**30**(1):81–8.

151. Nelson WA, Gardent PB, Shulman E, Splaine ME. Preventing ethics conflicts and improving healthcare quality through system redesign. *Quality & Safety in Health Care*. 2010;**19**(6):526–30.

152. Cholbi M. Moral expertise and the credentials problem. *Ethical Theory & Moral Practice*. 2007;**10**:323–34.

153. Rasmussen LM, ed. *Ethics Expertise: History, Contemporary Perspectives, and Applications*. Dordrecht: Springer; 2005.

154. Weinstein BD. What is an expert? *Theoretical Medicine*. 1993;**14**:57–73.

155. Weinstein BD. The possibility of ethical expertise. *Theoretical Medicine*. 1994;**15**:61–75.

156. Fiester A. Why the clinical ethics we teach fails patients. *Academic Medicine: Journal of the Association of American Medical Colleges*. 2007;**82**(7):684–9.

157. Kinghorn W. Medical education as moral formation: an Aristotelian account of medical professionalism. *Perspectives in Biology and Medicine.* 2010;**53**(1):87–105.

158. Bryan C, Babelay A. Building character: a model for reflective practice. *Academic Medicine.* 2009;**84**(9):1283–8.

159. Buyx A, Maxwell B, Supper H, Schöne-Seifert B. Medical ethics teaching. *Wiener Klinische Wochenschrift.* 2008; **120**(21–22):655–64.

160. Eckles R, Meslin E, Gaffney M, Helft P. Medical ethics education: where are we? Where should we be going? A review. *Academic Medicine.* 2005;**80**(12): 1143–52.

161. Fox E, Arnold R, Brody B. Medical ethics education: past, present, and future. *Academic Medicine.* 1995;**70**(9):761–9.

162. Bloom BS, ed. *Taxonomy of Educational Objectives. The Classification of Educational Goals: Handbook 1, Cognitive Domain.* New York: Longmans; 1956.

163. Stirrat G, Johnston C, Gillon R, Boyd K. Medical ethics and law for doctors of tomorrow: the 1998 Consensus Statement updated. *Journal of Medical Ethics.* 2010; **36**(1):55–60.

164. Mattick K, Bligh J. Undergraduate ethics teaching: revisiting the Consensus Statement. *Medical Education.* 2006;**40**:329–32.

165. Report 1, *Learning Objectives for Medical Student Education, Guidelines for Medical Schools.* Washington DC: Association of American Medical Colleges; 1998.

166. Persad GC, Elder L, Sedig L, Flores L, Emanuel EJ. The current state of medical school education in bioethics, health law, and health economics. *Journal of Law, Medicine and Ethics.* Spring 2008; Religions and Cultures of East and West: Perspectives on Bioethics:89–94.

167. Soleymani Lehmann L, Kasoff WS, Koch P, Federman DD. A survey of medical ethics education at U.S. and Canadian medical schools. *Academic Medicine: Journal of the Association of American Medical Colleges.* 2004;**79**(7):682–9.

168. DuBois J, Burkemper J. Ethics education in U.S. medical schools: a study of syllabi. *Academic Medicine: Journal of the Association of American Medical Colleges.* 2002;**77**:432–7.

169. Christakis DA, Feudtner C. Ethics in a short white coat: the ethical dilemmas that medical students confront. *Academic Medicine.* 1993;**68**(4):249–54.

170. Thomasma DC, Kushner T. *Ward Ethics.* Cambridge: Cambridge University Press; 2001.

171. McDougall R, Sokol DK. The ethical junior: a typology of ethical problems faced by house officers. *Journal of the Royal Society of Medicine.* 2008;**101**:67–70.

172. André J. Learning to see: moral growth during medical training. *Journal of Medical Ethics.* 1992;**18**:148–52.

173. Leget C, Olthuis G. Compassion as a basis for ethics in medical education. *Journal of Medical Ethics.* 2007;**33**:617–20.

174. Kumagai A. A conceptual framework for the use of illness narratives in medical education. *Academic Medicine.* 2008; **83**(7):653–8.

175. Cowley C. The dangers of medical ethics. *Journal of Medical Ethics.* 2005;**31**:739–42.

176. Mills S, Bryden D. A practical approach to teaching medical ethics. *Journal of Medical Ethics.* 2010;**36**(1):50–4.

177. Kelly E, Nisker J. Increasing bioethics education in preclinical medical curricula: what ethical dilemmas do clinical clerks experience? *Academic Medicine.* 2009; **84**(4):498–504.

178. McCullough M. A skills-based approach to teach clinical ethics. *Academic Medicine.* 2009;**84**(2):154.

179. White A, Gallagher T, Krauss M, Garbutt J, Waterman A, Dunagan W, *et al.* The attitudes and experiences of trainees regarding disclosing medical errors to patients. *Academic Medicine.* 2008; **83**(3):250–6.

180. Molewijk A, Abma T, Stolper M, Widdershoven G. Teaching ethics in the clinic. The theory and practice of moral

case deliberation. *Journal of Medical Ethics.* 2008;**34**(2):120–4.

181. Thulesius H, Sallin K, Lynoe N, Löfmark R. Proximity morality in medical school – medical students forming physician morality 'on the job': grounded theory analysis of a student survey. *BMC Medical Education.* 2007;7.

182. Campbell AV, Chin J, Voo T-C. How can we know that ethics education produces ethical doctors? *Medical Teacher.* 2007;**29**:431–6.

183. Fryer-Edwards K, Wilkins M, Baernstein A, Braddock 3rd C. Bringing ethics education to the clinical years: ward ethics sessions at the University of Washington. *Academic Medicine.* 2006;**81**(7):626–31.

184. Pauls M, Ackroyd-Stolarz S. Identifying bioethics learning needs: a survey of Canadian emergency medicine residents. *Academic Emergency Medicine.* 2006; **13**(6):645–52.

185. Singer PA. Strengthening the role of ethics in medical education. *Canadian Medical Association Journal.* 2003;**168**(7):854–5.

186. Sokol DK. William Osler and the jubjub of ethics; or how to teach medical ethics in the 21st century. *Journal of the Royal Society of Medicine.* 2007;**100**:544–6.

187. *Demonstrating Personal Qualities: Acting with Integrity.* NHS Institute for Innovation and Improvement [accessed 16/03/11]; Available from: http://www.institute.nhs.uk/assessment_tool/personal_qualities/personal_qualities_-_acting_with_integrity.html.

188. Lane DS, Ross V. Defining competencies and performance indicators for physicians in medical management. *American Journal of Preventive Medicine.* 1998;**14**(3):229–36.

189. Levertov D. 'Variation on a Theme by Rilke' *The Book of Hours* (Book 1, Poem 1, Stanza 1). *Breathing the Water.* New York: New Directions; 1987.

(a)

fig a – BEFORE

Dum de dum...

(b)

fig b – AFTER

Well I never...

Steven Appleby 2006

"A man who carries a cat by the tail learns something he can learn in no other way."

Mark Twain

Appendix 1: How the research was done

This research began as an inquiry into the moral quandaries that medical leaders confronted, and the ways that medical leaders reasoned about them. It certainly remained a study of moral quandaries; but the focus of inquiry shifted towards moral narrative and behavioural propriety, rather than moral reasoning. How did this happen?

The complexities of designing worthwhile social research reflect a world that the poet Louis MacNiece described as 'crazier and more of it than we think/Incorrigibly plural'. In this appendix, I explain how the arguments and conclusions of previous chapters have been shaped by the decisions I made in the course of planning and conducting the research. I endeavour to justify the research design, discuss its method and explain its conduct. I then clarify the methodological framework for the study, and the status of the conclusions that may be drawn from it.

Journal articles reporting empirical research typically describe the research process in terse and formal terms that give novices little insight into how qualitative research actually proceeds. I offer more detail and, I think, candour here. By doing so I hope to supply an account that will enlighten newcomers to the field as much as persuade experienced readers that my research procedures have yielded findings of value.

The research process

I start by recalling the specific questions that underlay the field research, and then explain how the research strategy, methods of data collection and methods of data analysis addressed them.

The field research was designed to supply data about the nature of healthcare organizational ethical challenges in the UK, and data on how medical leaders faced those challenges. Embedded in the field research questions were a set of starting assumptions about what organizational ethics entailed. Focussed on moral analysis and moral reasoning, and making reference to contextual factors as a somewhat secondary consideration, they now look rather quaint. Here, nevertheless, was the question that took me into the field:

How do medical professionals in leadership roles make sense of and manage the moral quandaries arising out of their role responsibilities?

And these were the four secondary questions that underpinned it:

(i)   What organizational moral quandaries do medical leaders recognize, and why?

(ii) How do they analyse these issues, and what approaches to moral reasoning do they draw upon?

(iii) What contextual factors seem to shape their actions, and how do they manage those?

(iv) What is their subjective, personal experience of moral leadership and moral challenge?

The original research questions were thus exploratory, descriptive and directed at achieving understanding. The literature of healthcare organizational ethics was primarily normative, so it was fitting to first explore the range of moral challenges that informants believed they faced. I assumed that in 'doing ethics' they would be doing moral analysis and moral reasoning, so I wanted to understand their orientation, and to attend to the social complexity in which these organizational ethical problems were buried. I hoped that it would be possible to produce a 'thick description' [1,2][1] of the moral phenomena that the study identified, accounting for the context in which moral phenomena arose, grasping the intentions and subjective meanings that underpinned moral action and appreciating the processes through which 'ethics' was done in healthcare organizational life. Paying attention to the moral phenomena that the study data revealed meant, however, reconsidering the place of individual moral reasoning in organizational ethical activity.

Deciding what to investigate: locating 'the ethical'

One of the difficulties intrinsic to empirical study of moral or ethical reasoning and moral or ethical action is ascertaining the boundaries of these normatively and socially constructed categories. Quite simply, how are we to recognize the phenomenon to which we are referring: what issues should be treated as 'being ethical'; and what behaviours should be treated as 'doing ethics'? These questions return us to the conceptual concerns that occupied us in Chapter 7, where we compared philosophical and sociological approaches to bioethics. Each of these implies a different point of entry into empirical inquiry.

Holm's study of the 'moral attitudes and the moral reasoning' [3(p4)] of healthcare professionals exemplifies how empirical inquiry into healthcare ethics may proceed

from a theoretical-juridical philosophical perspective. Holm defined the phenomenon that he intended to study by reference to three major traditions of normative theorizing: deontological moral theory, consequentialist theory and virtue theory. Thus,

> a consideration is classified as an ethical consideration if it a) refers to a non-legal or not solely legal norm, duty, obligation or right; or b) refers to consequences (well-being, happiness etc.) for some specifiable person or groups of persons; or c) refers to what kind of person one ought to be or what virtues one ought to have. [3(p85)]

Holm's was not a study of the 'actual actions' [3(p4)] of nurses and doctors, but of the reasoning that underpinned their action. He did not, therefore, stipulate what would count as ethical behaviour for the purposes of his study. Holm was, nevertheless, interested in how organizational forums, such as case conferences and routine collegial conferring, influenced ethical decision-making. Ethical behaviours are thus defined, by implication, as the behaviours surrounding ethical decision-making.

Entering into empirical inquiry on the basis of a theoretical-juridical definition of morality allows, as it did in Holm's study, for comparisons between 'lay medical' and 'professional philosophical' moral reasoning [3(p131–5)].[2] The sociological 'decisional realities' studies, exemplified by Reneé Anspach's elegant study *Deciding Who Lives: Fateful Choices in the Intensive Care Nursery*, adopt a not dissimilar approach [4,5]. Those studies aim to explore the similarities and expose the differences between bioethical prescription and real-life decision processes.

---

[1] The notion of thick description was developed by Clifford Geertz drawing on Gilbert Ryle. Since the publication of Geertz's much-quoted essay, the notion of 'thick description' appears in peril of losing its theoretical specificity, being treated as simply a detailed account. In Geertz's interpretative terms it means placing social facts within the context of action, focussing on the intentions of actors and the meanings they assign to their experience, and considering the processes through which social action and interaction are sustained. See references 1 and 2.

[2] E.g. Holm found that healthcare professionals' assumption of 'protective responsibility' bore strong affinity with the philosophy of Martin Buber and Hans Jonas. See reference 3, pp. 131–5.

They are thus embedded in professional and philosophical consensus on what counts as a bioethical issue, and they share with moral philosophy the tendency to associate ethical behaviour with, essentially, reasoning and decision-making.

Although adherents to theoretical-juridical models of morality are concerned to delineate the boundaries of the moral and the non-moral, this is not essential to all moral theorizing. Virtue ethics, narrative ethics and care ethics all countenance a degree of ambiguity or opacity. The expressive-collaborative model, Walker argues, does not entail any 'sharp, principled, or noncircular demarcation of moral responsibilities' [6]. The boundaries of the ethical are open-textured, she suggests, noting our tendency to refer to 'the moral' when the stakes are high, when failing to meet a responsibility seems to reflect upon a person's character, or when there are no formal mechanisms through which to enforce important responsibilities.

Treating moral responsibilities as a matter of intersubjective negotiation, the expressive-collaborative model accepts that what we perceive as a moral issue will be socially defined. This is an assumption shared by the Durkheimian studies of occupational morality that were considered in Chapter 7, including Bosk's inquiry into the norms that appeared to govern surgical training. Occupational morality studies are concerned with how morality is defined by and within specific practices. They see 'the ethical' in 'the complex of ideas and sentiments, [the] ways of seeing and [of] feeling, the certain intellectual and moral framework' of occupations [7(p5)]. As befits a study of occupational morality, and taking his cue from the data, Bosk thus defined moral failure as failure to conscientiously discharge role obligations [7(p51)]. What counted as 'being ethical', and what counted as 'doing ethics', both fell to be determined by the goals of the practice and the claims of the profession.

Which of these starting points was the more appropriate for a study of organizational ethical experience? It was not my intention to assess participants' moral outlook or moral understanding against any prior moral framework or moral theory. The research was exploratory, and there was no clear consensus on what did or should count as an organizational ethical issue. Neither did I have any particular sociological axe to grind. This was not intended to be a study in mechanisms of professional social control, as was Bosk's, and I was not persuaded that healthcare ethics might usefully be reduced to professional status conflict, as Chambliss suggests. So it made sense to define 'the ethical' by reference to 'insider' views, and to treat as an 'ethical issue' whatever an involved insider believed warranted discussion as an 'ethical issue'. The research thus rests on deliberately hazy sensitizing categories, such as 'troubling issues' and 'moral quandaries'.

Endeavouring to develop an account of organizational ethics by working outwards from an insider perspective has, however, some serious limitations. There are complications of ethical perception, in that an insider providing information may not notice issues an observant outsider would think they 'ought' to notice; or they may fail to recognize the ethical dimension in issues that their peers would recognize as ethical [3(p100),8,9].[3] There are complications of data selection, in that an insider may wittingly or unwittingly withhold information the outsider would value; and the

---

[3] Different disciplines label this problem differently. Rest uses the term 'moral awareness' (see reference 8). Others writing in a social-cognitive framework use the term 'moral recognition'; see, for example, reference 9. Holm noted 'ethical perception' had received scant treatment in philosophy but the deficit was being addressed (see reference 3, p. 100).

outsider may contribute to data selection by wittingly or unwittingly directing the insider's attention to particular topics. And there are problems of interpretation, among them the difficulty that insiders may disagree among themselves or with outsiders about whether issues are ethical concerns, technical problems, occupational conflicts, political infighting or some other sort of concern [10]. Inevitably, then, this insider account of organizational ethics is highly contingent, radically incomplete and open to the objection that what it views as essentially ethical is not what the reader considers essentially ethical.

The associated question that has had to be considered as the analysis has developed is what behaviours should be treated as 'doing ethics'? Throughout the book I have challenged the view that 'doing ethics' is merely 'doing decision-making'. Subsequent chapters have set out an alternative account that is based on treating as moral or ethical conduct the behaviours through which actors pursue their moral or ethical goals. If we reject the theoretical-juridical model of morality, and any hard and fast distinction between moral and non-moral reasoning, we should also reject hard and fast distinctions between moral and non-moral behaviours. Thus moral reasoning is reasoning in the same way that (say) legal reasoning is reasoning, and ethical behaviour is behaviour in the same way that (say) criminal behaviour is behaviour. All are identifiable by reference to specific goals, whilst sharing many generic characteristics.

What seems to identify ethical behaviour as 'ethical' is a combination of its regulative ideals, in the form of normative expectations, and its mode of expression, in the form of clusters of behaviour recognizable as propriety. While some actions, such as empathetic listening, might be described as having an intrinsically ethical quality to them, for the most part 'doing ethics' is not some ethically unique way of behaving.

Deciding how to investigate: the choice of grounded theory

I selected grounded theory as my method because this seemed to offer the best way of achieving methodological congruence, that is, securing a close fit between the research aim, questions, approach to data collection and conduct of data analysis [11].

The first link in the chain of methodological congruence was created by affinity between the research aims and questions and the origins and end results of grounded theory. The purpose of the research was to ascertain the 'organizational ethical' situations in which participants found themselves, to discern how they understood and responded to those situations and to compile an account of organizational ethical action from their accounts of what they did.

Grounded theory is a means of constructing an account of the forms and processes of social life from the data of everyday experience. It is a useful strategy where there is a paucity of empirical data and a poverty of empirically informed explanation of a phenomenon. In its classic form, grounded theory bears traces of both the positivist sociology that inspired Glaser, and the symbolic interactionism that influenced Strauss [12–14].[4] It has consequently been vulnerable to criticism from interpretivist perspectives, and it remains controversial how far it may be severed from its positivist origins and treated solely as a method. In Charmaz's strongly interpretive rendering, however, grounded theory suggested a flexible and credible set of principles and practices for deriving an 'insider' understanding of how medical leaders could 'create, enact and change meanings and

---

[4] Glaser and Strauss presented their classic statement in reference 12. The method was further developed in reference 13, which Glaser has criticized as tending to force data into preconceived categories; see reference 14.

actions' [15(p7)], in this case specifically ethical meanings and actions. As it turned out, the method both revealed and concealed unexpected aspects of ethical action. The 'narrative turn' the research took is strongly suggestive of its strengths and weaknesses as a research strategy, and this is the focus of later discussion.

The second link in the chain of methodological congruence was forged in the fit between grounded theory and the practical challenge of collecting data about medical leaders' moral experiences. Of three types of data that might be gathered (observational, interview and documentary) interview data were the only realistic source. 'Troubling issues' arise only intermittently, and when they do they are likely to concern sensitive matters. Observation of their management by medical leaders would have entailed a long period in the field shadowing several very senior figures, and remaining present when organizational and individual crises were under discussion. Achieving this level of access, and negotiating the ethical issues relating to others' informed consent and their interest in confidentiality, would have been well nigh impossible. Documents in the private domain (such as reports of Serious Untoward Incidents or full Board Papers) would be likely to be beyond reach. Documents in the public domain (such as Healthcare Commission Reports) would not reflect ordinary day-to-day difficulties, and would not provide direct access to 'insider' views.

Using interview data as the primary source, with some documentary data as a secondary source, seemed to allow for the 'what' and the 'how' of everyday moral leadership to be identified. That one aspect of the 'how' might only be retrieved through interview data became apparent during the study: one of the answers to the 'how' of organizational ethics is 'over a very considerable period of time and a wide group of actors'. Observing these extended interactions in the field would have taken several years.

Discussion of participants' probable action in response to researchers' scenarios has been a favourite tool of research in business and healthcare ethics [16]. I doubted, however, that vignettes would be a reliable means of simulating the context of day-to-day ethical responsiveness, or of accessing tacitly held moral convictions.

Vignette-based research into ethical orientation seems to me to be accompanied by a number of problems. First, it puts the ethical cart before the perceptual horse. Vignettes present the research subject with the results of another's ethical attention, another's perception and another's view of what is a salient fact. Responses can tell us little about how ethical issues are apprehended in everyday life, or of how sense-making proceeds. Additionally, long experience of learning and teaching law through case vignettes has taught me to be wary of using them to judge moral cognition. Those presented with them (including myself) can be transfixed by complex written problems that seem simpler or different when we have time for reflection. Further, solutions that have to be imagined wholesale, in advance, might be quite different from those that we discover when we act one step at a time. Finally, individual responses to a vignette presented to a group frequently change during group discussion. We know that individuals are responsive to group views about what is 'good' or 'right', which raises the question of what, in the nature of moral reasoning, scenario research can or should be testing. Should we treat as 'moral reasoning' what an individual thinks when they are on their own, or what an individual thinks after they have submitted their views to an audience of colleagues and peers?

These doubts suggest that, although the method has a long and reputable history in research, endeavouring to understand ethical action by interrogating individual responses to written scenarios has significant limitations [16].[5] As will be apparent to the reader who comes to the current chapter after reading the study findings, the data tend to reinforce these views about the value of scenario research for understanding how people really think about real moral life. The expressive, collaborative, socially situated ethical enactment that became the central subject of the study would not have emerged so clearly from scenario-based interviews.

The interviews were thus designed, as will be seen shortly, to be loosely structured and open-ended, and to focus on retrieving a detailed account of the recent ethical experience of the interviewee. Despite, or rather because of, the reliance of social research upon interview data, interviews have long been the subject of methodological controversy. I discuss these controversies below when I consider how the conceptual category of 'realizing moral narrative' emerged from the data.

Creating the data: interviewing, transcribing, sampling

One of the defining procedural components of grounded theory is that data are concurrently collected and analysed throughout the entire research process. Although some initial data must of course be gathered in order to get the analysis started, as the research proceeds it is analysis and the emerging theory that direct data collection. Theory construction demands, and data collection turns upon, theoretical sampling. This is the process of identifying and recruiting participants in whose diverse experience the theory will be grounded.

In grounded theory research, data collection and data analysis inform each other. The customary linear summary of research method (entry into the field, data sources, data collection, data analysis, results, discussion) is therefore somewhat misleading if it is construed as a descriptive account of the process. The real process is very much messier and more iterative. There are multiple entries into the field and exits into analysis, data sources are selected in response to analysis of data collected from previous data sources, and the results and topics for discussion erupt through the data at many different stages. The linear account is, however, logical and tidy, so this account of how the study data were constructed starts with information about entry into the field, moves from discussion of the content of interviews into data analysis, and concludes with theory-building and the theoretical sampling that supports it.

Interviewing

Prospective participants were approached in accordance with the protocol mandated by the NHS Research Ethics Committee that approved the study. Participants were sent a letter that described the aims of the study, and a pre-paid reply card that they were asked to return to me if they were willing to be contacted again. Included in this mailing was a token gift, a print of the cartoon that appears at the beginning of this section and which was specially commissioned for the study. The purpose of the cartoon was to draw attention to the letter, to reinforce the message that the research was an inquiry into experience, and to portray the researcher as someone who had empathy for the demands of the medical leadership role.

The reply card, and the stipulation that there should be no follow-up whatever unless the reply card was returned, was the stringent requirement imposed by the REC. It is an unusual one by comparison

---

[5] McMahon and Harvey concluded by questioning the value of scenario research, proposing that open-ended interviews would be more useful. See reference 16.

with commonly approved protocols for recruitment to an interview study that does not seek information about sensitive or distressing personal matters. As the reasons for imposing it were not made apparent, I can only guess that it reflects excessive deference to high-status doctors.

Entry into the field was further complicated by the gate-keeping role fulfilled by the Research and Development function of individual NHS organizations.[6] Research and Development departments are required to approve any and all research taking place within their organization. As each research participant was employed by a different NHS organization, each employing organization had to approve the research. In the end, twenty different NHS bodies independently approved this relatively harmless project.[7] The approval process raised something of a 'chicken and egg' problem in that theoretically an approach could not be made to the medical director of the organization unless the research was approved by their Trust, but it would be a waste of organizational resource to implement a thorough bureaucratic approval process unless the medical director wanted to participate. This conundrum was generally resolved by the R&D office making an approach on my behalf or allowing an approach subject to retrospective approval; but R&D officers were also reluctant to be seen to be 'bending the rules' when an approach was being made to their organization's lead clinician. R&D registration thus became a source of considerable delay, and it unavoidably affected the sampling process.

Once I received a reply card from a potential participant, I contacted them by telephone or email to explain issues of anonymity, confidentiality and consent, to see if they had any other issues they wanted to raise, and to arrange a meeting. Following that conversation or correspondence, I sent a follow-up letter to confirm arrangements for our meeting and in some cases to suggest a particular topic that I was interested in pursuing with them.

Each medical director was interviewed for between 60 minutes and 2 hours. All interviews but one were face–to-face, and took place either in the medical director's office at work or at the office of a national body with which they were associated. The sole exception was one interview carried out by telephone call to the medical director's office.[8] Informed consent was discussed at the beginning of the interview, and the promise of anonymity and the confidential nature of the interview were reiterated. Thereafter, interviews were in-depth and open-ended. The interviews were audio-recorded.

Four questions were on hand to initiate various stages of discussion, but were not always needed. One core question, however, an invitation to describe 'the most troubling issue you have had to deal with', was put to each interviewee, and always in the same words. Other questions were

---

[6] The longest interval between submitting an application and receiving approval was approximately six months.

[7] Some NHS organizations work as R&D consortia, which reduced the number of applications that had to be made. A minority of the organizations I approached designed their registration process to filter for risk, deemed this project low risk, and fast-tracked the application. Others imposed the full panoply of clinical trials risk management procedure, requiring an honorary contract and – in one case – an occupational health assessment. Only one organization took the view that as the point of R&D registration was to protect patients from risk and the organization from expenditure, my research need not be registered with them at all.

[8] Dr. Oxley (Goldenshire Primary Care Trust). It was considerably more difficult and I needed to check understanding more frequently, which disrupted the narrative.

phrased in a conversational idiom appropriate to the encounter.

> It would be helpful if you could start by telling me how you came to be a medical director at X Trust.
>
> Looking back over the past few years, what do you feel has been the most troubling issue that you have had to deal with?
>
> Could you assume I don't know anything, and tell me what you see as the ethical dimensions of that situation?
>
> It might seem very obvious to you, but could you tell me step by step what you actually did in response to that issue?

Some medical directors understandably sought clarification about what 'troubling issue' or 'ethical' meant. I replied that I was interested in understanding what they found to be a troubling aspect of their work, or what they classified as an ethical issue. Throughout the interview my responses ranged from active listening, laughter and empathic reflection, to detailed probing, an invitation to compare their outlook with that of other interviewees, and a request for comment on emergent categories.

Transcribing

The interviews were transcribed by the same professional transcriber experienced in preparing interview material for textual analysis, and according to an 'intelligent verbatim' protocol. This approach excluded 'ums' and 'ers' and background noise, but left 'you know' and similar devices intact. It also noted exceptional responses such as extensive laughter. I verified and corrected the transcript. I also returned to listen to the original recordings during data analysis where meanings seemed unclear, or where the text appeared to be at odds with my recall of the expressive meaning of spoken language. The final translation of conversations with my informants into units of text undergoing analysis was achieved using computer software, Atlas ti.

It is irrefutable that the conversion of moment-by-moment speech into first, an audio recording, second, a transcribed text, and third, a digital text, alters the data and invites a different treatment of them.[9] An audio recording offers the researcher opportunity to attend to language in a way that is impossible in field observations, but it retains none of the physical interaction that yields meaning in face-to-face encounters. An interview transcript affords opportunity for even closer analysis of language and linguistic structures, but in losing intonation and emotional expressiveness removes even more of the interaction cues. Computer software that encourages fragmentation and reassembly of many discrete units of data leads to a further recasting of the original meanings [19].[10]

Altering the data in this way invites the question (unanswerable within the scope of this paper) of whether the meanings that are detected in a recording or in a transcript could or would have been detected in interview conversation; and further, whether this matters. Is the 'truest' meaning of an interview interaction what the interviewer understood at the time; or what she subsequently comes to understand after twenty readings of a transcript? The assumption of grounded theory is, I think, the latter. But perhaps the language of everyday life is not designed for, and cannot bear the load of, interminable analysis. It may be that the meaning ascribed to transcript data is as much of a function of the transcript as it is of the original utterance.

Theoretical sampling

Theoretical sampling is one of the hallmarks of grounded theory. Its purpose is to gather data that will enable the researcher to further develop and more strongly ground concepts

---

9 See, for example, references 17 and 18, pp. 56–60.
10 My experience was consistent with Charmaz's assessment of computer-assisted qualitative data analysis. See reference 19.

and categories that are in the process of construction. (The approach to data analysis is described in greater detail below.) In the first phase, open sampling encourages exploration of 'persons, places and situations that will provide the greatest opportunity for discovery'. This is followed by relational and variational sampling, which is intended to elicit data that demonstrate variations in a concept or relationships among concepts. Finally, discriminate sampling seeks to generate data that validate or negate interpretations developed in preceding phases [13(p201–12)].

My initial sample of six potential participants was identified by reference to their reputation in their field. To give more specific detail could prejudice anonymity; however, it is safe to state that this sample included four men and two women medical directors leading district general hospital trusts, major teaching hospital trusts, or mental health trusts located across large metropolitan or smaller urban areas. Three of this sample responded and were included in the study.[11]

Working from the initial sample, I adopted a 'snowballing' technique to recruit further participants. Respondents were asked to recommend either colleagues whose outlook and experience was thought to be different from the interviewees' own, or, in some cases, colleagues whom they knew to have had a particular experience relevant to the emerging theory.[12] This technique elicited valuable introductions from interviewees to respected senior colleagues and secured a high rate of response, with all but two approaches resulting in a potential participant's inclusion in the study.

The aim of theoretical sampling is not to secure a representative sample from a population, nor to include all stakeholders, nor to seek to make a study more generalizable. The aim is to ensure that the data set includes whatever data are needed to elaborate a rich account of the key conceptual categories. As Hood has commented, 'theoretical sampling allows you to tighten ... the corkscrew or the hermeneutic spiral,' so that you end up with a theory that perfectly matches your data' [15(p101)]. A danger in theoretical sampling is thus that the researcher sets out to retrieve only confirmatory data. An important counterbalance is seeking to locate data that may introduce variation, disconfirm tentative assumptions or throw new light on the tentative conceptual categories [15(p101)].[13]

In this study, robust theoretical sampling was very difficult to achieve for three reasons: the difficulties in entering the field created by the ethical framework for research within the NHS; the snowball sampling technique; and significant conceptual revision late in the study.

The open sampling phase was designed to ensure variety of respondents and organizations, and it succeeded in doing so. However, significant delays in the R&D registration process meant that some participants approached early on during open sampling were not interviewed until the closing stages of the study. The same applied to some interviewees identified early in relational or variational sampling. Moreover, the scope for rigorous relational

---

[11] One professional group volunteered to distribute materials to some members. No responses were received through this avenue, and those materials may not have been circulated. Depending on whether this group is counted as non-respondents, between a half and three-quarters of those approached agreed to participate.

[12] E.g. colleagues who had developed policies on managing innovation.

[13] As Charmaz argues, the logic of theoretical sampling makes 'negative' cases ambiguous: 'negative' findings may become new properties of a category, or a new category. See reference 15, p. 101.

or variational sampling was limited by reliance on snowball recruitment. I was dependent upon interviewees in order to select and recruit further participants. This did result in variation, but with one or two exceptions data collection was perhaps closer to open data gathering than to relational or variational sampling. A degree of discriminate sampling was achieved, through recruiting five PCT medical directors late in the study. This permitted some testing of concepts that were thought to be specific to the acute hospital or mental health trust setting.

A further obstacle to theoretical sampling arose out of the late development of the core conceptual category of 'realizing moral narrative'. Its discovery is discussed below but it arose from some conceptual reconfiguration three-quarters of the way through the planned study. Without limitation of time or resource, conceptual revision in a grounded theory study should not prevent relational, variational or discriminate sampling from taking place. Following the reanalysis of data, one would simply continue to recruit participants to the study as necessary. Where time and resource are limited, however, major conceptual revision becomes a significant problem. This suggests a very real practical deterrent to developing robust grounded theory: any conceptual impediment to forward momentum can be extremely costly.

The logic of theoretical sampling continues into the notion of theoretical saturation. In principle, the researcher should continue to collect data until the categories are saturated, that is, until fresh data cease to reveal new properties in core categories. Clearly, then, theoretical saturation is as much a property of the emergent theory as it is a property in the data. Whether a category is saturated depends upon whether further theoretical sampling is capable of yielding variant data for further conceptual refinement. It is not necessarily reached when data appear to tell the same story, because this may merely indicate that better theoretical sampling or tighter analysis is needed [20].

It has been commented of grounded theory research that theoretical saturation is more often proclaimed than proved [21]. I shall resist that temptation. Whilst sufficient data were gathered to make this study a worthwhile and original contribution, I have little doubt that continuing data collection would yield greater insight into how moral narrative is negotiated, and into different organizational ethical challenges. That is work for the future.

Moving towards a theory: data analysis and the emergence of moral narrative

This study used an abductive research strategy, in which theory is developed by working 'upwards' from units of study data that include lay conceptions of social life [13(p136–7), 15(p103),22].[14]

---

[14] I touched upon the differences between deductive, inductive and abductive methods in the Epilogue to Chapters 4 and 5. There is disagreement about the reasoning process of grounded theory, perhaps because grounded theory is adopted as a strategy by researchers whose ontological assumptions are different. Strauss and Corbin characterize their procedures as 'moving between induction and deduction' (see reference 13, pp. 136–7). Constructivist researcher Charmaz eschews grounded theory's positivist roots and claims to reason abductively: 'reasoning about experience for making theoretical conjectures and then checking them through further experience. Abductive reasoning about the data starts with the data and subsequently moves toward hypothesis formation'. See reference 15, p. 103. She notes that Strauss was heavily influenced by C.S. Peirce, who developed the concept of abductive reasoning. Blaikie claims grounded theory is not abductive: 'much more a process of the researcher 'inventing' and imposing concepts on the data ... the various forms of coding

I started by adopting a process central to classic grounded theory, breaking the study data down into very small units to conduct a systematic 'micro-analysis' of its meaning. Coding and tentative theory-building began as soon as data were collected. These very small units for microanalysis consisted of single words, phrases or single lines of interview data [13(p65)].[15] The first phase of open coding involved examining and interpreting units of data in order to identify the characteristics of the phenomena they represented. This initial open coding identified concepts, relatively discrete units of social action described by respondents. Some concepts, referred to as *in vivo* concepts, were striking lay interpretations that seemed to present themselves 'fully formed'. Other concepts expressed my interpretation of a respondent's statement.

Grounded theory proposes a process of constant comparison to yield insight into the features that phenomena have in common, to identify where they differ, and to begin to group concepts together into categories.[16] The intention is, as concepts continue to be built up into categories, to elevate the most significant categories into one or more core conceptual categories. These core conceptual categories constitute the focal point of the 'theory'. I adopted a process of continuously

coding, reviewing concepts and categories, exploring similarities and differences between concepts and categories, and testing emergent categories.

From here, the story I intended to be able to tell was of a core conceptual category emerging in accordance with the idealized grounded theory process. This is not, however, how it was. In fact the core conceptual category – realizing moral narrative – emerged quite late. It was the result of a niggling sense that by breaking the data down for coding purposes, and doggedly developing ideas that had emerged early in data analysis, I might be missing the point of what I was subsequently hearing.

I am not the only researcher to have wondered whether the coding process I had adopted was in fact obscuring as much as it was revealing. It is rather rare, and therefore very refreshing, to read self-critical accounts of qualitative research processes, so Carolyn Ellis's gave me some succour at the time:

> In my book, I concentrated on . . .
> institutions and interactional patterns that
> 'order the lives of the people', because that's
> how a 'good' sociologist is supposed to
> construct the world . . . . Often, however,
> I saw as many exceptions and variations as
> I saw evidence for patterns. Nevertheless,
> my grounded theory approach forced me
> to concentrate on patterned responses . . . .
> When some detail didn't fit into a pattern,
> I explained it away . . . I convinced myself
> of the accuracy of what I said by pushing and
> squeezing all the details into my emerging
> categories. Although these categories had
> explanatory value, they presented life as
> lived much more categorically than actual
> day-to-day experiences warranted. [23]

are a search for technical concepts that will organize and make sense of the data . . . there appears to be little attempt to derive them from lay concepts, or to tie them to lay concepts'. See reference 22. This description may fit more positivist strands in grounded theory but would be rejected by Charmaz.

[15] 'Doing microanalysis compels the analyst to listen closely to what the interviewees are saying and how they are saying it . . . . This prevents us from jumping precipitously to our own theoretical conclusions.' See reference 13, p. 65.

[16] Discussions of grounded theory tend to use the words concept and category interchangeably. I follow Charmaz in using 'conceptual category' to refer to overarching concepts.

With my seventeenth interview as yet uncoded, I decided to adopt a different approach to analysing what Dr. Quentin Quinn had told me. My aim was to see what would emerge if I could code it without making use of any existing concepts. In the course of that exercise, one of Dr. Quinn's phrases stood out: 'we speak the same language'. In context, he was describing a productive working relationship with a highly respected colleague. But there was something more in that phrase 'we speak the same language'. Reviewing the interview as a whole, it became apparent that he had told several mini-stories about 'speaking the same language'. Sometimes this meant sharing the same priorities. Sometimes it meant sharing a moral outlook. Sometimes it meant taking the trouble to explain yourself to others, or to listen as others explained themselves to you. Sometimes it meant making compatible moral judgements. Negotiating understanding between different linguistic communities – between managers, patients, doctors, politicians, awkward colleagues – was the vital precondition to getting difficult things done. Moreover, where a 'different language' remained unintelligible in the face of all attempts to understand it, it was a sign of a potential trouble.

When I went back to re-examine earlier data, and the codes and categories into which I had sorted it, it began to become clear what the point was that I had been missing. What those codes and categories contained were reports of people engaging in narrative-making activity with each other. They were crammed with details of narrative interaction. What I was being told was everything that had to be said and done by some, and heard and seen by others, so that people could eventually come to share a moral understanding.

What was equally striking was how I was being told about this narrative-making activity. It was through the recounting of moral narratives that I was being told how shared moral narratives were made. I had found out the slow, experiential way what other narrative researchers had already discovered: that 'traditional approaches to qualitative analysis often fracture these texts in the service of interpretation and generalization by taking bits and pieces, snippets of a response edited out of context. They eliminate the sequential and structural features that characterize narrative accounts' [18(p3)].

As I reviewed the clusters of codes and quotations that microanalysis had created, I began to appreciate a nice irony. Scanning down the serried lists of codes and categories that appeared on the computer screen, it was possible to see them for what they were: narrative-making components. In their serried lists it was impossible to see where they had come from: moral narratives. The process of microanalysis, the tearing apart of narrative, had both concealed and revealed the core conceptual category.

Strauss and Corbin's account of grounded theory describes open coding as a process of breaking down the data, to be followed by axial coding, when data are to be put back together in new ways. At the axial coding stage Strauss and Corbin encourage the analyst to 'reassembl[e] data that were fractured during open coding' [13(p124)]. Now that I was beginning to understand them, I wanted to preserve the coherence in these narratives of moral action and narratives of self. To me, this has meant reassembling their structure and meaning as integrated moral narratives, accounts of both the world and the self.

The meaning in interview narratives, and the ontological status of 'moral narrative'

What is the status of the interview data, and can they support the claims that I have made? In a letter to a colleague, the sociologist Herbert Blumer remarked, 'The central problem of social science, which ostensibly is trying to understand human behaviour, is the problem of communication' [24(p163)].[17] His comment shares the recursive irony of a student slogan that apparently adorned the streets of Paris in 1968, 'IT IS FORBIDDEN

TO FORBID'.[18] Who is to know exactly what Blumer meant when he wrote that the central problem was the problem of communication? Maines suggests, 'Blumer understood that human conduct ... is communicative in its fundamental nature' [24(p163)]. If we are to understand, therefore, how humans conduct social life we must understand at every level – macro, meso and micro – how humans communicate with one another. Humans' interactive, communicative behaviour is social life.

There is, however, another sense in which the social sciences must confront the problem of communication. It is how we are to understand what 'informants' communicate to 'researchers' when researchers ask informants to report on social life.

What happens when an ethicist seeks information from a medical director for research purposes [25]?[19] The answer to the question helps to determine what meaning we may ascribe to the interview data. Are the findings merely an artefact of the research design, with data taking the form of a moral narrative because they were elicited in the form of a moral narrative? Are these narratives simply a display of the narrator's self-justificatory moral objectives? Or are they a report on the world as it is? These questions raise methodological concerns going to the internal validity of the research, and take us into vexing issues of ontology and epistemology.

In summary, the answers are as follows. First, the medical directors spontaneously organized many of their explanations and descriptions as narratives. When they described in detail how they had managed troubling situations, their explanation took the form of a moral narrative of the type described in Chapter 6. Second, these narratives were not innocent of persuasive intent but shaped by participants' desires to give a good account of themselves. In the context of the interview they were intended to communicate personal meaning as well as experience; they were explanations that projected a preferred moral self. Third, I propose that medical directors' moral narratives correspond to (but are not isomorphic with) the world of experience. By this I mean that the moral narratives that medical directors recounted are the residual 'thought objects' of the narrative interactions that they have experienced in the world. To the extent that they report a process of a moral narrating, it is their experience, as they understood it, that they recall. They supply neither an exhaustive nor an undistorted account of moral narrating. The interview narratives were a 'living history', both reliable and unreliable in the way that all history must be.

I now consider these answers in greater detail.

The presence of moral narrative

Why did my informants recount (moral) narratives? A simple answer would be that they did so because this is how humans organize meaning and communicate their experience. The founding assumption of an array of narrative research methods is that:

> A primary way individuals make sense
> of experience is by casting it in narrative
> form .... Precisely because they are essential
> meaning-making structures, narratives must
> be preserved, not fractured, by investigators,
> who must respect respondents' ways of
> constructing meaning and analyze how
> it is accomplished. [18(p4)]

For Mishler classic objectivist methods of interview research, such as standardized questions, served only to suppress spontaneously occurring narrative accounts [26].

---

[17] Letter from Herbert Blumer to Robert Park; 1939, in reference 24, p. 163.

[18] Recalled in a BBC Radio 4 broadcast '1968: Myth or Reality', 29 April 2008.

[19] Cf. reference 25: 'What happens during the moment when a sociologist seeks information from someone else for sociological purposes?'

To get better data on the authentic experience of interviewees, researchers ought to offer them the opportunity to do what they would do 'naturally' outside an 'artificial' and constraining interview context. Unstructured, in-depth interviews are a means, according to Mishler, by which the interviewer can 'empower respondents ... to find and speak in their own "voices"' [26(p118)]. These voices would generate narrative accounts otherwise repressed by the controlling, interrogative approach that had dominated quantitative research interviews and infiltrated positivistic qualitative research.

It is not essential to my argument to join Mishler and other narrative researchers in seeing narrative as a means of accessing fully authentic selves [27]. My claim is that narrative emerged in the interviews because the interviewees found it the most appropriate way to recount their experience, an experience that was, in turn, an experience of narrative. This requires a little further consideration.

Elliot has cautioned that even researchers interested in eliciting and hearing stories or other narratives [18(p18)][20] may fail to do so. She has suggested that not only must interview questions be open-ended and framed in everyday language if narrative is to emerge, but they should also invite the interviewee to focus on specific times and situations [28,29]. Reviewing the skills the narrative interviewer needs, she notes it is

widely recognized ... that the subjects of research are eager to comply with the wishes of the researchers and to provide the type of responses the researcher is looking for. If the researcher implicitly communicates that narrative responses are not what is wanted ... this in some senses 'trains' the respondent to provide a different type of information. [30]

The notion of 'training' the respondent can be turned on its head; perhaps narrative interviews are the result of interviewers coaching their interviewees to offer up narrative? Elliot's discussion thus begs the question whether a narrative response to questions is any more 'natural' than any other sort of response.

Early supporters of narrative research frequently treated the ubiquity of narrative in social life as self-evident. Researchers claimed that the narratives that erupted into their interviews were not idiosyncratic responses to an artificial situation, but were comparable to the narratives that arose spontaneously in social life [31,32]. There is now an accumulating evidence base that supports this view, illustrating naturally occurring narrative behaviour in diverse settings from commercial corporations to self-help health groups [33–35].[21,22]

More significantly, narration is a familiar component of medical practice, extensively documented and discussed. A few examples: the 'history-taking' that converts patients' experience into formal medical narrative [36,37], the importance of the patients' own personal narrative [38], the dark humour and horror stories of medical education [39], and the narratives that serve as conduits of nursing expertise [40]. Wherever else in society narrative erupts, and for whatever reason, narrative is omnipresent in medical practice. We would expect, then, to find among expert doctors many consummate narrators. This may mean that they narrated because this is

---

[20] Riessman is clear that stories are not the only narrative genre: she elicited 'habitual narratives (when events happen over and over and consequently there is no peak in the action), hypothetical narratives (which depict events that did not happen), and topic centred narratives (snapshots of past events that are linked thematically'. See reference 18, p. 18.

[21] Cf. naturalistic decision-making research, which uses story to analyse expertise. See reference 33.
[22] References 34 and 35 are both studies of natural settings.

what doctors do; it may mean that they narrated because this is how experience is recalled; it may mean they narrated because morality is enacted through narrative. There is reason enough in the data to consider the last proposition to be plausible.

While narratives may seem ubiquitous, it is clear that narratives are used for some communicative purposes but not for others. Many communicative interactions do not call for narrative organization. If someone asks me to tell them the time, I do not respond by telling a story about clocks. It seems equally to be the case however that some forms of human communication demand a narrative pattern. If stopping to tell an inquirer the time makes me late for an appointment, I may endeavour to exculpate myself by offering a narrative explanation to the person I kept waiting. If I am a skilled social actor (a skilled narrator) the narrative is one that will present me as morally praiseworthy: 'The poor child looked so worried, I couldn't not stop. And then I missed the bus'. Just as this exculpatory story assumed a narrative pattern, so too did moral communications in the data. Accounts of troubling events took on the form of moral narratives.

Narrating a preferred moral self

My example of framing a narrative so as to anticipate and answer reproach echoes the point made by Riessman in the introduction to this discussion: narratives both communicate meaning and recount experience. So how ought we to interpret what we are told? What in a narrative should we construe as primarily a communication of personal meaning, and what in narrative should we treat as a report on experience?

Just as we might expect medical directors to exhibit their virtuosity as narrators, we might also expect them to display their virtue through their narrative. We need now to consider the personal moral meanings that may have been embedded in the narratives that the interview encounter produced. To recall the question that opened this discussion: what happens when an ethicist seeks information from a medical director for research purposes? A part of the answer is that the interview narrative is a vehicle for the presentation of a preferred moral self. This 'preferred self' was often (but not always) a moral activist, the protagonist at the centre of the moral narrative. He or she appeared in references to moral virtues, moral doubts and moral anxieties. How much of the interview narrative is an account of an internal self, and how much an account of an external reality?

The validity of interview data has been widely debated across the domain of social research, and it is unsurprising that the field of narrative research has itself come to reflect these patterns of discord. In positivist social research, 'impression management', 'conformist respondents', 'interviewer effects' and other intrusions into reportage irreversibly contaminate interview data. At the other extreme, strongly interpretivist social research has treated the 'contaminations' in the data as the data that are truly worth studying, for what they unintentionally and obliquely reveal. It is not that interview effects result in contaminated data, it is that 'interview effects' constitute different data. Similarly, some narrative researchers treat narrative as a superior way of retrieving data about individuals' lived experience of an external reality, consistent with 'realist' or 'weak' constructivist approaches. Others treat narrative as a superior way of retrieving data about individuals' subjective interpretations and meanings, reflecting ethnomethodological or 'strong' social constructivist orientations. The former treat interview narratives as internally valid data that express a communicative interaction with an interviewer. The latter treat interview narratives as internally valid data giving access to an understanding the social world of the interviewee.

Although there are theorists at the extreme ends of the spectrum who view the naturalist/realist and ethnographic/strong constructionist approaches to interview data as mutually exclusive, qualitative researchers more commonly endeavour to steer a course between the two [41]. Holstein and Gubrium, for instance, give a constructionist account of analyzing the 'active interview' in which the goal:

> is to show how interview responses are produced in the interaction between interviewer and respondent, without losing sight of the meanings produced or the circumstances that condition the meaning-making process. The analytic objective is not merely to describe the situated production of talk, but to show how what is being said relates to the experiences and lives being studied. [42,43][23]

It would be hard to refute Dingwall and Murphy's 'subtle realist' contention that all interviews are occasions for impression management [44], and absurd to disagree with them that the effects of this need to be taken into account. As they point out, 'all parties – informants and interviewers alike – strive to present themselves as competent, sane, and moral persons to those with whom they are interacting' [45(p86)]. In an inquiry into actual ethical practice, we would expect interviewees to wish to appear particularly competent, sane and moral. The question then is what impact this expectation should have on our construction of the interview narratives.

Stimson and Webb's seminal study of doctor-patient interaction was among the first to explore how interview narratives reflected interviewees' aims during their encounter with researchers [46]. Having been observed as passive and compliant in their medical consultation, Stimson and Webb's patient interviewees went on to recount 'atrocity

stories' about their doctors in the interview. In many of these stories the patients painted themselves as the protagonist, the doctor as the villain of the piece, and the moral of the tale as vindication of the patient's point of view. Stimson and Webb concluded that patients narrated their atrocity stories in an attempt to redress the inequality they felt in the doctor-patient relationship. Baruch drew a comparable conclusion in his analysis of the atrocity stories that emerged from a study of the parents of children suffering from cystic fibrosis [47]. He interpreted the parents' atrocity stories as narratives that allowed them to present themselves as morally good parents. They composed an account of events that addressed their feelings of guilt and responsibility, as much as it reported the history of their child's diagnosis.

What might have been at stake for participants in the present study? Participants were invited to describe a situation that was both 'troubling' and that they had 'dealt with'. As research into the experience of ostensibly powerful professionals, it is notably different from inquiries into doctor-patient inequality. My interviewees may have been seeking covertly to persuade me of something, but it was not that they were more important than institutions told them they were. They had the opportunity to offer up for scrutiny a creditable moral performance of their own choice, reducing the need to gloss personal or organizational difficulties. As a result, this study seems not to have suffered from the pretence that everything is well, a problem that Dingwall experienced in his interviews with child protection service directors [45(p85)]. Only one of the medical directors seemed to me to be unwilling to confess to personal or organizational troubles; others disclosed them, but sometimes requested that details be withheld. If participants harboured doubts about whether they were as effective as they believed they should be, this did not

---

[23] Reference 42 quoted in reference 43.

deter them from presenting a frank, and occasionally unflattering, portrait of themselves and their milieu. So if they had no need to narrate a reversal of power or retrospectively rectify their failures, did other concerns nevertheless pervade the interviewees' talk?

For some, the interview undoubtedly supplied a rare opportunity to acknowledge the burdens of office (we noted the significance of acknowledgement in Chapter 5) without running the risk of losing respect. And for some, the interview was also an occasion to present their moral judgement as a Solomonic balance between the needs of patients and the claims of colleagues. They were at pains to portray themselves as at once attentive and compassionate towards patients, while wielding moral authority over colleagues in a manner more consensual than coercive. As they narrated it, when colleagues erred, interviewees would present a certain 'face': it was 'a countenance more in sorrow than in anger' [44,48].[24] Such judgements reflect, I think, a desire to reconcile their potentially conflicting loyalties to patients and peers, and to manage the personal and political vulnerabilities that these potentially conflicting loyalties produce. Clinician leaders become *primus inter pares*: simultaneously 'one of us' and 'one of them', an equal and a superior, a practitioner and a judge. To say that one has done what must be done, but done it with sincere regret, is a way of saying that one has balanced the moral demands of patients and colleagues without denying anything due to either. To appeal to the internal morality of medical practice, and to present oneself as an active but conscientious arbiter of agreed-upon standards is to stake a claim to the trust of both patients and fellow professionals.

---

[24] The term 'face' is Goffman's; see reference 44. The phrase is from *Hamlet* Act 1, Scene 2. See reference 48[1].

The evidence for moral narrating

I return one final time to my question: what happens when an ethicist seeks information from a medical director for research purposes? I argued in Chapter 6 that medical directors recounted narratives that were echoes of narrative interaction in the world. I hope that I have shown, convincingly, that moral narratives may be found in what my informants said. This takes me to the final part of my argument, which is that moral narrating appears also to be what my informants do when they are enacting ethics. What is the status of this claim? It rests upon the interpretivist (that is, constructivist) ontology and epistemology that the study has assumed.

I have argued that the oral moral narratives presented in the interview situation corresponded to interactive moral narratives that were a part of the medical directors' experience. In striving to make sense of what participants told me, I have differentiated between the narratives and meanings that were internal to our interaction, and the narratives and meanings that were a part of informants' external realities. Although as Riessman notes, informants' narrative accounts are 'constructed, creatively authored, rhetorical, replete with assumptions, and interpretive' [18(p5)] this does not imply that they afford no window onto a world that is 'out there'.

Ontology

What do I mean by the world 'out there'? Social reality is the social construction of social actors,

> in the basic sense that whatever it is that humans have in their societies – from economic structures to bureaucracies, courts, values, ideologies, racism, single parent families, romantic relationships, or whatever – human beings have created them somewhere along the line. [24(p228)]

This study is set in the complex social world constructed to manage the obdurate physical demands of failing or uncooperative bodies, and the perplexing social challenges of disordered or unhappy minds. It is a remarkable social achievement to create, routinize and maintain this particular world, and to preserve its moral order in the face of disruptive events. Disruption might be a contravention of the social order, such as an egregious failure to respect what is left of patients' dignity in this milieu; it could be a surprising turn of event in the material order, such as an unexpected death. Disruptions force themselves on actors' attention, and demand a response, requiring that sense be made of them. But actors notice the need for sensemaking because, for the most part, an agreed and settled sense has already been made.

Those who work in healthcare experience disruption because they hold normative expectations of how things really are, and about how things should really be, normative expectations that have been constituted in the process of human interaction and engagement with that complex social reality.

In this interpretivist ontology, social actors *make* the realm of the social (such as the social organization of the hospital) and they make *meaningful* the realm of the material (such as the body). By making the body meaningful we can, within limits, remake the body too: treat it, cure it, alter it, restore it. To treat social reality as a social construction in this way is not to treat meaning as transcendent, so that 'all that is solid melts into air' [49].[25] In the basic sense in which I use it, social constructivism recognizes both the contingent power of social forces and the non-contingent presence of material realities. Basic social constructivism acknowledges that a society's system of law, for example, operates as a social fact, but

that it could always have been constituted otherwise than how it is. Basic social constructivism is compatible with the subtle realist's warning that it would be unwise to fly at low altitude with a pilot who believes mountains are a social construct [45(p12)].

Institutions such as aviation and healthcare are social and linguistic achievements that work, because they create a fit between our cognition and the world beyond us. Aviation is a set of social constructs that succeeds, because it reflexively theorizes gravity and treats mountains as more than a mere matter of belief. Healthcare is a stable social construction that persists because it reflexively theorizes and manages health, treating body and mind in accordance with, but as more than merely, systems of meaning.

On this account, narrating is a means of constituting – that is, actively creating – social reality. It is also, as an interview artefact, a means of understanding how and what social reality has been created.

Epistemology

This study is an examination both of the social phenomenon – morality – that concerns moral philosophers, and of some philosophical conceptions of that social phenomenon. In Chapter 1 I noted that, for philosophers, the term 'morality' refers to a special compartment of lived experience, a social phenomenon; and the term 'ethics' refers to the normative study of this special compartment of lived experience. In the process of inquiring into how the compartment of lived experience felt to be morally loaded was lived, I found it necessary to reject some philosophical assumptions about the nature of moral experience. Theoretical-juridical moral theories (TJM) treat the lived experience of morality as a matter of making moral choices in accordance with moral rules, norms and consequences. Walker's expressive-collaborative

---

[25] The phrase seems to have originated in reference 49.

model (ECM) on the other hand treats the lived experience of morality as an ongoing negotiation of mutual responsibilities. I found moral experience to be more akin to the ECM than the TJM.

The social actors who live morality operate according to their models of the world: models that Schütz has called 'thought objects'. Social actors have their own schemes, perceptions, frameworks and assumptions through which they make sense of experience, formulate plans of action and offer a retrospective account of what they have done. It is these thought objects that have been studied here. I have then constructed further 'thought objects' (moral narrative, propriety, for example) that I believe faithfully represent those social actors' social reality. The narratives I have discussed are 'thought objects' serving not only the social actor but also, in this case, the social scientist.

> The thought objects constructed by the social scientist, in order to grasp this social reality, have to be founded upon the thought objects constructed by the common-sense thinking of men [sic], living their daily life within their social world. Thus, the constructs of the social sciences are, so to speak, constructs of the second degree, that is, constructs of the constructs made by the actors on the social scene. [22(p117),50]

Thus 'what happens when an ethicist seeks information from a medical director for research purposes' is that she gains access to some of the 'thought objects' medical leaders construct for the purposes of 'living their daily life within their social world'. Using those thought objects, she can begin to model the social interactions of everyday ethical life.

But what ethical reality can reliably be modelled from the 'thought objects' present in the data? A moral narrative in the interview transcript is an echo of life as it had been lived in the sense that it is a record of how one person interpreted and recalled

the life that they had experienced. The moral narratives of the interview are a fleeting glimpse, from individual informants' points of view, of what reality itself had seemed to be as they lived it.

The study participants' social realities may not have appeared to others to be what study participants thought they were. But in so far as the moral narratives recall how situations were defined as real, the 'Thomas theorem' applies: 'situations defined as real are real in their consequences' [51].[26] The moral narratives recall something of how sense was made of situations, what had been thought to be real, and what the effects were of making a certain sense of situations. The moral narratives in the interviews record a remembered and re-described life. It would be foolish to see in them anything approaching scientific truth, purportedly accurate, objective and exhaustive accounts of what actually happened. They are, however, echoes of ways of knowing and thus making the world.

The stories not told

The data presented an embarrassment of riches, and they contain many stories that remain untold in this account of ethical enactment. We should note here the other possibilities that these data presented.

First, the interpretations of the data are interpretations, albeit well grounded ones. Another researcher might have followed different cues in the interviews, formulated different concepts from initial data, pursued different theoretical conjectures in later interviews, and construed otherwise the emotional tenor and ethical implications of medical leaders' narratives. If the 'grand narrative' that I have derived from these data is grounded, coherent and plausible, there may nevertheless be others equally so.

Next, the data supplied valuable insight into aspects of these medical leaders'

---

[26] Cited in reference 51.

professional lives that have not received a great deal of attention here. All of the interviewees recounted in detail their experience of becoming a medical director, what they believed qualified them for the role, and the dynamics of power within their organizations. The account I have rendered in previous chapters hints at the significance of career biographies and organizational culture for medical leadership, but it has not been possible to fully develop these themes for reasons of space and balance.

Finally, this account of medical leadership is not exhaustive of the data. Some interviewees described ethical concerns that, in this study, were unique to them. I have made reference to some individual troubles, while others remain hidden from view. In a larger sample further participants might have echoed individual anxieties, elevating them to more substantial categories; or it might have been possible to conclude that minority views were idiosyncratic, and isolated experiences unusual. In this study, all that could be supposed was that some participants' outlook or experience was not widely shared by others in the sample. Their concerns have, however, assumed less prominence in the discussion.

The world will always be 'incorrigibly plural'. No method of inquiry can hold the social world still, and simple and singular. Nor should it, because that is not the world's nature. Ultimately, I make both a modest and an immodest claim for this research. Modestly, this study imperfectly captures something of the experience of moral leadership. Immodestly, in spite of its imperfections, I believe it has uncovered a certain 'reality' of morality absent from empirically ungrounded moral theories.

References

1. Ryle G. The Thinking of Thoughts; What is Le Penseur Doing?. Collected Papers. London: Hutchinson; 1971.

2. Geertz C. Thick description: toward an interpretative theory of culture. The Interpretation of Cultures. New York: Basic Books; 1973.

3. Holm S. Ethical Problems in Clinical Practice: The Ethical Reasoning of Healthcare Professionals. Manchester: Manchester University Press; 1997.

4. Anspach R, Mizrachi N. The field worker's fields: ethics, ethnography and medical sociology. In: de Vries R, Turner L, Orfali K, Bosk C, eds. The View From Here: Bioethics and the Social Sciences. Oxford: Blackwell; 2007, pp. 48–66.

5. Anspach RR. Deciding Who Lives: Fateful Choices in the Intensive Care Nursery. Berkeley: University of California Press; 1993.

6. Walker MU. Moral Understandings: A Feminist Study in Ethics. 2nd edn. New York: Oxford University Press; 2007, p. 103.

7. Bosk CL. Forgive and Remember: Managing Medical Failure. 2nd edn. Chicago: University of Chicago Press; 2003.

8. Rest J. Moral Development; Advances in Research and Theory. New York: Praeger; 1986.

9. Jones TM. Ethical Decision Making by Individuals in Organizations; An Issue Contingent Model. Academy of Management Review. 1991;16(2):366–95.

10. Chambliss DF. Beyond Caring: Hospitals, Nurses, and the Social Organization of Ethics. Chicago: Chicago University Press; 1996.

11. Morse J, Richards L. Read Me First: For a User's Guide to Qualitative Methods. London: Sage; 2002.

12. Glaser B, Strauss A. Discovery of Grounded Theory. Chicago: Aldine; 1967.

13. Strauss A, Corbin J. Basics of Qualitative Research: Techniques and Procedures for Developing Grounded Theory. Thousand Oaks, CA: Sage; 1998.

14. Glaser B. Basics of Grounded Theory Analysis. Mill Valley, CA: The Sociology Press; 1992.

15. Charmaz K. Constructing Grounded Theory: A Practical Guide through Qualitative Analysis. London: Sage; 2006.

16. McMahon JM, Harvey RJ. The effect of moral intensity on ethical judgment. *Journal of Business Ethics.* 2007;**72**:335–57.

17. Kvale S. *InterViews: An Introduction to Qualitative Research Interviewing.* Thousand Oaks, CA: Sage; 1996. pp. 166–70.

18. Riessman CK. *Narrative Analysis.* London: Sage; 1993.

19. Charmaz K. Grounded theory: objectivist and constructivist methods. In: Denzin NK, Lincoln YS, eds. *Handbook of Qualitative Research.* 2nd edn. London: Sage; 2000, pp. 509–35.

20. Dey I. *Grounding Grounded Theory.* San Diego: Academic Press; 1999, p. 257.

21. Morse J. The significance of saturation. *Qualitative Health Research.* 1995;**5**:147–9.

22. Blaikie N. *Designing Social Research: The Logic of Anticipation.* Cambridge: Polity Press; 2000.

23. Ellis C. Emotional and ethical quagmires in returning to the field. *Journal of Contemporary Ethnography.* 1995;**24**(1): 68–98.

24. Maines DR. *The Faultline of Consciousness.* New York: Aldine de Gruyter; 2001.

25. Maines DR. Narrative's moment and sociology's phenomena: toward a narrative sociology. *Sociological Quarterly.* 1993; **34**(1):17–38.

26. Mishler EG. *Research Interviewing: Context and Narrative.* Cambridge, MA: Harvard University Press; 1986.

27. Clandinin DJ, Connelly FM. *Narrative Inquiry: Experience and Story in Qualitative Research.* San Francisco: Jossey Bass; 2000.

28. Chase SE. Taking narrative seriously: consequences for method and theory in interview studies. In: Josselson R, Lieblich A, eds. *Interpreting Experience: The Narrative Study of Lives.* Thousand Oaks, CA: Sage; 1995.

29. Hollway W, Jefferson T. *Doing Qualitative Research Differently: Free Association, Narrative and the Interview Method.* London: Sage; 2000.

30. Elliott J. *Using Narrative in Social Research.* London: Sage; 2005, p. 31.

31. Cox SM. Stories in decisions: how at-risk individuals decide to request predictive testing for Huntingdon Disease. *Qualitative Sociology.* 2003;**26**:257–80.

32. Linde C. *Life Stories; The Creation of Coherence.* Oxford: Oxford University Press; 1993.

33. Klein G. *Sources of Power: How People Make Decisions.* Cambridge, MA: MIT Press; 1999.

34. Boje DM. The storytelling organization: a study of story performance in an office-supply firm. *Administrative Science Quarterly.* 1991;**36**:106–26.

35. Currie G, Brown AD. A narratological approach to understanding processes of organizing in a UK hospital. *Human Relations.* 2003;**56**(5):563–86.

36. Hunter KM. *How Doctors Think: Clinical Judgment and the Practice of Medicine.* New York: Oxford University Press; 2006.

37. Sinclair S. *Making Doctors: An Institutional Apprenticeship.* Oxford: Berg; 1997.

38. Greenhalgh T, Hurwitz B, eds. *Narrative Based Medicine.* London: BMJ Books; 1998.

39. Calman KC. *A Study of Storytelling, Humour and Learning in Medicine.* London: The Stationery Office; 2000.

40. Benner P. *From Novice to Expert: Excellence and Power in Clinical Nursing Practice.* Menlo Park, CA: Addison-Wesley 1984.

41. Seale C. Qualitative interviewing. In: Seale C, ed. *Researching Society and Culture.* London: Sage; 1998, pp. 202–16.

42. Holstein J, Gubrium J. Active interviewing. In: Silverman D, ed. *Qualitative Research: Theory, Method, and Practice.* London: Sage; 1997, pp. 113–29.

43. Silverman D. *Interpreting Qualitative Data: Methods for Analysing Talk, Text and Interaction.* London: Sage; 1993, 2001, p. 97.

44. Goffman E. *The Presentation of Self in Everyday Life.* London: Penguin; 1990.

45. Dingwall R, Murphy E. *Qualitative Methods and Health Policy Research.* New York: Aldine de Gruyter; 2003.

46. Stimson G, Webb N. *Going to See the Doctor*. London: Routledge & Kegan Paul; 1975.

47. Baruch G. Moral tales: parents stories of encounters with the health profession. *Sociology of Health and Illness*. 1981; 3(3):275–96.

48. Spencer TJB, ed. *The New Penguin Shakespeare*. London: Penguin; 1979.

49. Marx K, Engels F. *The Communist Manifesto*. 1848.

50. Schütz A. Concept and theory formation in the social sciences. In: Natanson MA, ed. *Philosophy of the Social Sciences*. New York: Random House; 1963, pp. 231–49.

51. Clarke AE. *Situational Analysis: Grounded Theory after the Postmodern Turn*. London: Sage; 2005, p. 7.

Appendix 2: Accountability for clinical performance: individuals and organizations

The framework for regulation, oversight, management, and accountability in respect of doctors' conduct has consisted of five overlapping domains:

1. Professional regulation by the General Medical Council (GMC) overseen by the Council for Healthcare Regulatory Excellence (CHRE; currently being renamed and given greater powers).
2. Employee management procedures applied to doctors employed by NHS Trusts.
3. Local regulatory framework applied to General Practitioners treating NHS patients in primary care.
4. Service provider regulation by the Care Quality Commission.
5. The common law, for example the crime of assault and the torts of battery and negligence.

The activities of NHS Trusts, professional regulators and lawyers are supported and augmented by the medical Royal Colleges, agencies including the National Clinical Assessment Service and the National Health Service Litigation Authority, and by doctors' own protective bodies such as the Medical Defence Union, the Medical Protection Society and the British Medical Association.

In this overview I concentrate on professional regulation, hospital employer procedures and regulation of primary care practitioners. Performance management practices are evolving further, owing to the long-delayed introduction of revalidation for doctors, in which the licence to practice will have to be renewed every five years; the abolition of the Primary Care Trusts which have played an important role in reviewing the performance of General Practitioners; and regulatory changes associated with NHS reorganization.

Professional self-regulation

The UK General Medical Council has responsibility for regulating individual professionals. Following completion of their bachelor's-level medical degree, newly qualified doctors receive provisional registration with the GMC while they undertake a year of supervised training and education in the Foundation Year One programme. On successful completion they are fully qualified and may apply for full registration.

Any doctor working in unsupervised medical practice in the UK must have full registration with the GMC. 'Unsupervised' does not mean without any further training; it means that their registration is no longer provisional, as it is during the Foundation One year, and they have acquired the right to prescribe medicines and to carry out procedures for which they have been trained. Since 2007 UK or International Medical Graduates new to full registration are required to work in so-called Approved Practice Settings. These are organizations whose management, governance and supervisory systems have been approved by the GMC. Most NHS hospitals are Approved Practice Settings.

As medical careers proceed, most doctors will train to become hospital specialists or General Practitioners. On qualifying, they enter onto either the specialist or GP registers held by the GMC. NHS Consultants in medical or surgical specialties are required to be included in the specialist register, and GPs are required to be included in the GP register. This requirement has implications for the employment of hospital specialists in particular, if they do not successfully revalidate (see below).

As well as its responsibility for maintaining the registers of practitioners and hearing complaints about those on the register, the GMC also regulates medical education and training. Its remit extends from the undergraduate years right through to specialist registration. As a regulator it sets out requirements for education and training that are then implemented by higher education providers and local NHS organizations. Providers are subject to periodic review of their education and training provision by the GMC. The medical Royal Colleges support specialist registration by playing a leading role in determining specialty standards, the content of specialty training and qualification in the specialty. Their standards and curricula are approved by the GMC.

Raising concerns about doctors

Members of the public may make complaints directly to the GMC, or referral may be made by an employing organization. All doctors are subject to organizational-level performance management procedures, and these are discussed below.

The Fitness to Practise (FTP) procedures

The legal framework for the FTP procedures is set out in the Medical Act 1983 and the Fitness to Practise Rules 2004. The GMC may seek to remove a doctor from the register on grounds of misconduct, deficient performance, physical or mental ill health, a criminal conviction or caution or a determination by another regulatory body either in the UK or overseas. Following the Shipman Inquiry it had been proposed to separate the investigation and adjudication function, with the GMC retaining the investigatory responsibilities and a separate body undertaking adjudication. Following consultation this plan was dropped in December 2010, so the GMC continues to carry out both functions.

Streaming stage

The initial stage of the Fitness to Practise procedure is an assessment by the GMC of the severity of the complaint.

Stream One complaints are those assessed as requiring immediate action by the GMC.

Stream Two complaints are those assessed as being more suitable for local resolution. These complaints are referred to the employing hospital or commissioning PCT, and the local body is responsible for deciding whether to investigate further.

If local procedures raise serious doubts about a doctor's fitness to practise, the case is referred back to the GMC. The GMC will conduct its own investigation and make a determination whether or not to invoke the FTP procedures.

Investigation stage

Stream One complaints are investigated by the GMC and may entail obtaining further documentary evidence or witness statements, commissioning an expert report on clinical concerns, conducting an assessment of the doctor's performance at work or commissioning an assessment of the doctor's health.

Where it is believed that a doctor should be suspended or restricted from practising pending the outcome of the investigation, the GMC may refer the case to an Interim Orders Panel.

At the end of the investigation the GMC may conclude the case with no further action, issue a warning, require the doctor to make undertakings regarding health or performance issues, or refer the case to a full FTP panel with powers to remove the doctor from the register.

Adjudication stage

Cases referred to an FTP panel may conclude in exoneration, a warning or a view that fitness to practise is impaired. Where fitness to practise is impaired, the GMC may impose conditions requiring the doctor to work under supervision or to give up certain areas of practice (e.g. treating children), suspend the doctor from the register so that they may not practise for a determined period, or remove the doctor from the register altogether.

Following an FTP hearing, the doctor has 28 days in which to appeal. The Council for Healthcare Regulatory Excellence has the right to request that a case be referred to the High Court if it is of the view that the GMC decision is unduly lenient.

Revalidation

In 2007 the Government published its response to the Shipman and other inquiries [1]. It proposed to move forward with processes for periodic revalidation of medical practitioner registration, processes that had been mooted for several decades. These developments will be of considerable significance for the future management of under-performing doctors.

Hitherto, once doctors were registered with the GMC they were registered for life unless they were actively removed from the register following Fitness to Practise proceedings. From 2012 (the implementation date has been delayed several times) doctors in practice will be required to revalidate their licence to practise every five years. Revalidation will be on the basis of satisfactory annual 'enhanced' appraisal, which will require evidence of continuing professional development as well as of continuing satisfactory performance. Doctors on the specialist register who are certified

to practise in a specialty will be required to demonstrate continuing satisfactory performance in their specialty or sub-specialty as well as general competence.

Revalidation will be accompanied by new structures. Responsible Officers (most likely the Trust Medical Director) will be required to make a recommendation for revalidation to the GMC, who will then make the formal decision to permit continued registration. A network of GMC Affiliates will be appointed to provide advice and supervision at regional level.

At the date of writing the full revalidation process is still under development by the GMC, the Department of Health and the medical Royal Colleges. It is expected that doctors who appear unlikely – on the basis of poor annual appraisal – to revalidate will be supported by their employers, and offered opportunity to work under supervision for a period of remediation. The need for remediation ought to be identified early through appraisal, and remedial support should begin well before the date for revalidation is due. Doctors who still fail to satisfy the Responsible Officer that revalidation should be supported would be referred to the GMC's fitness to practice procedures for investigation. As the GMC has a range of powers under its fitness to practise procedures they could decide to take no action (in which case the doctor would be revalidated), issue a warning, place conditions on registration, or suspend or erase the doctor from the register.

Employment procedures

The Department of Health published guidance on procedures governing doctors in NHS employment in 2003 (*High Professional Standards in the Modern N.H.S*) [2]. A subsequent document, *Directions on Disciplinary Procedures 2005*, required all NHS bodies in England to implement the agreed framework by June 2005 but significant elements had been widely introduced prior to this.

High Professional Standards governs the employment of doctors in NHS Trusts, and is treated as advisory for doctors employed by NHS Foundation Trusts. It is the current government's intention that all NHS Trusts should become Foundation Trusts (these are public hospitals with somewhat greater freedoms than standard NHS organizations and governance arrangements that include elected user 'governors').

High Professional Standards in the Modern NHS

High Professional Standards supplies detailed guidance on internal procedures and the discharge of core responsibilities covering: first response when a concern arises, including possible restriction of practise and exclusion; concerns relating to misconduct, including hearings and termination of employment; concerns relating to capability, including capability panel procedures; and concerns about a practitioner's health. (I do not deal here with issues relating to health.)

Special provisions apply to doctors in training. Where there are doubts about the competence of trainees in either the Foundation Programme or specialist training, these are to be treated initially as educational and training issues. They are taken up first within the framework of supervision in the employing organization and where difficulties remain, trainees should be referred to the NHS Postgraduate Deanery. It is a frequently voiced concern among doctors supervising trainees that performance issues may not be effectively managed at local level, and that trainees escape surveillance in the frequent moves from one training post to another. As with any other doctor, concerns about trainees' fitness to practise, as distinct from concerns about their competence, may be referred to the GMC.

First response to concerns, whether conduct or capability, including restrictions and exclusions

NHS Trusts are required to have a framework of procedures for handling serious concerns about both conduct (i.e. 'behavioural' offences) and capability (i.e. 'technical' failure). When serious concerns are raised they must be registered with the Chief Executive, a non-executive director must be designated to oversee the case, and where concerns relate to consultant-level staff the medical director should act as a 'case manager'.

The case manager is responsible for overseeing a preliminary investigation. They determine:

- whether protection of patients requires placing temporary restrictions on the scope of clinical practice, or whether a doctor should be excluded from work;
- whether to refer the practitioner to the National Clinical Assessment Service (NCAS), which is able to carry out an assessment of the clinician's performance or health;
- whether a formal investigation is required under conduct or capability procedures.

It is the case manager's responsibility to decide what procedural pathway should be followed (conduct or capability) and to appoint a formal investigator if required. This may be a clinician at the employing Trust or an outside organization. Some of the medical Royal Colleges also play a role in the assessment of practitioners and departments when concerns have been raised. The Royal College of Surgeons, for example, has a 'rapid response team' that may be invited to make a specialist assessment of circumstances.

Concerns relating to conduct: disciplinary procedures

NHS employers are expected to enforce a Code of Conduct that covers all staff, including doctors, and makes provision for disciplinary procedures, conduct hearings and grievance procedures. Misconduct is analytically distinct from, but may in practice be linked to, concerns about practitioner capability. Where cases involve both misconduct and capability issues, they are subject to capability procedures.

Misconduct is likely to fall into one or more of four categories: a refusal to comply with the reasonable requirements of the employer; an infringement of disciplinary rules, including conduct contravening GMC standards; the commission of a criminal offence outside the place of work; or otherwise inappropriate behaviour likely to compromise the service.

The guidance refers to the expectation that staff will not be dismissed for a first offence unless it is one of gross misconduct.

It is an employer's responsibility to consider whether a criminal offence, if proven, renders the doctor unsuitable for employment; and what action to take pending trial once charges have been laid.

Where terms of settlement are agreed on termination of employment following allegations of misconduct, these terms may not preclude further investigation or referral to the GMC.

Concerns about competence: capability procedures

The capability procedures are designed to address concerns about clinical performance that are not attributable to wilful misconduct: e.g. out-of-date clinical practice; inappropriate practice arising from lack of skill or knowledge; incompetence; inability to communicate; inappropriate delegation; poor team work. However, there is frequently some overlap and, where misconduct is a feature of the capability concerns, the capability procedures take precedence over misconduct procedures.

Managing capability concerns falls into the following phases:

- Initial investigation and referral to NCAS

After an initial investigation by the case manager the practitioner has a right to comment in writing. The case manager must consider whether local action such as retraining, counselling or performance review may resolve the situation.

Prior to instigating a capability panel, the employer is required to refer the practitioner to NCAS. Following NCAS assessment, the employer must implement any remedial action plan that is agreed with NCAS.

- A capability hearing and appeal procedure

Capability panels consist of three people, one of whom is a doctor not employed by the Trust. The practitioner under investigation may be represented, although it is not a legal hearing, so a legally qualified representative does not act in a legal capacity. The practitioner's performance is judged according to the typical standard of competence of the grade of doctor in question.

The panel may decide that no action is required; issue an oral warning to improve performance which is recorded and stays on file for six months; issue a written warning which stays on file for a year; issue a final written warning which stays on file for a year; or terminate the practitioner's contract.

The decision of the panel may be appealed against internally on grounds of due process, fairness and reasonability.

- Further action

The capability procedure itself terminates after the appeal stage. A practitioner may, however, pursue proceedings in an Employment Tribunal; and the organization may make a further referral to the GMC if they believe that the doctor's fitness to practise is impaired.

A system of 'Alert Letters' operates in order to inform other NHS bodies of practitioners believed to be a serious potential risk to patients or staff, and who may seek employment or access to premises elsewhere. Alert Letters are issued by the Regional Director of Public Health following an appropriate request.

High Professional Standards also includes guidance on managing concerns in respect of practitioner's health. These are not discussed here.

Regulation of General Practitioners

Changes to the system of local management of General Practitioners are a (probably unintended) consequence of new arrangements for commissioning healthcare. Because it will be GP-led Commissioning Consortia that replace Primary Care Trusts, the question arises how local regulation of GPs will proceed. This was a task that previously fell to PCTs and it is by no means obvious that GP-led commissioning bodies should now do it. At the current time, this responsibility is being reassigned to the 'Independent Commissioning Board', an element of the new NHS structures, and regional offices of the Board will probably conduct the necessary work. Despite the government's expressed intention to localize decision-making and give it to those on the front line, this move seems likely to remove responsibility for local regulation of GPs from those close enough to the ground to know what is going on. It is probably just as well, then, that the introduction of revalidation (above) will afford additional scrutiny. The 'balance of power' between NHS organizational mechanisms and professional regulatory mechanisms would seem to have tilted back in favour of professional regulation by the GMC.

The mechanisms I describe below were in force throughout the period of the study and remained the practice at the time of writing. The likelihood is that Primary

Medical Performers Lists will be retained but that the agencies responsible for maintaining them will change.

Primary Medical Performers Lists

The Department of Health issued guidance on managing Primary Medical Performers Lists in 2004 [3]. Any General Practitioner who wished to treat NHS patients in a primary care setting had to be registered with a Primary Care Trust as a 'primary medical performer'. The effect of registration on a single PCT's Performers List was to enable a doctor to perform primary medical services anywhere in England, not just in the area served by the PCT where they originally registered.

The Performers List Regulations apply to doctors who wish to be contracted to provide primary care services (e.g. as a sole practitioner or practice partner); and also to doctors employed by primary care provider organizations, including PCTs themselves. The aim of the List is to allow relevant agencies to deal with both conduct and capability issues. When it operated at PCT level it also made PCTs more accountable for the quality of GP services.

The Performers List has operated quite separately from (a) the contractual arrangements by which PCTs commissioned providers and (b) contracts of employment. PCTs therefore had two avenues by which to secure the performance of doctors they either contracted or employed. Whether doctors were providing services as an independent contractor, or whether they were directly employed by the PCT, a common avenue for regulating their performance was by recourse to the 'Performers List'. Alternatively, for GPs providing services as independent contractors, there was an alternative route via standard General Medical Services (GMS) and Personal Medical Services (PMS) contractual requirements. And then for GPs employed by the NHS (e.g. in primary care services provided alongside secondary care in hospitals) the alternative route is via the *High Professional Standards* framework set out above.

Of course GPs have remained subject to regulation by the GMC and participate in revalidation.

Powers and grounds of action

The behaviour of practitioners has been regulated through the Performers List by:

- refusing to admit practitioners to the list;
- admitting practitioners to the list subject to conditions;
- removing the practitioner from the list;
- imposing conditions on practitioners who wish to remain on the list; and
- suspending a practitioner from the list pending further action.

Legislation specifies five grounds for mandatory removal from the list:

- conviction in the United Kingdom of murder;
- conviction in the United Kingdom of a criminal offence, and a sentence to a term of imprisonment over six months;
- when the practitioner is subject to a national disqualification (see below);
- when the practitioner is no longer licensed as a member of the relevant healthcare profession;
- death (!).

Beyond the mandatory grounds entry to or removal from the list could occur on any of three discretionary grounds:

- efficiency – which covers competence, quality of performance, quality of management, and use of resources;
- fraud – not defined but treated as a common-sense term;
- suitability – which covers such issues as probity, satisfactory qualifications, personal conduct and character.

Where the failure is on efficiency or fraud grounds, the practitioner may be contingently removed from the list. Thus in efficiency cases the PCT could choose to impose conditions such as further training or supervision. Where there has been fraud or dishonesty, conditions may include limiting a doctor's access to public funds or making additional checks on claims.

Legislation has not permitted conditions to be imposed where suitability is in question. The effect of the law is that practitioners are either 'suitable' or 'unsuitable' but cannot be 'conditionally suitable'. The only option in suitability cases is therefore inclusion or exclusion from the List.

It has been possible for PCTs to make an application to impose a National Disqualification on the practitioner. The decision on national disqualification is made by the Family Health Services Appeal Authority (FHSAA), a tribunal independent of the Department of Health under the jurisdiction of the Lord Chancellor.

Doctors may withdraw themselves from the List, but not when there are proceedings for removal pending, or where the practitioner has already been suspended from the List.

Procedures

PCTs have been required to use standard procedures, which provided for both informal and formal resolution of Performers List issues. Recommended good practice was to appoint an executive member of the PCT Board to have responsibility for taking decisions to suspend or remove, and to have a senior member of staff who is not a member of the Board to act as an Investigating Officer.

- Investigation

The Investigating Officer is independent of any panel that makes decisions on List inclusion. They need not be a clinician but are expected to seek clinical advice. It is not obligatory to refer a doctor to NCAS prior to suspension, as is the case in an employment context.

- Panel hearing

Panels were expected to include the responsible executive Board member as Chair, a PCT non-executive Board Member or member of the Patient Forum, and a suitably qualified clinician.

The proceedings have not been open to the public, but the PCT or the Performer could request that observers be present. Witnesses could be called but were under no legal obligation to attend. Written and oral submissions from third parties could be included.

- Appeals

There has been no right of appeal against a mandatory removal from the list, although the decision could be challenged through the civil courts. Where entry on the list was refused or removed on discretionary grounds, or where conditions have been imposed, the practitioner has had a right of appeal to the FHSAA and from the FHSAA to the High Court.

Appeals are re-determinations of the original decision, so that the FHSAA could make any decision that a PCT could have made in the exercise of its discretion.

Notifications

Removal from the list entails notifying relevant parties: the Secretary of State for Health or equivalent in devolved jurisdictions, the GMC, the NCAS and the NHS counter-fraud body (when appropriate), locum agencies or out-of-hours cooperatives. An Alert Letter served to interested parties is a supplement to the usual notifications where it is believed the practitioner could pose a serious risk to patients or staff.

Relationship to GMC procedures

Registration with the GMC is a condition of inclusion on the List, so that mandatory removal from the Performers List

automatically follows removal from the Medical Register.

Where the GMC has made an Interim Order suspending the doctor from the Medical Register, suspension from the Performers List is encouraged.

Regulating at the organizational level

This area is also undergoing change following the election of the coalition government. We have seen that concerns about individual practitioners are managed through the GMC, employers and Performers List Regulations. Where the issue is a systemic one concerning organizational failure it falls under the remit of the Care Quality Commission (CQC) or the foundation trust regulator Monitor. If the issue concerns care quality it is dealt with by the CQC, and if it concerns governance or financial irregularities in a foundation trust it is dealt with by the Monitor. Here I deal only with concerns about care quality.

The Care Quality Commission was created in 2009 by a merger of the Healthcare Commission, the Commission for Social Care Inspection (which regulated facilities such as care homes) and the Mental Health Act Commission (which supervised the application of the Mental Health Act particularly in respect of compulsory detention).

Alongside its planned programme of regulatory work, the CQC inherited the powers of the Healthcare Commission to conduct an inquiry in response to allegations of major failings within a hospital or primary care organization. The HCC processes for responding to possible major problems fell into three stages. When it first received a referral, HCC carried out an 'initial consideration' to review the concerns and determine whether they fell within HCC criteria for investigation. The 'initial consideration' could result in:

- termination of the inquiry, and no action is required by the Trust;
- a decision to conduct an 'intervention', that is, is a limited inquiry;
- a decision to conduct a full investigation.

An 'intervention' could subsequently become a full investigation where serious concerns came to light. Either an intervention or an investigation could result in proceedings against individual doctors initiated either by the GMC or by the employer organization.

References

1. White Paper. *Trust Assurance and Safety: The Regulation of Health Professionals in the 21st Century*: Department of Health; 2007.

2. *High Professional Standards in the Modern N.H.S; a framework for the initial handling of concerns about doctors and dentists in the N.H.S*: Department of Health; 2003.

3. Primary Medical Performers Lists: *Delivering Quality in Primary Care. Advice for Primary Care Trusts on List Management*: Department of Health; 2004.

Appendix 3: A brief guide to commonly used ethical frameworks

'The Four Principles'; aka 'the Georgetown mantra'

Healthcare professionals frequently refer to 'principlism' because it is widely taught in medical schools, and often permeates specialty curricula. It was developed by leading US bioethicists Tom Beauchamp (of Georgetown University) and James Childress. They argue that their framework encompasses all the moral considerations that are relevant to healthcare, that it is universally applicable, and that it reflects a common morality. In the UK its main proponent has been the distinguished and influential medical ethicist Raanan Gillon.

The principles are:

Respect for patient autonomy. This means that where possible decisions should be made so as to protect and promote patients' exercise of deliberated self-rule. Patients should be supported to make their own decisions, and where they are unable to decide (because they lack capacity, for example) everything possible should be done to promote future capacity or to act consistently with their known views.

Non-maleficence. This appears at first to be a negative duty: to refrain from doing anything that will harm patients, often recalled in the Latin phrase *primum non nocere*. However, it also implies taking strenuous steps to ensure that patients do not incur harm in medical settings, for example by using theatre checklists to ensure patient safety during surgical operations.

Beneficence. This appears at first to be a positive duty: act so as to promote patients' overall well-being. It also implies, though, sometimes not acting, for example adopting a stance of 'watchful waiting' or 'masterly

inaction' in order to best manage a patient's condition.

Justice. Justice in this context means, primarily, to adjudicate fairly between competing claims and to treat patients as equal to one another.

The four principles are viewed as prima facie principles, meaning that each principle is binding unless it conflicts with another moral principle. If there is a conflict, the moral agent has to choose between the principles. This prima facie quality of the principles is what has given rise to much of the criticism of the 'Georgetown mantra'. Critics argue that decision-making is easy when there is no conflict between principles, and when decisions are easy the framework is unnecessary. Conversely decisions are difficult when principles conflict, and in these situations the 'four principles' framework affords little assistance because it does not provide grounds for choosing between the principles. Beauchamp and Childress have attempted to circumvent the criticism by providing criteria for when principles conflict, and Gillon has argued that the first principle – respect for autonomy – is the 'first among equals' [1].

Consequentialism; of which the best-known theory is Utilitarianism

Consequentialism is an approach to moral decision-making in which the good or bad consequences of one's actions determine what is right. The best-known consequentialist theory is utilitarianism. Utilitarianism has become such a familiar part of secular thinking that it is difficult to hold in mind that in its time it represented a genuine revolution in moral thought, challenging the moral grip of the church and status distinctions in society. It was first proposed by Jeremy Bentham in the nineteenth century and ably developed and defended by his acolyte John Stuart Mill. Utilitarians defend the principle that the best solution is that which achieves the greatest good for the greatest number of people. Utilitarianism proposes that the right thing to do is that which will have the consequence of maximizing the achievement of 'worthwhile' pleasure, and minimizing pain and suffering among sentient beings.

The notion of 'worthwhile' pleasure reflects Mill's view that it was probably better to be a human being discontented than to be a pig happy, or Socrates dissatisfied than a fool satisfied [2]; Mill distinguished between higher pleasures such as learning and lower pleasures such as sexual debauch. It should be remembered too that the pain that is inflicted as we pursue happiness has to be taken into consideration. In addition, utilitarianism is radically impartial in arguing that every sentient being is entitled to consideration when we calculate the good.

Among the most obvious criticisms of utilitarianism is that it is extremely difficult to calculate the consequences of one's actions, and to do so one act at a time. This led to the development of two branches of utilitarianism: act utilitarianism, which stuck to the proposition that each act's consequences had to be weighed; and rule utilitarianism, which accepted that over time society would develop moral rules that reflected the probable consequences of certain ways of acting, and that utilitarians should stick by such rules [3,4]. The problem with rule utilitarianism is that it begins to look like deontology (see below) and begs the question of when it might be right to break the rules.

If taken to its logical conclusion, utilitarianism can be very morally demanding. It requires of us that we give as much weight to the impact of our actions on those we don't know as on those whom we care about. Emphasizing

that the pain of sentient beings is of moral relevance, utilitarian thinking has also underpinned the animal rights movement [5].

Deontology; of which the best-known secular proponent is Immanuel Kant

Whereas consequentialism involves deciding what is right by assessing how good the consequences of our actions will be for everyone affected, deontological theories command obedience to absolute rules or duties irrespective of the consequences. It is following the rule that is right, in and of itself. Religious duties are broadly deontological, but the most celebrated secular deontologist is Immanuel Kant.

Kant argued that humans should decide what to do by considering an overarching principle he named the 'Categorical Imperative'. According to the categorical imperative, you should act in such a way that if you formulated a universal law that was binding on everyone, at all times, your act would be compatible with it. (As Kant put it, 'Act only according to that maxim by which you can at the same time will that it should become a universal law' [6(p12)].) Unhelpfully, perhaps, Kant wrote different versions of the Categorical Imperative; he also exhorted us always to treat humans as an end in themselves, not as a means to an end. ('So act as to treat humanity, whether in your own person or in that of any other, never solely as a means but always also as an end' [6(p19)].)

Whichever version is used for guidance, the point of calling the imperative 'categorical' is to emphasize that categorical imperatives supply an absolute and unbreachable moral 'law' that must be followed however unpleasant the consequences that might ensue. For example, Kant argued that a categorical rule that permitted lying would be self-contradictory: if everyone lied then no one would know what was true. For Kant, lying entailed the 'obliteration of one's dignity as a human being'. The problem with the notion of the rule being absolute, however, is that Kant was then driven to defend the view that it would be wrong to lie to murderers who asked you if their intended victim had run into the house behind you [7]. In a famous debate with critics, he claimed that as we could never predict with absolute certainty the consequences of our act (perhaps by lying you would inadvertently deliver the victim into the murders' hands when he ran away out back) it was better to follow the rule. Only by following a good rule could you be confident you were acting well.

This argument does not convince many consequentialists, who simply assert that where bad consequences will reasonably certainly follow, it cannot be good to abide by the rule. There is a further criticism of Kantian ethics that we may illustrate through the rule against lying. It is this: whether or not an action could agreeably support a universal rule all depends on how you describe the action. To Kant, a lie was a lie. To Elizabeth Anscombe, a thoughtful critic of Kant, a lie could be 'a lie in such and such circumstances' [8(p2)]. Thus a reasonable rule might stipulate that 'It is permissible to lie when doing so would save someone's life'. She thought this limited permission to lie would be justified and would not undermine the possibility of honesty. But is it permissible, for example, to lie to a patient to save their life? If so, the possibility of honesty and trust in medicine would be severely compromised.

It is sometimes said that the 'universalization principle' is somewhat akin to the 'Golden Rule' or 'ethic of reciprocity', commanding that you should treat others as you would wish to be treated yourself. While the golden rule is not a bad rule to live by, it is not quite the same as the Categorical Imperative. Kant pointed out that a judge sentencing a criminal would not wish to be treated in the way that the judge was about to treat the offender.

Virtue ethics; derived from Aristotle, revived in the late twentieth century

Virtue ethics is one of the most venerable approaches to ethics, but it went rather out of fashion in scholarly circles in the nineteenth and early twentieth centuries. Starting with Plato and Aristotle, it began to enjoy a revival from about the 1950s. Virtue ethics proposes that good decisions come from the character of the person deciding what to do. An ethical person will cultivate his or her character, will hold in mind the goal of accomplishing a morally good life in which they flourish as a human person, and will hopefully grow wiser with age and practice. This peremptory summary points the way to one of the commonest criticisms of virtue ethics, that it is somewhat self-centred and focuses on 'keeping one's hands clean' at the expense of doing good in the world by accepting moral compromise.

Many contemporary commentators are in agreement with Alasdair MacIntyre that if we want to know what is virtuous, we should look at what needs to be done to achieve the goods 'internal' to a practice. The goods internal to a practice are the underlying purposes and aims of the practice itself, rather than any ancillary advantages to be gained from pursuing it. In the practice of medicine, 'internal' goods are, for example, the prevention of ill health, cure of disease, alleviation of pain, the advancement of medical science. The 'external' goods are such things as financial reward and the esteem of peers.

Following this course of reasoning, the leading US bioethicist Pellegrino [9] has argued that the primary virtues of a doctor could be said to be:

(i) fidelity to trust and promise
(ii) benevolence
(iii) intellectual honesty
(iv) compassion and caring
(v) prudence
(vi) justice
(vii) effacement of self-interest (putting the patient before your bill)

Further reading

Rachels J. *The Elements of Moral Philosophy*. 4th edn. London: McGraw Hill; 2003.

Benn P. *Ethics*. Abingdon: Routledge; 1998.

Harris J. *The Value of Life*. London: Routledge; 1985.

Holland S. *Bioethics: A Philosophical Introduction*. Cambridge: Polity; 2003.

Hursthouse R. Virtue theory and abortion. *Philosophy & Public Affairs*. 1991;**20**(3):223–46.

References

1. Gillon R. Ethics needs principles – four can encompass the rest – and respect for autonomy should be 'first among equals'. *Journal of Medical Ethics*. 2003;**29**(5):307–12.

2. Mill JS. *Utilitarianism*. Crisp R, ed. Oxford: Oxford University Press; 1998, p. 57

3. Smart JJC. Extreme and restricted utilitarianism. *Philosophical Quarterly*. 1956;**6**:344–54.

4. Smart JJC. Outline of a system of utilitarian ethics. In: Smart JJC, Williams B, eds. *Utilitarianism: For and Against*. Cambridge: Cambridge University Press; 1973, pp. 3–74.

5. Singer P. *Taking Life: Animals. Practical Ethics*. Cambridge: Cambridge University Press; 1993, pp. 110–34.

6. Kant I. Groundwork of the Metaphysics of Morals (1785). In: Darwall S, Gregor M, eds. *Deontology*. Cambridge: Cambridge University Press; 2003, pp. 11–20.

7. Kant I. On a Supposed Right to Lie from Altruistic Motives (1797). *Critique of Practical Reason and Other Works on the Theory of Ethics*. 6th edn. London: 1909, pp. 361–3.

8. Anscombe E. Modern moral philosophy. *Philosophy*. 1958;**33**(124):1–19.

9. Pellegrino ED, Thomasma DC. *The Virtues in Medical Practice*. New York: Oxford University Press; 1993.

Index

Printed in the United States
By Bookmasters